REFERENCE EDITION

Pediatric ESAP™ 2021-2022

Endocrine Society's
Pediatric Endocrine Self-Assessment Program
Questions, Answers, and Discussions

Liuska M. Pesce, MD, Program Chair (2020-present)
Clinical Associate Professor
Pediatric Thyroid Clinic Director
Stead Family Children's Hospital
Division of Pediatric Endocrinology and Diabetes
University of Iowa Carver College of Medicine

Paola A. Palma Sisto, MD, Program Chair (2017-2021)
Associate Professor
Medical College of Wisconsin
Children's Hospital of Wisconsin

Li Chan, MD
Reader in Molecular Endocrinology
and Metabolism
Honorary Consultant in
Paediatric Endocrinology
Centre for Endocrinology
William Harvey Research Institute

Cem S. Demirci, MD
Pediatric Endocrinology
Director, T1DM Program
Connecticut Children's Medical Center
Assistant Professor of Pediatrics
Chase Family Chair in Juvenile Diabetes
University of Connecticut
School of Medicine

Oscar Escobar, MD
Associate Professor
University of Pittsburgh
School of Medicine
UPMC Children's Hospital of Pittsburg

Reema L. Habiby, MD
Associate Professor of Pediatrics
Northwestern University
Feinberg School of Medicine
Ann & Robert H. Lurie Children's
Hospital of Chicago

Ryan S. Miller, MD
Assistant Professor
University of Maryland
School of Medicine

Ron Newfield, MD
Clinical Professor
University of California – San Diego
Rady Children's Hospital San Diego

Sripriya Raman, MD
Pediatric Endocrinologist
K S Pediatrics

Christine M. Trapp, MD
Pediatric Endocrinology, Connecticut
Children's Medical Center
Associate Fellowship Director,
Pediatric Endocrinology
Assistant Professor of Pediatrics,
University of Connecticut
School of Medicine

Halley Wasserman, MD
Assistant Professor of Pediatrics
Cincinnati Children's Hospital
Medical Center
University of Cincinnati
College of Medicine

Ari Wassner, MD
Medical Director, Thyroid Center
Director, Endocrinology
Fellowship Training Program
Assistant Professor of Pediatrics
Boston Children's Hospital
Harvard Medical School

Abbie L. Young, MS, CGC, ELS(D)
Medical Editor

Endocrine Society
2055 L Street NW, Suite 600, Washington, DC 20036
1-888-ENDOCRINE • www.endocrine.org

ENDOCRINE
SOCIETY
Hormone Science to Health

ENDOCRINE SOCIETY

Hormone Science to Health

The Endocrine Society is the world's largest, oldest, and most active organization working to advance the clinical practice of endocrinology and hormone research. Founded in 1916, the Society now has more than 18,000 global members across a range of disciplines. The Society has earned an international reputation for excellence in the quality of its peer-reviewed journals, educational resources, meetings, and programs that improve public health through the practice and science of endocrinology.

Visit us at:
education.endocrine.org
endocrine.org

Other Publications:
endocrine.org/publications

For updates to the professional development books between editions:
https://www.endocrine.org/bookupdates

On the Cover: @ Freepik. Pediatrician writing prescription (by annastills).

OVERVIEW

The Pediatric Endocrine Self-Assessment Program (Pediatric ESAP™) is a self-study curriculum specifically designed for endocrinologists seeking a self-assessment and a broad review of pediatric endocrinology. Pediatric ESAP consists of approximately 100 multiple-choice questions in all areas of pediatric endocrinology, diabetes, growth, and metabolism. There is extensive discussion of each correct answer and references.

The Pediatric ESAP reference book is intended primarily for consultation and self-assessment of knowledge relating to endocrinology. As a reference book, educational credits are not available upon completion of the multiple-choice questions included. For information on educational products that include educational credit, please visit endocrine.org/store.

LEARNING OBJECTIVES

Pediatric ESAP 2021-2022 will allow learners to assess their knowledge of all aspects of pediatric endocrinology. Upon completion of this educational activity, participants will be able to:

- Recognize clinical manifestations of pediatric endocrine, growth, and metabolic disorders and select among current options for diagnosis, management, and therapy.
- Identify risk factors for endocrine and metabolic disorders in pediatric patients and develop strategies for prevention.
- Evaluate pediatric endocrine and metabolic manifestations of systemic disorders.
- Use current, evidence-based clinical guidelines and treatment recommendations to guide diagnosis and treatment of pediatric endocrine and metabolic disorders.

TARGET AUDIENCE

Pediatric ESAP is a self-study curriculum aimed at physicians seeking certification or recertification in pediatric endocrinology, program directors interested in a testing and training instrument, and clinicians seeking a self-assessment and broad review of pediatric endocrinology.

STATEMENT OF INDEPENDENCE

The Endocrine Society has a policy of ensuring that the content and quality of this educational activity are balanced, independent, objective, and scientifically rigorous. The scientific content of this activity was developed under the supervision of the Endocrine Society's Pediatric ESAP Faculty.

DISCLOSURE POLICY

The faculty, committee members, and staff who are in position to control the content of this activity are required to disclose to the Endocrine Society and to learners any relevant financial relationship(s) of the individual or spouse/partner that have occurred within the last 12 months with any commercial interest(s) whose products or services are related to the CME content. Financial relationships are defined by remuneration in any amount from the commercial interest(s) in the form of grants; research support; consulting fees; salary; ownership interest (eg, stocks, stock options, or ownership interest excluding diversified mutual funds); honoraria or other payments for participation in speakers' bureaus, advisory boards, or boards of directors; or other financial benefits. The intent of this disclosure is not to prevent CME planners with relevant financial relationships from planning or delivering content, but rather to provide learners with information that allows them to make their own judgments of whether these financial relationships may have influenced the educational activity with regard to exposition or conclusion.

The Endocrine Society has reviewed all disclosures and resolved or managed all identified conflicts of interest, as applicable.

The following faculty reported relevant financial relationship(s): **Ryan S. Miller, MD,** is an NIH grantee. **Ron Newfield, MD,** is a principal investigator for Spruce and Neurocrine for new medications; a consultant for Spruce; a consultant and member of the Independent Safety Committee for Ascendis; a principal investigator for Merck; and a principal investigator for Zealand for dasiglucagon. **Ari Wassner, MD,** is a topic peer reviewer for UpToDate (thyroid). **Liuska M. Pesce, MD,** has a spouse who is a consultant for VIDAS Diagnostics and GlaxoSmithKline.

The following faculty reported no relevant financial relationships: **Paola A. Palma Sisto, MD; Cem S. Demirci, MD; Oscar Escobar, MD; Reema L. Habiby, MD; Sripriya Raman, MD; Christine M. Trapp, MD; Halley Wasserman, MD; Li Chan, MD.**

The medical editor for this program, **Abbie L. Young, MS, CGC, ELS(D),** reported no relevant financial relationships.

The Endocrine Society staff associated with the development of this program reported no relevant financial relationships.

DISCLAIMERS

The information presented in this activity represents the opinion of the faculty and is not necessarily the official position of the Endocrine Society.

USE OF PROFESSIONAL JUDGMENT:

The educational content in this self-assessment test relates to basic principles of diagnosis and therapy and does not substitute for individual patient assessment based on the health care provider's examination of the patient and consideration of laboratory data and other factors unique to the patient. Standards in medicine change as new data become available.

DRUGS AND DOSAGES:

When prescribing medications, the physician is advised to check the product information sheet accompanying each drug to verify conditions of use and to identify any changes in drug dosage schedule or contraindications.

POLICY ON UNLABELED/OFF-LABEL USE

The Endocrine Society has determined that disclosure of unlabeled/off-label or investigational use of commercial product(s) is informative for audiences and therefore requires this information to be disclosed to the learners at the beginning of the presentation. Uses of specific therapeutic agents, devices, and other products discussed in this educational activity may not be the same as those indicated in product labeling approved by the Food and Drug Administration (FDA). The Endocrine Society requires that any discussions of such "off-label" use be based on scientific research that conforms to generally accepted standards of experimental design, data collection, and data analysis. Before recommending or prescribing any therapeutic agent or device, learners should review the complete prescribing information, including indications, contraindications, warnings, precautions, and adverse events.

ACKNOWLEDGMENT OF COMMERCIAL SUPPORT

This activity is not supported by educational grant(s) or other funds from any commercial supporter.

PUBLICATION DATE: February 2021

Common Abbreviations Used in Pediatric ESAP

ACTH -- corticotropin

ACE inhibitor---------------angiotensin-converting enzyme inhibitor

ALT --alanine aminotransferase

AST ---------------------------------- aspartate aminotransferase

BMI --body mass index

CNS--- central nervous system

CT-- computed tomography

DHEA --dehydroepiandrosterone

DHEA-S----------------------------dehydroepiandrosterone sulfate

DNA -- deoxyribonucleic acid

DPP-4 inhibitor --------------------- dipeptidyl-peptidase 4 inhibitor

DXA---------------------------------- dual-energy x-ray absorptiometry

FDA---------------------------------- Food and Drug Administration

FGF-23 ---------------------------------- fibroblast growth factor 23

FNA-- fine-needle aspiration

FSH -------------------------------------- follicle-stimulating hormone

GH -- growth hormone

GHRH------------------------- growth hormone–releasing hormone

GLP-1 receptor agonist-----glucagonlike peptide 1 receptor agonist

GnRH --------------------------------- gonadotropin-releasing hormone

hCG --------------------------------- human chorionic gonadotropin

HDL--- high-density lipoprotein

HIV------------------------------------human immunodeficiency virus

HMG-CoA reductase inhibitor ---
   3-hydroxy-3-methylglutaryl coenzyme A reductase inhibitor

IGF-1------------------------------------- insulinlike growth factor 1

LDL -- low-density lipoprotein

LH ---luteinizing hormone

MCV ---------------------------------- mean corpuscular volume

MIBG------------------------------------ meta-iodobenzylguanidine

MRI ------------------------------------- magnetic resonance imaging

NPH insulin ---------------------neutral protamine Hagedorn insulin

PCSK9 inhibitor ----proprotein convertase subtilisin/kexin 9 inhibitor

PET ---------------------------------- positron emission tomography

PSA --- prostate-specific antigen

PTH --- parathyroid hormone

PTHrP----------------------- parathyroid hormone–related protein

SGLT-2 inhibitor ---------- sodium-glucose cotransporter 2 inhibitor

SHBG --------------------------------sex hormone–binding globulin

T_3 -- triiodothyronine

T_4 -- thyroxine

TPO antibodies -------------------------thyroperoxidase antibodies

TRH--------------------------------- thyrotropin-releasing hormone

TRAb -------------------------------------TSH-receptor antibodies

TSH -- thyrotropin

VLDL--------------------------------- very low-density lipoprotein

PEDIATRIC ENDOCRINE SELF-ASSESSMENT PROGRAM 2021-2022

Part I

1 A 4-and-7/12-year-old boy born to Scottish parents presents to the emergency department with recurrent bouts of vomiting and diarrhea over the past year. While in the emergency department, he has a seizure and is noted to be hypoglycemic (blood glucose = 14.4 mg/dL [0.8 mmol/L]). He is given a glucose and fluid bolus and is maintained on an intravenous dextrose and saline solution.

He was born at term and was treated for neonatal jaundice. His parents describe him as being a sickly child who "catches everything," but because he has always grown well, they have not been concerned. He has no skin problems or infections.

On physical examination, the child is hyperpigmented. His weight is at the 50th percentile, and height is greater than the 90th percentile. His midparental range is between the 25th and 50th percentile. Bone age is advanced to 8.2 years. Blood pressure is normal, and he is clinically prepubertal.

Blood tests confirm that serum cortisol is undetectable and plasma ACTH is high.

Laboratory test results:
Random serum cortisol = <1.8 µg/dL (4.3-9.4 µg/dL) (SI: <50 nmol/L [120-620 nmol/L])
Plasma ACTH = 4310 pg/mL (6-48 pg/mL) (SI: 948.2 pmol/L [1.3-10.6 pmol/L])
Sodium = 140 mEq/L (136-144 mEq/L) (SI: 140 mmol/L [136-144 mmol/L])
Potassium = 4.8 mEq/L (3.2-5.2 mEq/L) (SI: 4.8 mmol/L [3.2-5.2 mmol/L])
Plasma renin activity = 3.5 ng/mL per h (0.6-3.8 ng/mL per h)
Aldosterone = 6.7 ng/dL (3.6-16.2 ng/dL) (SI: 185 pmol/L [100-450 pmol/L])
17-Hydroxyprogesterone = 33.0 ng/dL (<92.4 nmol/L) (SI: 1.0 nmol/L [<2.8 nmol/L])
Androstenedione = <10.0 ng/dL (10.0-16.9 ng/dL) (SI: <0.35 nmol/L [0.35-0.59 nmol/L])
Calcium = 9.2 mg/dL (8.4-10.0 mg/dL) (SI: 2.3 mmol/L [2.1-2.5 mmol/L])
TSH = 4.0 mIU/L (0.5-4.8 mIU/L)
Free T$_4$ = 1.1 ng/dL (0.9-1.6 ng/dL) (SI: 13.8 pmol/L [12.0-20.6 pmol/L])
Adrenal antibodies, negative
Very long-chain fatty acids, normal

Which of the following is the most likely diagnosis?
   A.   Addison disease
   B.   Familial glucocorticoid deficiency
   C.   Congenital adrenal hypoplasia
   D.   Congenital adrenal hyperplasia
   E.   X-linked adrenoleukodystrophy

2 A 2-year-old boy presents to the emergency department with left eye esotropia 1 week after a fall from standing height. MRI shows dilated optic nerve sheaths bilaterally, optic nerve tortuosity, and mild flattening of the posterior globes consistent with clinical papilledema. He has an unusual head shape. A 3-dimensional reconstruction CT shows complete fusion of the sagittal suture with associated dolichocephaly.

On physical examination, he has short stature (height <5th percentile), mild genu varum deformity, and a waddling gait. His hands and feet are normal. He has no dental abnormalities. His medical history is otherwise unremarkable. He was breastfed without vitamin D supplementation until 1 year of life. He started walking at age 15 months, and his parents have noticed the waddling gait since that time. X-rays are consistent with rachitic changes at the knees.

These physical examination characteristics are most concerning for which of the following underlying skeletal disorders?
   A.   X-linked hypophosphatemic rickets
   B.   Hypophosphatasia
   C.   Hypochondroplasia
   D.   Severe vitamin D deficiency
   E.   Apert syndrome

3 A 13-year-old girl with type 1 diabetes mellitus treated with multiple daily insulin injections uses a continuous glucose monitor efficiently for her daily glycemic management. She plans to eat dry cereal for her afternoon snack when she comes home from school. The food label for this cereal is displayed (*see image*). She carefully measures 2 servings of one-third cup (total two-thirds cup) in a bowl. Her continuous glucose monitor reads 92 mg/dL (5.1 mmol/L) with a flat arrow. Her insulin-to-carbohydrate ratio in the afternoon is 1:6 (1 unit for every 6 g carbohydrate).

How many units (rounded to the nearest whole unit) of rapid-acting insulin she should inject before consuming this snack?
- A. 10 units
- B. 9 units
- C. 8 units
- D. 7 units
- E. She should eat her snack and monitor her glucose via continuous glucose monitoring to decide

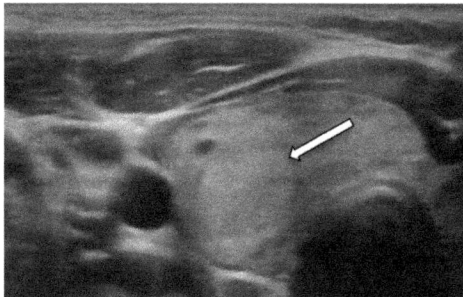

Nutrition Facts	
11 servings per container	
Serving size	1/3 cup dry (40g)

Amount per serving	
Calories	**150**

	% Daily Value*
Total Fat 3g	4%
Saturated Fat 0g	0%
Trans Fat 0g	
Cholesterol 0mg	0%
Sodium 0mg	0%
Total Carbohydrate 27g	10%
Dietary Fiber 5g	18%
Soluble Fiber 2g	
Insoluble Fiber 3g	
Total Sugars 0g	
Includes 0g Added Sugars	0%
Protein 7g	
Vitamin D 0mcg	0%
Calcium 22mg	2%
Iron 2mg	10%
Potassium 180mg	4%

*The % Daily Value tells you how much a nutrient in a serving of food contributes to a daily diet. 2000 calories a day is used for general nutrition advice.

Calories per gram:
Fat 9 • Carbohydrate 4 • Protein 4

4 A 12-year-old girl with primary hypothyroidism secondary to chronic lymphocytic thyroiditis (negative thyroglobulin antibodies) is seen for evaluation of thyroid nodules. Neck ultrasonography documents a solid right nodule measuring 1.8 × 1 × 1 cm and a less well-defined, smaller nodule on the left lobe measuring 1.2 × 0.8 × 0.8 cm (*see images*).

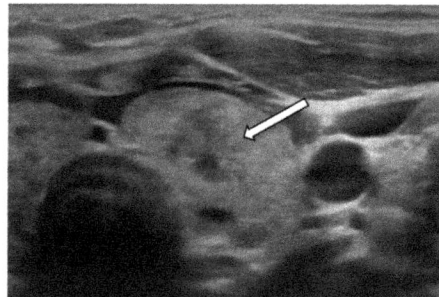

Ultrasound-guided FNA reveals a benign nodule on the right lobe and atypia of unclear significance in the left lobe. Options for treatment are discussed, and the family decides to proceed with total thyroidectomy.

Pathologic examination documents a right follicular adenoma and a 0.9-cm left lobe papillary thyroid carcinoma, classic type, confined to the thyroid without lymphovascular invasion. Lymph nodes are negative for tumor (3 on the left, 4 on the right, and 13 in the left central neck). Staging is assigned as pT1a pN0 (where p stands for pathological examination of surgical specimen, T1a refers to tumor ≤1 cm limited to the thyroid, and N0 refers to nonregional lymph node metastasis).

Two weeks after surgery, the family comes for a follow-up visit to discuss further management.

Which of the following is the best management plan?
- A. Perform ^{123}I scan and measure stimulated thyroglobulin following levothyroxine withdrawal and low-iodine diet
- B. Optimize levothyroxine treatment to maintain TSH between 0.5 and 1.0 mIU/L and follow-up with thyroglobulin measurement (while on levothyroxine) 12 weeks after surgery
- C. Treat with ^{131}I following levothyroxine withdrawal and low-iodine diet and perform posttreatment scan 4 to 7 days after treatment
- D. Optimize levothyroxine treatment to maintain TSH between 0.1 and 0.5 mIU/L and measure thyroglobulin (while on levothyroxine) 6 weeks after surgery
- E. Optimize levothyroxine to maintain TSH between 0.5 and 4.5 mIU/L and measure thyroglobulin (while on levothyroxine) 12 weeks after surgery

5 A 5-week-old male newborn is referred by his pediatrician for evaluation of gynecomastia. He was born at 40 weeks' gestation, birth weight was 7 lb 12 oz (3520 g), and there were no complications during pregnancy or delivery. His parents report that they first noticed breast tissue at about 1 week of age. The tissue has been increasing in size and getting firmer, and they have noticed milky discharge on 2 occasions. His diet is primarily breast milk with some formula supplementation. His parents state that he has had no known contact with hormone preparations, and they use a standard baby wash for baths.

On physical examination, his length is at the 60th percentile and weight is at the 90th percentile. He appears well, and examination findings are normal except for very firm, mobile breast tissue bilaterally, measuring 7 to 8 cm. There are no midline defects, and there is no discharge from the nipples.

Laboratory test results:
β-hCG = <1 mIU/mL (0-3 mIU/mL) (SI: <1 IU/L [0-3 IU/L])
TSH = 6.38 mIU/L (0.72-11.00 mIU/L)
Free T$_4$ = 1.46 ng/dL (0.48-2.34 ng/dL) (SI: 18.8 pmol/L [6.2-30.1 pmol/L])
Prolactin = 108.5 ng/mL ($\leq$10 ng/mL) (SI: 4.7 nmol/L [$\leq$0.4 nmol/L])
Karyotype = 46,XY

Which of the following is the best next step in this patient's management?
A. Perform MRI of the brain and pituitary gland
B. Measure LH, FSH, and testosterone
C. Measure prolactin again in 2 to 4 weeks
D. Start dopamine agonist therapy
E. Order genetic testing of the *MEN1* gene

6 A 17-year-old girl is followed in endocrinology clinic for thyroid hormone and GH replacement. Medulloblastoma was diagnosed at age 9 years. She had total tumor resection and received craniospinal radiation therapy (2340 cGy to the craniospinal axis plus a boost of 1260 cGy to the posterior fossa and 1980 cGy to the tumor bed) followed by 8 months of chemotherapy with cisplatin, cyclophosphamide, and lomustine. At her initial endocrine visit at age 11 years, her parents reported that she had not changed shoe size in 2 to 3 years. Subsequently, TSH and GH deficiencies were diagnosed, and she was prescribed appropriate replacement therapy. Her linear growth improved. At age 13 years, primary ovarian insufficiency was diagnosed, and hormone replacement therapy was initiated. GH therapy was stopped at age 16 years when she underwent menarche. At that time, her growth velocity was less than 2 cm/y. An IGF-1 measurement 2 months after stopping GH therapy was normal. She continues to take levothyroxine and an oral contraceptive pill with very good adherence.

Laboratory test results (sample drawn 2 weeks ago):
Free T$_4$ = 1.4 ng/dL (0.8-1.8 ng/dL) (SI: 18.0 pmol/L [10.3-23.2 pmol/L])
IGF-1 = 310 ng/mL (208-619 ng/mL) (SI: 40.6 nmol/L [27.2-81.1 nmol/L])
Cortisol (8 AM) = 17 μg/dL (SI: 469.0 nmol/L)
Hemoglobin A$_{1c}$ = 5.1% (4.0%-5.6%) (32 mmol/mol [20-38 mmol/mol])
Glucose = 91 mg/dL (70-100 mg/dL) (SI: 5.1 mmol/L [3.9-5.6 mmol/L])

At today's clinic visit, the patient describes tiredness and weakness with day-to-day activities. She participates in ballet and jazz 2 hours per week, but she is considering dropping these classes, as her energy level is low. She does well in school. Menses are regular. She drinks about 2 L of water every day and wakes up 1 to 2 times each night to urinate. She has no other symptoms. Her height and weight charts are shown (*see images*).

CDC Stature-for-age, 2 - 20 years, Girls

CDC Weight-for-age, 2 - 20 years, Girls

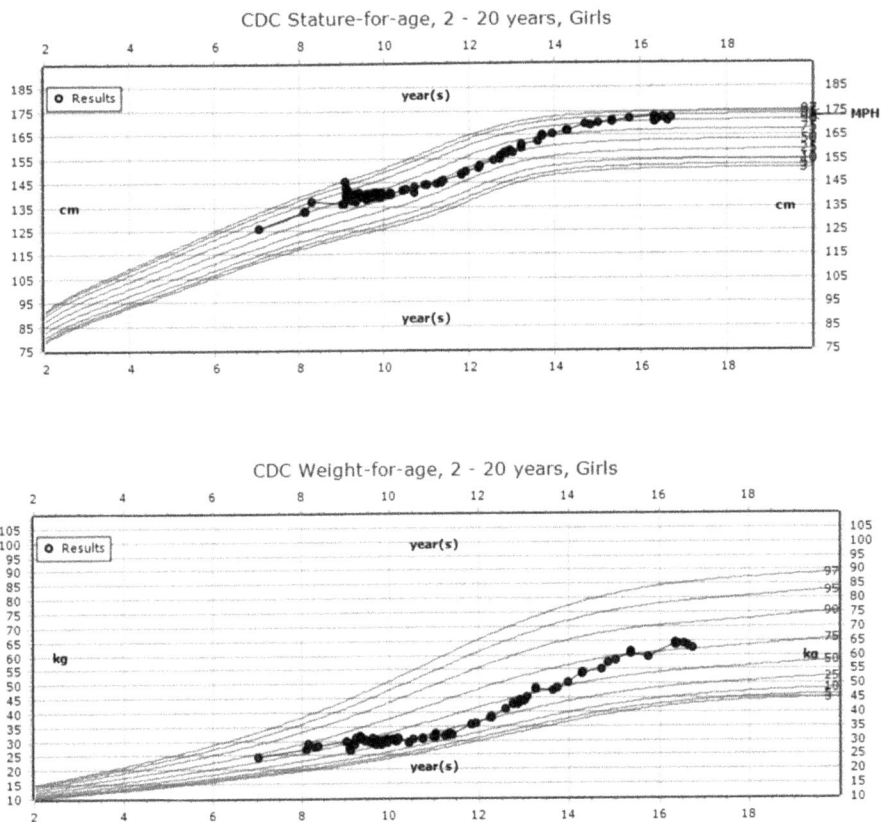

On physical examination, her vital signs and examination findings are normal.

Which of the following is the best next step in this patient's management?
- A. Measure first-morning urine osmolality, serum osmolality, and serum sodium levels to screen for diabetes insipidus
- B. Perform a low-dose cosyntropin-stimulation test to screen for central adrenal insufficiency
- C. Perform an arginine/glucagon GH-stimulation test; if abnormal, restart GH therapy at a dosage of 2.5 mg daily and titrate based on IGF-1 levels
- D. Perform a glucagon-stimulation test; if abnormal, start GH therapy at a dosage of 1.0 mg daily and titrate based on IGF-1 levels
- E. Reassure the patient and family that there is no need for further workup since her laboratory test results are normal

7 An 11-month-old boy presents with failure to thrive. The child was born full term at home after an uncomplicated pregnancy. He was breastfed exclusively until age 4 months at which time cereal and fruit juice were introduced. He continues to breastfeed every 2 to 3 hours during the day and eats cereal (3 tablespoons) and fruit juice (4 oz) twice daily. Family history is unremarkable. He is the first child for this family. Both parents are tall and the midparental height is at the 90th percentile.

On physical examination, his length and weight are at the 3rd percentile. His pulse rate is 100 beats/min, and respiratory rate is 38 breaths/min. Examination findings are remarkable for a prominent abdomen and hepatosplenomegaly.

Laboratory test results:
Plasma glucose = 45 mg/dL (65-109 mg/dL) (SI: 2.5 mmol/L [3.61-6.05 mmol/L])
Lactate = 18.0 mg/dL (2-27 mg/dL) (SI: 2.0 mmol/L [0.22-2.98 mmol/L])
Triglycerides = 1000 mg/dL (30-104 mg/dL) (SI: 11.3 mmol/L [0.34-1.18 mmol/L])

ALT = 70 U/L (10-40 U/L) (SI: 1.17 µkat/L [0.17-0.67µkat/L])
AST = 80 U/L (10-40 U/L) (SI: 1.34 µkat/L [0.17-0.67 µkat/L])
Creatine kinase = 350 U/L (10-90 U/L) (SI: 5.85 µkat/L [0.17-1.5 µkat/L])

Which of the following is the most likely explanation for this child's presentation?
A. Glycogen debrancher deficiency
B. Phosphofructokinase deficiency
C. Glucose-6-phosphatase deficiency
D. Liver phosphorylase deficiency
E. Glucose transporter 2 deficiency

8 An 8-year-old girl presents for evaluation of poor growth. She was born at 39 weeks' gestation with a birth weight of 6 lb 1 oz (2750 g) after an uncomplicated pregnancy. Growth charts from her pediatrician show that her length drifted to between the 5th and the 10th percentiles by 1 year of age and further decreased to below the 3rd percentile thereafter. Her weight has remained between the 3rd and 10th percentiles with minimal fluctuations. She has been otherwise healthy.

Her parents are first cousins. Her father's height is 68 in (172.2 cm) (–0.58 SDS), and mother's height is 60 in (153 cm) (–1.59 SDS). Her 5-year-old brother also comes for evaluation because of similar linear growth deceleration noted since age 3 years.

On physical examination, she has no evidence of major dysmorphic features. Her height is 45.6 in (116 cm) (–2.08 SDS), and weight is 44 lb (20 kg) (–1.67 SDS). She is prepubertal. Her arm span is 46 in (117 cm). Lower extremities show no bowing.

Laboratory test results:
IGF-1 = 825 ng/mL (112-276 ng/mL) (SI: 108.1 nmol/L [14.7-36.2 nmol/L])
IGF-2 = 758 ng/mL (334-642 ng/mL) (SI: 758 µg/L [334-642 µg/L])
IGFBP-3 = 5.9 mg/L (2.1-4.2 mg/L)
GH-binding protein = 638 pmol/L (267-1638 pmol/L)
GH (obtained in the morning after 12-hour fast) = 18.0 ng/mL (0.7-6.0 ng/mL) (SI: 18.0 µg/L [0.7-6.0 µg/L])
Thyroid function, normal

Bone age is interpreted to be 7 years, 10 months by the method of Greulich and Pyle.

Which of the following pathogenic variants most likely explains this child's growth failure and short stature?
A. Loss-of-function pathogenic variant in the *GHR* gene (growth hormone receptor)
B. Gain-of-function pathogenic variant in the *GHR* gene (growth hormone receptor)
C. Loss-of-function pathogenic variant in the *IGF1R* gene (IGF-1 receptor)
D. Loss-of-function pathogenic variant in the *STAT5B* gene (signal transducer and activator of transcription 5B)
E. Loss-of-function pathogenic variant in the *PAPPA2* gene (pappalysin 2)

9 An 8-day-old male newborn is referred because of an abnormal newborn screen for congenital hypothyroidism. His weight is 7 lb 1 oz (3200 g). His mother has no known thyroid disease. On physical examination, he is not jaundiced. His examination findings are normal.

Newborn screening (sample drawn at 20 hours of life) documents a TSH value of 222.7 mIU/L (<29 mIU/L).

Results of confirmatory testing:

Measurement	Day of life 4	Day of life 8 (different assay for TSH)
TSH (reference range: 0.34-5.60 mIU/L)	>100 mIU/L	42.1 mIU/L
Free T$_4$ (reference range: 0.6-1.6 ng/dL [SI: 7.7-20.6 pmol/L])	2.1 ng/dL (SI: 27.0 pmol/L)	...
Total T$_4$ (reference range, 4.3-12.5 µg/dL [SI: 55.3-160.9 nmol/L])	...	12.6 µg/dL (SI: 162.2 nmol/L)
T$_3$ uptake (reference range: 25%-35%)	...	24%

Technetium nuclear scanning on day of life 10 shows a normal-appearing, eutopic thyroid gland.

Which of the following is the best next step in this patient's management?
A. Measure TSH and T$_4$ in 1 week (off levothyroxine) and measure the mother's TSH and T$_4$
B. Measure calcium and PTH
C. Start levothyroxine
D. Assess the mother's thyroid antibodies
E. Order thyroid ultrasonography

10 A 15-year-old boy has been admitted to the hospital with tonic clonic seizure, which was self-limiting (lasted 5 minutes). Afterward, he was sweaty and confused. There were no obvious triggers for the seizure.

He has a 2- to 3-year history of monthly bitemporal headaches, lasting approximately 1 hour, which are eased with acetaminophen. He takes no prescription medications or illicit drugs. Over the past 6 weeks, his headaches have been much more severe and have been associated with palpitations and significant sweating.

He was born at 30 weeks' gestation and spent a short period in neonatal intensive care unit without long-term health problems. His vaccinations are up-to-date, and all developmental milestones are normal. His paternal grandfather has hypertension, which was diagnosed in his 50s. No other relevant family history is noted.

Findings on cardiovascular, respiratory, abdominal, and cutaneous examination are normal. Findings on thyroid examination are unremarkable and no goiter is palpable. His height is at the 50th percentile, and weight is at the 90th percentile.

On the day of admission, he has 2 more seizures. The first lasts 90 seconds (self-terminating) and the second requires intravenous lorazepam, which is given after 4 minutes. He is then intubated, ventilated, and transferred to the intensive care unit. Blood pressure is 165/84 mm Hg, and pulse rate is 105 beats/min.

Laboratory test results:
Sodium = 134 mEq/L (133-146 mEq/L) (SI: 134 mmol/L [133-146 mmol/L])
Potassium = 3.4 mEq/L (3.9-5.3 mEq/L) (SI: 3.4 mmol/L [3.9-5.3 mmol/L])
Serum urea nitrogen = 17.9 mg/dL (7.0-21.8 mg/dL) (SI: 6.4 mmol/L [2.5-7.8 mmol/L])
Creatinine = 0.9 mg/dL (0.5-1.0 mg/dL) (SI: 80 mmol/L [45-84 mmol/L])
Glucose = 139 mg/dL (70-99 mg/dL) (SI: 7.7 mmol/L [3.9-5.5 mmol/L])
TSH = 4.5 mIU/L (0.5-4.8 mIU/L)
Free T$_4$ = 1.1 ng/dL (0.9-1.6 ng/dL) (SI: 14.0 pmol/L [12.0-20.6 pmol/L])

Which of the following would be the most useful diagnostic investigation now?
   A. Echocardiography
   B. Head MRI
   C. Measurement of urinary or plasma metanephrines
   D. MIBG scan
   E. Abdominal CT

11 A 14-year-old girl presents with menstrual irregularity and occasional galactorrhea. Her parents report that she has always been tall for her age. They note that between the ages of 11 and 11.5 years, she grew 4 in (10.2 cm) to a height of 67 in (170.2 cm). She has no headaches. Her midparental target height is 63 in (160 cm). Her family history is noncontributory.

On physical examination, her blood pressure is 107/70 mm Hg and pulse rate is 87 beats/min. Her height is 70.9 in (180 cm) (99.8th percentile), weight is 162.4 lb (73.8 kg) (95.5th percentile), and BMI is 22.7 kg/m². She has mild coarsening of her facial features. Her breasts are Tanner stage 5 and there is easily expressible galactorrhea. Findings on neurologic examination are normal.

Laboratory test results (8 AM):
   Prolactin = 127 ng/mL (2-10 ng/mL) (SI: 5.5 nmol/L [0.1-0.4 nmol/L])
   LH = 2.4 mIU/mL (0.02-12.0 mIU/mL) (SI: 2.4 IU/L [0.02-12.0 IU/L])
   FSH = 3.5 mIU/mL (1.8-11.2 mIU/mL) (SI: 3.5 IU/L [1.8-11.2 IU/L])
   Estradiol = 16 pg/mL (34-170 pg/mL) (SI: 58.7 pmol/L [124.8-624.1 pmol/L])
   Free T_4 = 1.1 ng/dL (0.98-1.63 ng/dL) (SI: 14.2 pmol/L [12.6-21.0 pmol/L])
   TSH = 2.03 mIU/L (0.5-5.0 mIU/L)
   Cortisol = 10.9 µg/dL (8.0-19.0 µg/dL) (SI: 300.7 nmol/L [220.7-524.2 nmol/L])
   IGF-1 = 880 ng/mL (220-574 ng/mL) (SI: 115.3 nmol/L [28.8-75.2 nmol/L])
   GH = 15.2 ng/mL (0.06-4.30 ng/mL) (SI: 15.2 µg/L [0.06-4.30 µg/L])

GH levels failed to suppress on oral glucose tolerance testing. MRI reveals a 1.2 × 1.2-cm lobulated, peripherally enhancing cystic sellar/suprasellar lesion causing mild mass effect and elevation of the optic chiasm. She undergoes transsphenoidal resection of the mass. Her cortisol and thyroid levels measured 1 month postoperatively are normal, but oral glucose tolerance testing following surgery shows continued failure of GH levels to suppress. She is subsequently treated with subcutaneous octreotide. After 3 months of therapy, laboratory tests are performed (8 AM):

   Free T_4 = 0.97 ng/dL (0.98-1.63 ng/dL) (SI: 12.5 pmol/L [12.6-21.0 pmol/L])
   TSH = 0.27 mIU/L (0.5-5.0 mIU/L)
   Prolactin = 10 ng/mL (2-10 ng/mL) (SI: 0.43 nmol/L [0.09-0.43 nmol/L])
   GH = 1.17 ng/mL (0.06-4.30 ng/mL) (SI: 1.17 µg/L [0.06-4.30 µg/L])
   IGF-1 = 266 ng/mL (220-574 ng/mL) (SI: 34.8 nmol/L [28.8-75.2 nmol/L])

Which of the following is the most likely etiology of her abnormal thyroid function tests?
   A. Destruction of thyrotropes by the tumor
   B. Effect of surgical resection
   C. Effect of the somatostatin analogue
   D. Late effects of hyperprolactinemia
   E. GH excess

12 A 3-and-6/12-year-old boy is referred to endocrine clinic for evaluation of short stature. He was born at 40 weeks' gestation, with a birth weight of 6 lb 14 oz (3120 g). He is developmentally appropriate for his age. His height is at less than the 3rd percentile, and weight is at the 10th percentile. His midparental target height is at the 75th percentile.

On physical examination, you notice that he is short and has a protruding abdomen. He is initially happy and cooperative, but he quickly becomes irritable and agitated, making it hard for you to finish the examination.

A fingerstick blood glucose measurement is 54 mg/dL (3.0 mmol/L). You send him to the lab right away, and the following results are documented:

Plasma glucose = 52 mg/dL (70-120 mg/dL) (SI: 2.9 mmol/L [3.9-6.7 mmol/L])

Bicarbonate = 12 mEq/L (22-26 mEq/L) (SI: 12 mmol/L [22-26 mmol/L])

Lactate = 32.4 mg/dL (9-22 mg/dL) (SI: 3.6 mmol/L [0.9-2.4 mmol/L])

β-Hydroxybutyrate = 1.1 mg/dL (SI: 108 μmol/L)

Insulin, undetectable

GH = 1.8 ng/mL (SI: 1.8 μg/L)

Cortisol = 8.9 μg/dL (SI: 245.5 nmol/L)

Which of the following is the best next step in this patient's evaluation?
A. Measure uric acid, order a lipid panel, and refer to a metabolic nutritionist
B. Perform cosyntropin-stimulation testing
C. Perform brain MRI and additional laboratory tests to screen for hypopituitarism
D. Discuss the importance of frequent feeds and follow-up in 6 months
E. Perform GH-stimulation testing

13 A 7-year-old girl is referred for evaluation of low BMI. Her medical history is unremarkable and she is asymptomatic.

On physical examination, her height is at the 75th percentile, weight is at the 25th percentile, and BMI is 13.15 kg/m² (Z-score, –2.38). Her blood pressure is 98/61 mm Hg, and pulse rate is 93 beats/min. Examination findings are normal.

Her father has a history of bilateral pheochromocytoma diagnosed at age 41 years, and he was found to have a pathogenic variant in the *RET* proto-oncogene (C634R). You recommend *RET* genetic testing and the patient is found to have the same pathogenic variant.

Which of the following is characteristic of this patient's condition?
A. High risk for hyperparathyroidism; screening is recommended now
B. High risk for pheochromocytoma; screening is recommended now
C. History of Hirschsprung disease; screening for cutaneous lichen amyloidosis is recommended
D. High risk for aggressive medullary thyroid carcinoma; total thyroidectomy is recommended now
E. Marfanoid habitus; high risk for metastatic medullary thyroid carcinoma and ophthalmologic and skeletal manifestations; screening is recommended now

14 An 8-and-3/12-year-old girl presents for evaluation of breast development and vaginal bleeding. Her parents first noted breast development just before age 8 years. She began developing axillary hair and pubic hair at age 7 years. Her pediatrician is also concerned about short stature. The patient had an episode of vaginal bleeding 1 month ago, which lasted 6 days. Three weeks later, she had another episode of vaginal bleeding. She has no headaches or abdominal pain. She has not had a change in shoe or clothing size in the past year. Her energy level is normal. She does not take any medications or use any creams or lotions. Her midparental target height is 62 in (157.5 cm).

On physical examination, her blood pressure is 81/57 mm Hg and pulse rate is 59 beats/min. Her height is 45.6 in (115.8 cm) (1st percentile; Z-score, –2.37), weight is 54.1 lb (24.6 kg) (33rd percentile; Z-score, –0.45), and BMI is 18.3 kg/m² (83.8th percentile, Z-score, 0.99). She has some periorbital edema. Breasts are Tanner stage 2, and pubic hair is Tanner stage 2. The labia minora are prominent. Her visual fields are normal to confrontation. Her thyroid gland is small to normal in size. Her skin is dry with hypertrichosis over her back. Findings on abdominal examination are normal.

Bone age is 6 years.

Pelvic ultrasonography shows a postmenarchal uterus. The endometrial stripe measures 0.7 cm. The right ovary is enlarged and measures 6.1 × 3.9 × 5.5 cm with a volume of 67 mL. It contains multiple enlarged cysts or follicles, the largest measuring up to 4 cm. The left ovary is normal in size and measures 3.3 × 1.2 × 2.1 cm with a volume of 7.1 mL. Like the right ovary, the left ovary contains multiple enlarged cysts or follicles.

Which of the following most likely represents her laboratory results?

Answer	LH	TSH	hCG
A.	↑	Normal	Normal
B.	↓	↑↑	Normal
C.	↓	Normal	Normal
D.	↓	↑	↑
E.	↓	↓	Normal

15 A 3-year-old girl with a history of congenital sodium-losing diarrhea (also known as trichohepatoenteric syndrome) (homozygous *SPINT2* pathogenic variants) with dependence on parenteral nutrition for 80% of her caloric needs presents to the emergency department after 1 month of increasing fatigue and lethargy. She has had no vomiting, changes in stool pattern, or fevers. Laboratory test results prior to the onset of these acute symptoms have been normal. She has a history of hypothyroidism secondary to iodine deficiency and has been off levothyroxine for 3 months following normalization of urine iodine levels with potassium-iodine supplementation.

On physical examination in the emergency department, she is a tired-appearing girl with dry, brittle hair and dry skin. She has tachycardia, muscle spasms, and cramping. Her thyroid gland is normal on examination.

Laboratory test results:
    Potassium = 3.4 mEq/L (3.3-4.7 mEq/L) (SI: 3.4 mmol/L [3.3-4.7 mmol/L])
    Carbon dioxide = 29 mEq/L (17-31 mEq/L) (SI: 29 mmol/L (17-31 mmol/L])
    Creatinine = 0.32 mg/dL (0.17-0.42 mg/dL) (SI: 28.3 μmol/L [15.0-37.1 μmol/L])
    Calcium = 7.0 mg/dL (8.5-10.1 mg/dL) (SI: 1.8 mmol/L [2.1-2.5 mmol/L])
    Phosphate = 5.4 mg/dL (3.7-6.5 mg/dL) (SI: 1.7 mmol/L [1.2-2.1 mmol/L])
    Magnesium = 0.8 mg/dL (1.7-2.4 mg/dL) (SI: 0.3 mmol/L [0.7-1.0 mmol/L])
    Albumin = 3.1 g/dL (3.5-4.7 g/dL) (SI: 31 g/L [35-47 g/L])
    PTH = 40 pg/mL (15-87 pg/mL) (SI: 40 ng/L [15-87 ng/L])

Urinary electrolytes show low excretion of calcium and magnesium.

In the emergency department, she is given infusions of calcium chloride and magnesium sulfate. Her symptoms improve and her condition remains stable with ongoing magnesium supplementation only. Review of her medical record reveals no previous episodes of hypocalcemia or hypomagnesemia.

Which of the following is the most likely cause of her presentation?
    A. Impaired magnesium absorption due to pathogenic variants in the *TRPM6* gene
    B. Calcium deficiency secondary to hypoparathyroidism
    C. Iodine deficiency causing hypothyroidism
    D. Magnesium deficiency secondary to inadequate supplementation
    E. Gitelman syndrome

16 A 16-year-old African American girl with obesity (BMI = 31 kg/m²) presents for evaluation of oligomenorrhea and hirsutism. She has a family history of type 2 diabetes mellitus in her father and maternal grandfather and similar menstrual issues in a paternal aunt.

On physical examination, you note central obesity, facial hirsutism, acne, and marked acanthosis nigricans. Her fasting blood glucose concentration is 101 mg/dL (70-110 mg/dL) (SI: 5.61 mmol/L [3.89-6.11 mmol/L]). Her blood pressure is 134/86 mm Hg.

An elevated concentration of which of the following laboratory values would be the greatest predictor of cardiovascular disease risk in this child?
- A. Insulin
- B. LDL cholesterol
- C. Triglycerides
- D. Apolipoprotein B
- E. HDL cholesterol

17 A 15-year-old girl noticed a mass in her left neck 2 months ago. Her primary care physician ordered thyroid function tests, as well as thyroid ultrasonography. She is euthyroid. Thyroid ultrasonography reveals 2 nodules in the left lobe and no cervical adenopathy. One nodule is in the lower lobe and is 3.2 cm in largest dimension, relatively round, and has a mixed solid and cystic composition. It has normal edges, no increased blood flow, and no visible microcalcifications. The second nodule is in the upper pole and measures 1.1 cm. It is solid, hypoechoic, and has a taller-than-wide shape. There is increased blood flow and a possible microcalcification.

Findings on physical examination are unremarkable except for a left lower lobe thyroid nodule that is not very hard. There is no palpable cervical adenopathy.

Which of the following is the best next step in this patient's management?
- A. Referral to a surgeon for a left hemithyroidectomy
- B. Measurement of TPO antibodies and thyroglobulin antibodies
- C. FNA biopsy of the 3.2-cm nodule
- D. FNA biopsy of the 1.1-cm nodule
- E. FNA biopsy of both nodules

18 You are asked to evaluate a 17-year-old girl for secondary amenorrhea. She had onset of menarche at age 13 years and is uncertain whether her periods have ever been regular. She reports having had no menses for the past 7 months. She states that she is not sexually active, has never had galactorrhea, and has not experienced hot flashes. She has mild acne and no excessive body hair. She is concerned that she has gained a lot of weight over the past year.

She has a significant psychiatric history. Current medications are risperidone, benztropine, clonidine, and lithium carbonate.

On physical examination, her height is 67.3 in (171 cm) (89th percentile), weight is 229.7 lb (104.4 kg) (>99th percentile), and BMI is 36 kg/m² (98th percentile). She has mild darkening and thickening of the skin on her neck and mild hirsutism (Ferriman-Gallwey score = 8). There is no virilization. Examination findings are otherwise normal.

Laboratory test results:
TSH = 2.98 mIU/L (0.45-4.50 mIU/L)
Free T₄ = 1.17 ng/dL (0.93-1.60 ng/dL) (SI: 15.1 pmol/L [12.0-20.6 pmol/L])
β-hCG = <1 mIU/mL (0-5 mIU/mL) (SI: <1 IU/L [0-5 IU/L])
DHEA-S = 502.2 μg/dL (110.0-433.2 μg/dL) (SI: 13.6 μmol/L [3.0-11.7 μmol/L])
FSH = 6.2 mIU/mL (1.7-21.5 mIU/mL) (SI: 6.2 IU/L [1.7-21.5 IU/L])
LH = 18.6 mIU/mL (1.0-12.6 mIU/mL) (SI: 18.6 IU/L [1.0-12.6 IU/L])

Estradiol = 43.6 pg/mL (12.5-211.0 pg/mL) (SI: 160.1 pmol/L [45.9-774.6 pmol/L])
Free testosterone = 4.2 pg/mL (0.5-3.9 pg/mL) (SI: 0.15 nmol/L [0.02-0.14 nmol/L])
Prolactin = 124.9 ng/mL (4.8-23.3 ng/mL) (SI: 5.4 nmol/L [0.2-1.0 nmol/L])

Which of the following is the best next step in this patient's management?
A. Perform MRI of the brain and pituitary
B. Perform cosyntropin-stimulation testing to evaluate for nonclassic CAH
C. Perform progestin withdrawal challenge
D. Provide reassurance that risperidone is the most likely cause and continue to monitor
E. Discuss switching from risperidone to another atypical antipsychotic agent with her psychiatrist

19 A 16-year-old male high school athlete with type 1 diabetes mellitus decides to lift weights in preparation for football season. He administers multiple daily insulin injections via insulin pen devices and monitors his blood glucose with a conventional glucose meter. He recalls having episodes of hypoglycemia when he was cycling in the spring. Therefore, before his weight-lifting sessions, he consumes 15 to 20 g of carbohydrate in a protein bar without any insulin coverage because he is afraid of experiencing hypoglycemia during exercise. When he monitors his blood glucose before and after the weight-lifting sessions, he notices higher blood glucose values even if he does not consume the protein bar. He wonders why this would happen and poses the question to you during a clinic visit.

Which of the following is the best advice?
A. Suspect erroneous measurements of blood glucose; advise to monitor before, during, and after exercise and report back in 1 week
B. Advise increasing his daily basal insulin by 20%
C. Recommend increasing the insulin bolus for the meal before lifting weights
D. Recommend a small insulin bolus before lifting weights
E. Reassure the patient and recommend no changes in insulin dosage

20 A 10-and-5/12-year-old boy is referred by his pediatrician for evaluation of short stature and abnormal thyroid function test results:

Total T_4 = 3.3 µg/dL (3.8-12.0 µg/dL) (SI: 42.5 nmol/L [48.9-154.4 nmol/L])
TSH = 6.7 mIU/L (0.5-4.3 mIU/L)

The patient was born at 40 weeks' gestation with a birth weight of 8 lb 5 oz (3770 g) after an uncomplicated pregnancy. There is a vague history of seizures in the neonatal period. He has developmental delay and was diagnosed with attention-deficit/hyperactivity disorder at age 5 years. He has outbursts of aggressive behavior and is under the care of a psychiatrist. He takes several medications, including methylphenidate, quetiapine, and guanfacine. Hypothyroidism was diagnosed at age 1 year, and he received levothyroxine at a dosage of 25 mcg daily until he was 3-and-5/12 years old when his medication ran out. At a follow-up visit when he was 3-and-10/12 years old, his thyroid function was normal after 5 months of not receiving levothyroxine. Therefore, levothyroxine was not restarted. He lives with his grandmother (his legal guardian). The family history is not fully obtainable. His father's height is 67 in (170.2 cm), and his mother's height is 60 in (152.4 cm). Midparental target height is 66 ± 4 in (168 ± 10 cm).

On physical examination, his height is 53 in (134.6 cm) (SDS, −1.94), weight is 87.3 lb (39.7 kg) (SDS, +0.84), and BMI is 24.2 kg/m² (97th percentile; SDS, +1.98). He is obese and has a stocky build. Vital signs are normal. Six-year molars are present. No thyroid gland enlargement is noted. Pubic hair and genitalia are Tanner stage 1. Testicular volume is 2 to 3 mL bilaterally.

Bone age is interpreted to be markedly advanced at 15 years at a chronologic age of 10 years 5 months with fusion of epiphyses of all distal phalanges.

Laboratory test results:

Calcium = 8.0 mg/dL (8.8-10.8 mg/dL) (SI: 2.0 mmol/L [2.2-2.7 mmol/L])

Phosphate = 6.2 mg/dL (2.3-4.5 mg/dL) (SI: 2.0 mmol/L [0.7-1.5 mmol/L])

Total protein = 8.5 g/dL (6.0-8.0 g/dL) (SI: 85 g/L [60-80 g/L])

Albumin = 5.0 g/dL (3.8-5.4 g/dL) (SI: 50 g/L [38-54 g/L])

Alkaline phosphatase = 181 U/L (<400 IU/L) (SI: 3.0 μkat/L [<6.7 μkat/L])

AST = 46.0 U/L (<40.0 U/L) (SI: 0.77 μkat/L [<0.67 μkat/L])

ALT = 24.0 U/L (<40.0 U/L) (SI: 0.40 μkat/L [<0.67 μkat/L])

Free T_4 = 0.79 ng/dL (0.8-1.7 ng/dL) (SI: 10.2 pmol/L [10.3-21.9 pmol/L])

TSH = 5.9 mIU/L (0.7-5.7 mIU/L)

Total T_3 = 109.0 ng/dL (123.0-211.0 ng/dL) (SI: 1.7 nmol/L [1.9-3.2 nmol/L])

PTH = 169 pg/mL (10-65 pg/mL) (SI: 169 ng/L [10-65 ng/L])

Which additional physical findings would you expect to find on examination?

A. Almond-shaped eyes

B. Focal dysplasia of the distal radial physis

C. Widely-spaced eyes and low-set ears

D. Hemihypertrophy

E. Shortened fourth metacarpals and metatarsals

21 A 13-year-old boy presents to the emergency department with nonspecific chest pain, aches, and pains. His blood pressure is documented to be 170/90 mm Hg. Initial laboratory testing documents hypokalemia with a serum potassium concentration of 2.8 mEq/L (2.8 mmol/L). There is no family history of hypertension. He is initially seen by a cardiologist, who prescribes antihypertensive therapy. Despite this, he remains hypertensive with a systolic blood pressure of 140 to 150 mm Hg and a diastolic blood pressure of 90 to 100 mm Hg. He is referred to the pediatric endocrine department for further assessment.

Laboratory test results:

Serum aldosterone = 54.1 ng/dL (1.4-17.3 ng/dL) (SI: 1500 pmol/L [40-480 pmol/L])

Plasma renin activity = <0.15 ng/mL per h (0.5-2.6 ng/mL per h)

Findings on adrenal CT and MRI are reportedly normal.

Which of the following is the most likely diagnosis?

A. Renal artery stenosis

B. Congenital adrenal hyperplasia

C. Liddle syndrome

D. Adrenal adenoma

E. Licorice root ingestion

22 An 11-year-old girl is referred by her pediatrician because of poor growth. Review of her growth chart shows that she was tracking along the 95th percentile for height and the 50th percentile for weight from 4 to 8 years of age. In the last 3 years, her height has crossed multiple percentile lines (downward trend), whereas she has continued to have normal weight gain. Today, she is at the 33rd percentile for height and the 42nd percentile for weight. Chronic myeloid leukemia was diagnosed at age 8 years, and she started chemotherapy at that time. She did not receive any radiation therapy. She is followed by oncology and has been responding well to the oral pill (dasatinib) she takes every day. She is otherwise doing well.

On physical examination, breast development is Tanner stage 1 and pubic hair is Tanner stage 2. Her midparental target height is at the 90th percentile.

Baseline laboratory test results (sample drawn last week) document normal complete blood cell count, basal metabolic panel, IGF-1, IGFBP-3, free T_4, and TSH.

Which of the following is the best next step in this patient's management?
   A. Discuss the adverse effects of her cancer therapy and have her return for follow-up in 6 months
   B. Start levothyroxine and assess growth response in 6 months
   C. Order a GH-stimulation test and start GH therapy
   D. Explain that her growth will continue to deteriorate and she will most likely have short stature as an adult
   E. Perform DXA to evaluate bone health

23 A 30-day-old boy born at 25 weeks' gestation with a birth weight of 1 lb 6 oz (640 g) is noted to have temperature instability in the neonatal intensive care unit. Intravenous antibiotics are started, and cultures are negative. He has a history of pulmonary hypertension. He is intubated and his condition has otherwise been stable. He is tolerating feedings. Results of newborn screening (sample drawn at 48 hours of life) are normal. His mother has no history of thyroid disorders and takes no thyroid medications.

Thyroid hormone levels obtained at day of life 30:
   TSH = 22 mIU/L (0.5-6.5 mIU/L)
   Free T_4 = 0.9 ng/dL (0.8-2.2 ng/dL) (SI: 11.6 pmol/L [10.3-28.3 pmol/L])

Results of newborn screening (sample drawn at 48 hours of life) are normal. His mother has no history of thyroid disorders and takes no thyroid medications.

Which of the following is the best recommendation in this patient's management?
   A. Repeat TSH and free T_4 measurement in 4 weeks
   B. Measure thyroid antibodies in the mother
   C. Measure TSH, free T_4 by equilibrium dialysis, and total T_3 in 2 days
   D. Reassure the neonatologist that the results are most likely transient and due to recovery from nonthyroidal illness; recommend no intervention
   E. Start thyroid hormone replacement and measure TSH and free T_4 again in 2 weeks

24 An 11-year-old girl presents with headaches and vision changes. Brain MRI shows a 3.8 × 2.9 × 3.1-cm, heterogeneous, multicystic-appearing, heterogeneously enhancing mass within the suprasellar region consistent with a craniopharyngioma and hydrocephalus. She is taken to the operating room for endoscopic fenestration of the cyst with placement of a ventricular catheter. She does well postoperatively.

   Over the next year, she has an increase in the cystic component of the tumor and requires another surgery. Complications include a middle cerebral artery infarct, panhypopituitarism, central diabetes insipidus, and hypothalamic obesity. Her condition is well controlled on levothyroxine, hydrocortisone, and twice-daily oral desmopressin. On follow-up scans, there is further increase in the size of the cystic component of the tumor with compression of the optic nerve, necessitating another surgery. Her sodium and free T_4 levels are normal on replacement therapies before surgery, and she receives stress doses of hydrocortisone perioperatively and postoperatively. She is maintained on intravenous normal saline fluids, but by postoperative day 2 she is alert and hungry and is allowed to eat and drink ad lib, so intravenous fluids are discontinued. Her home desmopressin regimen of 0.2 mg orally twice daily is then initiated.

Laboratory test results:

Measurement	Postoperative day 2	Postoperative day 3	Reference range
Serum sodium	139 mEq/L (SI: 139 mmol/L)	153 mEq/L (SI: 153 mmol/L)	136-149 mEq/L (SI: 136-149 mmol/L)
Serum potassium	4.0 mEq/L (SI: 4.0 mmol/L)	3.8 mEq/L (SI: 3.8 mmol/L)	3.9-5.7 mEq/L (SI: 3.9-5.7 mmol/L)
Serum chloride	102 mEq/L (SI: 102 mmol/L)	115 mEq/L (SI: 115 mmol/L)	98-108 mEq/L (SI: 98-108 mmol/L)
Serum carbon dioxide	20.5 mEq/L (SI: 20.5 mmol/L)	18 mEq/L (SI: 18 mmol/L)	23-30 mEq/L (SI: 23-30 mmol/L)
Serum urea nitrogen	16 mg/dL (SI: 5.7 mmol/L)	15 mg/dL (SI: 5.4 mmol/L)	7-18 mg/dL (SI: 2.5-6.4 mmol/L)
Creatinine	0.54 mg/dL (SI: 47.7 µmol/L)	0.67 mg/dL (SI: 59.2 µmol/L)	0.25-1.14 mg/dL (SI: 22.1-100.8 µmol/L)
Plasma glucose	150 mg/dL (SI: 8.3 mmol/L)	140 mg/dL (SI: 7.8 mmol/L)	70-110 mg/dL (SI: 3.9-6.1 mmol/L)
Free T_4	1.27 ng/dL (SI: 16.3 pmol/L)	...	0.97-1.67 ng/dL (SI: 12.5-21.5 pmol/L)

Which of the following is the most likely cause of her hypernatremia?
A. Excessive administration of normal saline fluids
B. Adipsia
C. Stress doses of hydrocortisone worsening the diabetes insipidus
D. Hyperglycemia causing dehydration
E. Insufficient desmopressin dosage

25 A primary care physician is calling to inform you that a 14-year-old girl with type 1 diabetes mellitus under your care has asthma exacerbation and is being treated with prednisone, 2 mg/kg per day divided twice daily for 5 days. When on the same prednisone dosage in the past, she developed hyperglycemia with glucose values in the range of 300 to 400 mg/dL (16.7-22.2 mmol/L) and mild-to-moderate ketonuria. She will receive her first prednisone dose tomorrow morning. She is currently on insulin pump therapy, and her most recent hemoglobin A_{1c} value was 7.2% (55 mmol/mol).

What, if any, initial changes in the pump settings do you recommend to control her blood glucose while she is taking glucocorticoids?
A. Increase all correction/insulin sensitivity factors by 30% now
B. Increase all basal rates by 30% now
C. Increase insulin-to-carbohydrate ratios by 30% now
D. Increase all basal rates by 30% within 6 to 12 hours after initiating prednisone
E. Check blood glucose every 3 hours and correct hyperglycemia as needed without adjusting insulin pump settings

26 A 12-and-6/12-year-old girl is referred for evaluation of short stature. She was originally seen by an adult endocrinologist closer to home at age 8 years because of poor growth. At that time, laboratory test results (comprehensive metabolic panel, complete blood cell count, thyroid function tests) and bone age were normal.

On physical examination today, her height is 49 in (124.5 cm) (<1st percentile, –2.9 SD), weight is 118.8 lb (54 kg) (85th percentile), and BMI is at the 98th percentile. Her vital signs are normal. She has macrocephaly and mild retrognathia. Her arms and legs appear short. She has mild brachydactyly. She does not have scoliosis. Breasts and pubic hair are Tanner stage 5.

Her mother reports that she grew 1.5 cm in the last year. Breast development and pubic hair growth started at age 9 years, and menarche was at age 11 years. She has spontaneous regular menses. She has a history of frequent ear infections. There are no developmental delays. Review of systems is otherwise normal. Her midparental target height is 64 in (162.6 cm) (close to the 50th percentile). There is no family history of short stature.

The patient is very anxious about her growth potential.

Which of the following is the most likely explanation for her short stature?
A. Maternal uniparental disomy of chromosome 15
B. Mosaic Turner syndrome
C. Activating pathogenic variant in the *FGFR3* gene
D. Inactivating pathogenic variant in the maternal allele of the *GNAS* gene
E. Pathogenic variant in the *FMR1* gene

27 You are asked to evaluate a 7-week-old newborn for hypospadias. The baby was born at 31 weeks' gestation to a 40-year-old mother with chronic hypertension. Family history is notable for chordee in the patient's 22-year-old half-brother. The pregnancy was notable for maternal gestational diabetes, preeclampsia, and breech presentation. Birth weight was 2 lb 11 oz (1222 g [appropriate for gestational age]). Prenatal karyotype was documented to be 46,XY. FISH for *SRY* performed on day 2 of life was normal.

The baby's course in the neonatal intensive care unit was unremarkable, with normal electrolytes, no respiratory distress, and quick transition to full oral feeds.

On physical examination, the baby appears well. Phallus length is 1.9 cm. There is perineal hypospadias, chordee, and bifid scrotum. Gonads are palpable in the inguinal canals.

Laboratory test results (sample drawn at 5 weeks of age):
Sodium = 139 mEq/L (134-144 mEq/L) (SI: 139 mmol/L [134-144 mmol/L])
Potassium = 5.2 mEq/L (3.5-5.2 mEq/L) (SI: 5.2 mmol/L [3.5-5.2 mmol/L])
Serum urea nitrogen = 3 mg/dL (5-18 mg/dL) (SI: 1.1 mmol/L [1.8-6.4 mmol/L])
Creatinine = 0.29 mg/dL (0.30-0.59 mg/dL) (SI: 25.6 μmol/L [26.5-52.2 μmol/L])
FSH = 6.6 mIU/L (3.0-6.0 mIU/L) (SI: 6.6 IU/L [3.0-6.0 IU/L])
LH = 3.2 mIU/L (<0.02-5.0 mIU/L) (SI: 3.2 IU/L [<0.02-5.0 IU/L])
17-Hydroxypregnenolone = 325 ng/dL (229-3104 ng/dL) (SI: 9.8 nmol/L [6.9-93.4 nmol/L])
17-Hydroxyprogesterone = 179.6 ng/dL (0-200 ng/dL) (SI: 5.4 nmol/L [0-6.1 nmol/L])
Total testosterone = 169 ng/dL (≤201 ng/dL) (SI: 5.86 nmol/L [≤6.97 nmol/L])
Dihydrotestosterone = 46.6 ng/dL (12-85 ng/dL) (SI: 1.6 nmol/L [0.4-2.9 nmol/L])

Which of the following diagnoses is most consistent with this patient's examination and laboratory findings?
A. 5α-Reductase deficiency
B. 3β-Hydroxysteroid dehydrogenase deficiency
C. Swyer syndrome (gonadal dysgenesis)
D. Partial androgen insensitivity syndrome
E. Pathogenic variant in the *LHCGR* gene

28 A 17-year-old boy presents with concerns about lipid abnormalities. His LDL-cholesterol concentration is 225 mg/dL (5.83 mmol/L). His paternal grandfather and paternal uncle died early of cardiovascular disease. Treatment is initiated with atorvastatin, 10 mg daily, which lowers the patient's LDL-cholesterol concentration to 140 mg/dL (3.63 mmol/L) over a 6-month period. His mother calls this morning because he is experiencing mild discomfort in his calves. Yesterday he had soccer tryouts, during which he was physically active.

Laboratory test results:
    Creatine kinase = 198 U/L (15-105 U/L) (SI: 3.3 μkat/L [0.3-1.8 μkat/L])
    ALT = 54 U/L (<55 U/L) (SI: 0.90 μkat/L [<0.92 μkat/L])
    AST = 34 U/L (<35 U/L) (SI: 0.57 μkat/L [<0.58 μkat/L])
    Creatinine = 0.7 mg/dL (0.5-1.0 mg/dL) (SI: 61.9 μmol/L [44.2-88.4 μmol/L])

Atorvastatin is continued and his symptoms resolve. One month later, he returns with new pain in his calves. He just started soccer 1 week ago.

Results of repeated laboratory tests:
    Creatine kinase = 250 U/L (15-105 U/L) (SI: 4.18 μkat/L [0.25-1.75 μkat/L])
    ALT = 55 U/L (<55 U/L) (SI: 0.92 μkat/L [<0.92 μkat/L])
    AST = 28 U/L (<35 U/L) (SI: 0.47 μkat/L [<0.58 μkat/L])
    Creatinine = 0.7 mg/dL (0.5-1.0 mg/dL) (SI: 61.9 μmol/L [44.2-88.4 μmol/L])

Bearing in mind current recommendations regarding statin treatment in children, which of the following is the best next step?
    A. Continue atorvastatin and measure creatine kinase in 2 days
    B. Stop atorvastatin; wait 2 weeks and then reintroduce atorvastatin and assess for symptoms
    C. Stop atorvastatin and pursue nonstatin cholesterol treatment
    D. Admit him to the hospital for observation and treatment of muscle damage
    E. Order MRI of his legs

29 A 17-and-4/12-year-old girl has been followed for Hashimoto thyroiditis, diagnosed at age 14-and-9/12 years on the basis of elevated TPO antibodies.

Laboratory test results at age 14-and-6/12 years:
    TSH = <0.003 mIU/L (0.5-4.3 mIU/L)
    Total T_4 = 11.4 μg/dL (4.5-12.0 μg/dL) (SI: 146.7 nmol/L [57.9-154.4 nmol/L])

At age 14-and-9/12 years, she was evaluated by an endocrinologist. She had no goiter or bruit. At that time, her TSH was no longer suppressed (0.39 mIU/L) and the following laboratory values were documented:
    Total T_4 = 7.6 μg/dL (4.5-12.0 μg/dL) (SI: 97.8 nmol/L [57.9-154.4 nmol/L])
    Total T_3 = 124 ng/dL (84-179 ng/dL) (SI: 1.9 nmol/L [1.3-2.8 nmol/L])
    TPO antibodies = 42 IU/mL (<9 IU/mL)
    Thyroid-stimulating immunoglobulin, negative
    Thyroglobulin antibodies, negative

She remained euthyroid and has never required levothyroxine. However, current routine laboratory test results (at age 17-and-4/12 years) show she is hyperthyroid:
    TSH = 0.01 mIU/L (0.5-4.3 mIU/L)
    Free T_4 = 2.3 ng/dL (0.9-1.4 ng/dL) (SI: 29.6 pmol/L [11.6-18.0 pmol/L])
    Total T_4 = 17.0 μg/dL (4.5-12.0 μg/dL) (SI: 218.8 nmol/L [57.9-154.4 nmol/L])
    Total T_3 = 288 ng/dL (86-192 ng/dL) (SI: 4.4 nmol/L [1.3-3.0 nmol/L])

She is asymptomatic (no heat intolerance, loose stools, or palpitations), but she has lost 7.3 lb (3.3 kg) in the previous 5 months. She has no pain in her neck or jaw.

On physical examination today, her blood pressure is 116/73 mm Hg and pulse rate is 112 to 116 beats/min. She has a small, diffuse goiter (3.5 cm) without a bruit. She has no thyroid nodules, no tenderness to palpation, no lymphadenopathy in her neck, no proptosis, and no tremor. The rest of her examination findings are unremarkable.

One week later, laboratory tests show that she is still hyperthyroid with similar thyroid function. A celiac panel is negative, she has a normal erythrocyte sedimentation rate, and thyroid-stimulating immunoglobulin is 280% (<140%).

Which of the following is the most likely diagnosis?
- A. Hashitoxicosis
- B. Silent subacute thyroiditis
- C. Graves disease
- D. Hot nodule
- E. Exogenous ingestion of levothyroxine

30 You are evaluating an 8-and-2/12-year-old boy for signs of early pubertal development. He has a history of medulloblastoma diagnosed at age 6 years and was treated with cranial radiation to the hypothalamic-pituitary area. He received a total of 20 Gy of radiation therapy. Before the tumor was diagnosed, his linear growth had been steadily progressing along the 25th percentile. At his 8-year well-child check, his pediatrician noted evidence of testicular and penile enlargement and referred him to you for evaluation. His medical history and family history are noncontributory.

On physical examination, his height is 49.6 in (126 cm), which plots at the 25th percentile (SDS, –0.65). His weight is 58.5 lb (26.6 kg), which plots at the 8th percentile (SDS, –1.35). His arm span is 50 in (127 cm). Vital signs are normal. He has no dysmorphic features. His thyroid gland is not enlarged. Findings on neurologic examination are grossly intact. Pubic hair is early Tanner stage 2. Testicular volume is 6 mL bilaterally, and his stretched penile length is 10 cm (mean penile length for 8- to 9-year-old boys is 6.3 cm). The rest of the physical examination findings are unremarkable.

Bone age is interpreted to be 10 years and 0 months at the chronologic age of 8 years and 2 months according to the Greulich and Pyle method.

Laboratory test results:
Testosterone (8 AM) (by liquid chromatography/tandem mass spectrometry = 121 ng/dL (SI: 4.2 nmol/L)
 (Tanner stage 1: <3-10 ng/dL [SI: <0.1-0.4 nmol/L]; Tanner stage 2: 18-150 ng/dL [SI: 0.6-5.2 nmol/L])
LH (ultrasensitive) = 1.5 mIU/mL (SI: 1.5 IU/L) (Tanner stage 1: <0.02-0.3 mIU/mL [SI: <0.02-0.3 IU/L];
 Tanner stage 2: 0.2-4.9 mIU/mL [SI: 0.2-4.9 IU/L])
IGF-1 = 125 ng/mL (SI: 16.4 nmol/L) (7- to 8-year-old males: 113-261 ng/mL [SI: 14.8-34.2 nmol/L];
 9- to 10-year-old males: 123-275 ng/mL [SI: 16.1-36.0 nmol/L])
Cortisol (8 AM) = 9 μg/dL (7-25 μg/dL) (SI: 248.3 nmol/L [193.1-689.7 nmol/L])

Which of the following is the best next step in this patient's evaluation?
- A. GnRH-stimulation test
- B. Low-dose cosyntropin-stimulation test
- C. GH-stimulation test
- D. Brain MRI with and without contrast
- E. Testicular ultrasonography

31 A 12-year-old girl presents to the outpatient clinic with a history of chronic fatigue, attention-deficit/hyperactivity disorder, irritability, and depression. She had a kidney stone 1 year ago, and laboratory testing at that time showed the following:

Serum calcium = 10.1 mg/dL (8.5-10.0 mg/dL) (SI: 2.5 mmol/L [2.1-2.5 mmol/L])
Phosphate = 2.5 mg/dL (2.8-5.1 mg/dL) (SI: 0.8 mmol/L [0.9-1.6 mmol/L])
PTH = 54 pg/mL (15-87 pg/mL) (SI: 54 ng/L [15-87 ng/L])
Urine calcium-to-creatinine ratio = 0.175

Hypercalciuria was diagnosed, and she was started on a thiazide diuretic. DXA of the lumbar spine documented a height-adjusted Z-score of –0.7.

In clinic today, the patient is well hydrated. She takes no other medications. There is no family history of calcium balance disorders.

Current laboratory test results:
    Serum calcium = 11.1 mg/dL (8.5-10.0 mg/dL) (SI: 2.8 mmol/L [2.1-2.5 mmol/L])
    Phosphate = 2.4 mg/dL (2.8-5.1 mg/dL) (SI: 0.8 mmol/L [0.9-1.6 mmol/L])
    PTH = 73 pg/mL (15-87 pg/mL) (SI: 73 ng/L [15-87 ng/L])
    25-Hydroxyvitamin D = 25 ng/mL (20.0-60.0 ng/mL) (SI: 62.5 nmol/L [49.9-149.8 nmol/L])
    Urinary calcium-to-creatinine ratio = 0.217

Which of the following is the best next step to determine the etiology of her condition?
A. Order genetic testing for a pathogenic variant in the *CASR* gene
B. Perform parathyroid ultrasonography
C. Perform a ^{99}Tc sestamibi scan
D. Perform DXA of the one-third distal radius
E. Stop the thiazide diuretic and repeat the laboratory tests

32 A 12-year-old girl presents for evaluation of poor growth. She was born full-term and had a normal birth weight. Her mother reports that she grew normally until 1 year ago when she began to have headaches and daily abdominal pain, feeling full after very small meals. She underwent a complete gastroenterologic workup, including endoscopy and colonoscopy, which were unrevealing. She lost more than 20 lb (9.1 kg) in the past year. She was subsequently admitted to a partial psychiatric hospitalization program. Midparental height is 63 in (160 cm). Her mother had menarche at age 15 years, and her father underwent puberty at age 16 years. Her medications include cyproheptadine, risperidone, and sertraline.

On physical examination, she is a pale, thin, quiet girl. Her blood pressure is 90/59 mm Hg, and pulse rate is 89 beats/min. Her height is 57.5 in (149 cm) (37th percentile), and weight is 68.2 lb (31 kg) (5th percentile) (BMI = 14 kg/m^2). Her breasts are Tanner stage 1, and pubic hair is Tanner stage 2. Findings on neurologic examination are normal.

Her growth chart is shown (*see image*).

Laboratory test results:
    Random GH = 8.4 ng/mL
        (0.06-4.3 ng/mL) (SI: 8.4 μg/L
        [0.06-4.3 μg/L])
    IGF-1= 98 ng/mL (104-665 ng/mL)
        (SI: 12.8 nmol/L [13.6-87.1 nmol/L])

Bone age is interpreted to be 10 years.

Which of the following is the most likely cause of her growth delay?
A. Craniopharyngioma
B. GH insensitivity syndrome
C. Addison disease
D. Constitutional delay of growth and maturity
E. Undernutrition

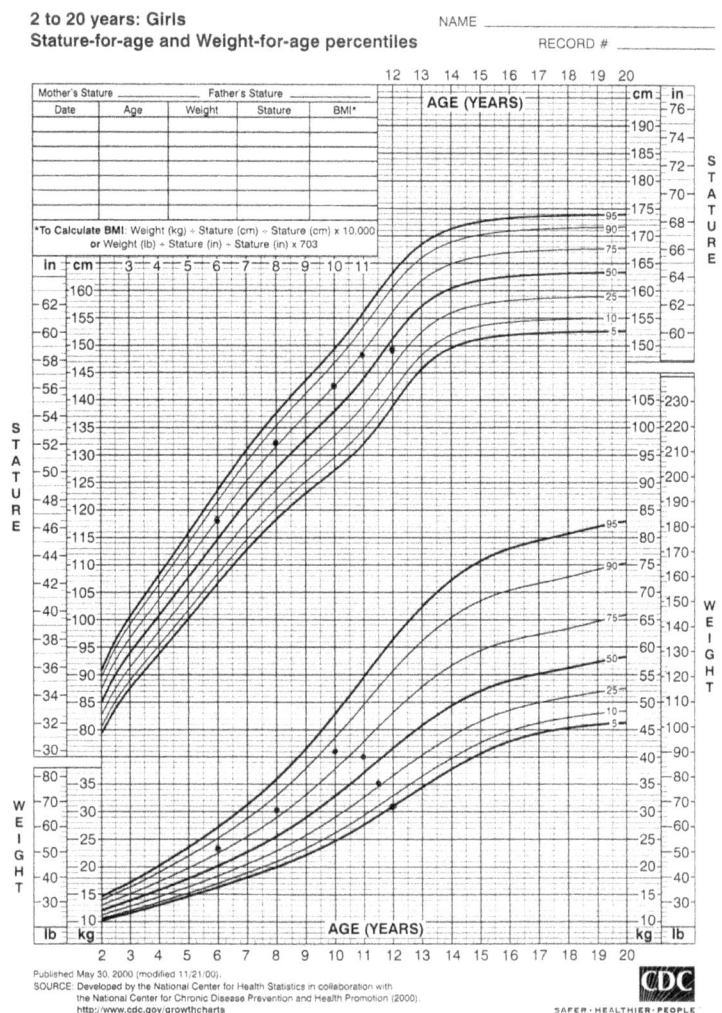

2 to 20 years: Girls
Stature-for-age and Weight-for-age percentiles

33 A 14-year-old boy with Silver-Rusell syndrome has recently moved to the area and is presenting for continuation of care. He was born at 37 weeks' gestation, with a birth weight of 4 lb 8 oz (2050 g) (small for gestational age) and birth length of 17.7 in (45 cm). His clinical course in infancy was complicated by feeding difficulties and recurrent hypoglycemia, particularly with illness, requiring hospital admission. He was evaluated by a geneticist and was found to have a methylation defect involving chromosome 11p15. He started GH therapy at age 4 years, and he developed signs of pubarche at age 7 years. He had a histrelin implant placed 2 years ago, and it was removed last year. His midparental target height is 70 in (177.8 cm), and his father has a history of constitutional growth delay.

His height is 62 in (157.5 cm) (25th percentile), and weight is 100.8 lb (45.8 kg) (31st percentile). On physical examination, he has Tanner stage 3 pubic hair and a testicular volume of 3 mL bilaterally. His height velocity over the past year has decreased from 5.6 cm/y to 4.6 cm/y.

Laboratory test results:
 IGF-1 = 546 ng/mL (148-551 ng/mL) (SI: 71.5 nmol/L [19.4-72.2 nmol/L])
 TSH = 1.78 mIU/L (0.450-4.500 mIU/L)
 Free T$_4$ = 1.26 ng/dL (0.8-1.8 ng/dL) (SI: 16.2 pmol/L [10.3-23.2 pmol/L])
 Total testosterone = 4.7 ng/dL (≤1000 ng/dL) (SI: 0.16 nmol/L [≤34.7 nmol/L])
 LH = 0.69 mIU/mL (0.31-5.29 mIU/mL) (SI: 0.69 IU/L [0.31-5.29 IU/L])

Bone age is 13 years.
 Laboratory testing 1 year ago was notable for a total testosterone concentration of 6.0 ng/dL (0.21 nmol/L) and LH concentration of 1.1 mIU/mL (1.1 IU/L).

Which of the following is the best interpretation of these data?
 A. Poor adherence to treatment resulting in slow growth
 B. Gonadotropin deficiency causing failed pubertal progression and slow growth
 C. Constitutional growth delay
 D. Retained portion of histrelin implant, which is continuing to suppress puberty
 E. Early epiphyseal closure causing slow growth

34 A 10-year-old boy with Down syndrome presents to the emergency department with a history of decreased activity, excessive sleep, increased appetite, rapid weight gain, and frequent episodes of tonic clonic seizures. He has a history of a ventricular septal defect repaired surgically.

On physical examination, his height is 51.6 in (131 cm) (5th percentile; −1.2 SDS) (50th-75th percentile for Down syndrome), weight is 121 lb (55 kg) (97th percentile; 2.21 SDS), and BMI is 32.2 kg/m^2 (99th percentile; 2.5 SDS).

On arrival to the emergency department, his blood glucose concentration is 40 mg/dL (2.2 mmol/L).

Laboratory test results (critical sample):
 Insulin = 119.8 µIU/mL (2.6-24.9 µIU/mL) (SI: 832.0 pmol/L [17.8-173.0 pmol/L])
 C-peptide = 7.6 ng/mL (0.8-3.1 ng/mL) (SI: 2.5 nmol/L [0.26-1.03 nmol/L])
 GH = <0.1 ng/mL (0-10 ng/mL) (SI: <0.1 µg/L [0-10 µg/L])
 Cortisol = 8.7 µg/dL (6.2-19.4 µg/dL) (SI: 241 nmol/L [171-536 nmol/L])
 Ammonia = 41 µmol/L (0-55 µmol/L)
 β-Hydroxybutyrate = <4.2 mg/dL (<4.2 mg/dL) (SI: <400 µmol/L [<400 µmol/L])
 Acylcarnitine profile, negative

He requires a high-concentration intravenous dextrose infusion with a glucose infusion rate greater than 20 mg/kg per min. Intravenous fluid infusion is interrupted to draw a second critical sample within 35 minutes, and the patient's blood glucose concentration is less than 30 mg/dL (<1.7 mmol/L). Other results from the second critical sample:

 Insulin = 47.4 µIU/mL (SI: 329 pmol/L)
 C-peptide = 4.8 ng/mL (SI: 1.58 nmol/L)
 GH = 4 ng/mL (SI: 4 µg/L)

Cortisol = 10.7 μg/dL (SI: 294 nmol/L)

Ammonia = 56 μmol/L

β-Hydroxybutyrate = <4.2 mg/dL (SI: <400 μmol/L)

Which of the following is the best next step in this patient's management?
A. Sulfonylurea screen
B. MRI of the pancreas
C. Diazoxide challenge
D. Another critical sample before ordering an imaging study
E. Genetic testing

35 A 4-and-9/12-year-old boy presents for initial evaluation of poor growth and short stature. He was born out of a second-degree consanguineous relationship at term gestation with a birth weight of 7 lb 11 oz (3500 g). Motor milestones have been delayed (started walking without support at age 3 years), but he has been reaching mental and social milestones appropriately. He describes leg pain while bearing weight and has an unstable gait with frequent falls. He has not sustained any fractures. His first tooth erupted at 18 months of age, and his primary dentition was completed at 4 and 6/12 years of age. He is a vegetarian. He has been taking vitamin D supplements for the last 4 months, as suggested by his pediatrician, with no symptomatic relief and no improvement in growth.

On physical examination, he is below the 3rd percentile for height and is at the 5th percentile for weight. His vital signs are normal. His physical appearance is shown in the photographs (*see images*).

Laboratory tests ordered by his pediatrician 2 weeks ago document the following results:

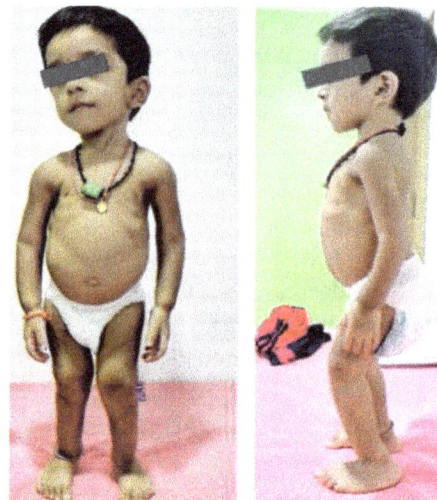

Serum calcium = 4.6 mg/dL (8.8-10.8 mg/dL) (SI: 1.2 mmol/L [2.2-2.7 mmol/L])

Serum phosphate = 3.1 mg/dL (3.8-5.8 mg/dL) (SI: 1.0 mmol/L [1.2-1.9 mmol/L])

Alkaline phosphatase = 1685 IU/L (100-320 IU/L) (SI: 28.1 μkat/L [1.7-5.3 μkat/L])

Total 25-hydroxyvitamin D = 88 ng/mL (30-100 ng/mL) (SI: 219.6 nmol/L [74.9-249.6 nmol/L])

25-Hydroxyvitamin D_2 = <5 ng/mL (SI: <12.5 nmol/L)

25-Hydroxyvitamin D_3 = 88 ng/mL (SI: 219.6 nmol/L)

1,25-Dihydroxyvitamin D = 25 pg/mL (15-90 pg/mL) (SI: 65.0 pmol/L [39-234 pmol/L])

PTH = 124 pg/mL (10-65 pg/mL) (SI: 124 ng/L [10-65 ng/L])

Which of the following is the most appropriate management for this patient?
A. Calcium supplementation and high-dosage ergocalciferol
B. Calcium supplementation and calcitriol
C. Phosphorus supplementation and calcitriol
D. Calcium supplementation alone and reevaluation in 3 months
E. Burosumab therapy

36 A 4-and-6/12-year-old girl with a recent diagnosis of hyperthyroidism secondary to Graves disease comes for initial consultation. She was seen by her primary care physician about 1 month ago for poor sleep and mood swings and was noted to have a pulse rate of 124 beats/min and blood pressure of 106/52 mm Hg. There is no history of recent illness or infections.

On physical examination, she has a nontender, symmetric goiter. She has no upper eyelid retraction, scleral erythema, or proptosis. Her weight is 44 lb (20 kg).

Laboratory test results:
 TSH = 0.005 mIU/L (0.27-4.2 mIU/L)
 Free T$_4$ = 2.5 ng/dL (0.9-1.7 ng/dL) (SI: 32.2 ng/dL [11.6-21.9 pmol/L])
 TPO antibodies = 479.9 IU/mL (<9.0 IU/mL) (SI: 479.9 kIU/L [<9.0 kIU/L])
 TSH-receptor antibodies = >40 IU/L (0-1.75 IU/L)

Laboratory test results (sample drawn at today's visit):
 TSH = <0.01 mIU/L
 Free T$_4$ = 2.2 ng/dL (0.9-1.7 ng/dL) (SI: 28.3 ng/dL [11.6-21.9 pmol/L])
 Total T$_3$ = 274 ng/dL (90-240 ng/dL) (SI: 4.2 nmol/L [1.4-3.7 nmol/L])
 Absolute neutrophil count (ANC) = 2.3 × 10^3/μL (4.0-6.5 × 10^3/μL)
 AST = 29 U/L (5-32 U/L) (SI: 0.48 μkat/L [0.08-0.53 μkat/L])
 ALT = 37 U/L (5-33 U/L) (SI: 0.62 μkat/L [0.08-0.55 μkat/L])

Methimazole is initiated at a dosage of 5 mg daily (0.3 mg/kg per day). Since she had abnormal ANC and liver enzymes before starting treatment, repeated levels are obtained for follow-up. Thyroid hormone levels improve over time and absolute neutrophil count remains stable. Liver enzymes change as follows:

Analyte	2 Weeks Later	4 Weeks Later
AST	37 U/L (SI: 0.6 μkat/L)	45 U/L (SI: 0.8 μkat/L)
ALT	72 U/L (SI: 1.2 μkat/L)	144 U/L (SI: 2.4 μkat/L)

Which of the following is the best next step in this patient's management?
 A. Discontinue methimazole and discuss thyroidectomy
 B. Discontinue methimazole and plan for radioactive iodine therapy
 C. Decrease the methimazole dosage and measure liver enzymes again in 2 weeks
 D. Order a comprehensive liver panel and refer to gastroenterology
 E. Decrease the methimazole dosage and refer to gastroenterology

37 A 16-day-old newborn is referred for endocrine evaluation following recurrent hypoglycemic episodes. He has 1 sister who is 30 months old and is reported to be healthy. His parents are nonconsanguineous and are of Romanian origin with no notable family history. His mother reports that her pregnancy with him was uneventful. He was born by vaginal delivery at 38 weeks' gestation with a birth weight of 6 lb 3 oz (2800 g). Apgar scores were 9/10, and assessment of cord gases documented a pH value of 7.42. He had respiratory arrest at 15 hours of life with a documented low glucose value. Over the next 14 days, he had recurrent hypoglycemic episodes. He required phototherapy for 72 hours because of jaundice.

Endocrinology consult is requested. On assessment, his weight is 7 lb 1 oz (3200 g), blood pressure is 78/42 mm Hg, and pulse rate is 140 beats/min. He appears jaundiced with no skin hyperpigmentation or hypopigmentation. No dysmorphic features are noted. Findings on cardiovascular and respiratory examinations are normal. He has normal male external genitalia, and both testes are palpable in the scrotum.

Laboratory test results (blood samples taken during a hypoglycemic episode):
 Glucose = 34.2 mg/dL (63-126 mg/dL) (SI: 1.9 mmol/L [3.5-7.0 mmol/L])
 Insulin = <1.0 μIU/mL (4.0-11.0 μIU/mL) (SI: <6.9 pmol/L [27.8-76.4 pmol/L]
 Sodium = 136 mEq/L (133-141 mEq/L) (SI: 136 mmol/L [133-141 mmol/L])
 Potassium = 5.6 mEq/L (4.3-6.2 mEq/L) (SI: 5.6 mmol/L [4.3-6.2 mmol/L])
 Lactic acid = 33.5 mg/dL (6.5-20.0 mg/dL) (SI: 3.7 mmol/L [0.72-2.22 mmol/L])
 Plasma ammonia = 85 μmol/L (10-150 μmol/L)

ACTH = 19.0 pg/mL (4.7-48.8 pg/mL) (SI: 4.2 pmol/L [1.0-10.7 pmol/L])

Cortisol = <1.0 µg/dL (7.8-26.2 µg/dL) (SI: <27.6 nmol/L [215.2-722.8 nmol/L])

GH = 14.4 ng/mL (5-50 ng/mL) (SI: 14.4 µg/L [5-50 µg/L])

Free T$_4$ = 1.02 ng/dL (0.55-1.65 ng/dL) (SI: 13.1 pmol/L [7.08-21.24 pmol/L])

TSH = 6.14 mIU/L (0.55-12.5 mIU/L)

Which of the following should be the next investigation?

A. Standard-dose cosyntropin-stimulation test

B. Low-dose cosyntropin-stimulation test

C. Brain and pituitary MRI

D. 17-Hydroxyprogesterone measurement

E. Adrenal ultrasonography

38 A 4-year-old girl is referred to you by her primary care physician for evaluation of short stature. She was born at 39 weeks' gestation with a birth weight of 5 lb 13 oz (2637 g) and a birth length of 18.5 in (47 cm). The pregnancy was uneventful.

On physical examination, she has no dysmorphic features, but she does have short stature. Her height is 36.2 in (92 cm) (SDS, –2.08), and weight is 27.5 lb (12.5 kg) (SDS, –2.05). Arm span is 34 in (86.4 cm).

Laboratory test results are normal, including IGF-1, IGFBP-3, thyroid function, liver function, kidney function, celiac screen, and inflammatory markers.

Her bone age is concordant with her chronologic age.

The family recently moved from a foreign country. Family history reveals that her parents are second cousins. Her father's height is 64 in (162.5 cm) (SD, –2.00). Her mother's height is 58 in (147.3 cm) (SD, –2.46). Neither parent has any dysmorphic features and both have normal intellect. The patient's 8-year-old full brother, who was born with normal proportions, has had abnormal growth noted from 1 year of age, and he now has severe short stature with a height SDS of –6.5. He has a prominent forehead, wide and depressed nasal bridge, prominent lips, short arms (especially fingers, hands, and forearms) and legs (especially feet and shanks), and normal intellect.

Which of the following are the most likely explanations for the short stature observed in this 4-year-old girl and her 8-year-old brother?

Answer	4-year-old patient	8-year-old brother
A.	Pseudoachondroplasia	Achondroplasia
B.	Heterozygous activating pathogenic variant in NPR2	Homozygous activating pathogenic variants in NPR2
C.	Heterozygous inactivating pathogenic variant in FGFR3	Homozygous inactivating pathogenic variants in FGFR3
D.	Turner syndrome	SHOX haploinsufficiency
E.	Heterozygous inactivating pathogenic variant in NPR2	Homozygous inactivating pathogenic variants in NPR2

39 A 13-year-old adolescent boy with a BMI of 38 kg/m^2 (142% above the 95th percentile) has been unable to lose weight over the last 2 years despite lifestyle modification efforts, including dietary changes and increased exercise. He has had normal vital signs at each visit. Sexual development is Tanner stage 3.

Recent laboratory test results:

Fasting glucose = 101 mg/dL (65-99 mg/dL) (SI: 5.61 mmol/L [3.6-5.5 mmol/L])

Total cholesterol = 211 mg/dL (<170 mg/dL) (SI: 5.46 mmol/L [<4.40 mmol/L])

HDL cholesterol = 45 mg/dL (>45 mg/dL) (SI: 1.16 mmol/L [>1.16 mmol/L])

Triglycerides = 199 mg/dL (<90 mg/dL) (SI: 2.25 mmol/L [<1.02 mmol/L])

Calculated LDL cholesterol = 125 mg/dL (<110 mg/dL) (SI: 3.24 mmol/L [<2.85 mmol/L])

Hemoglobin A$_{1c}$ = 5.7% (4.0%-5.6%) (39 mmol/mol [20-38 mmol/mol])

He asks your opinion regarding bariatric surgery, as his mother underwent sleeve gastrectomy 2 years ago. A bariatric surgeon at your center is experienced in performing this procedure in adolescents.

Which of the following findings must be considered to determine whether he qualifies for bariatric surgery?
- A. Degree of dyslipidemia
- B. Completion of pubertal growth
- C. Family history of bariatric surgery
- D. BMI percentile
- E. History participating in a formal weight-loss program

40 A nearly 15-year-old girl presents for evaluation of amenorrhea. Breast development started 2 years ago, but she thinks it has only minimally progressed. She developed pubic hair approximately 4 years ago. She is otherwise in good health and has no galactorrhea, dizziness, fatigue, or constipation. She is active in cross-country and track. There is a family history of late menarche (age 14-16 years) in her mother and other maternal relatives.

On physical examination, her height is 67.7 in (172 cm) (+1.56 SDS) and weight is 145 lb (65.9 kg) (+0.83 SDS). Midparental target height is 55.5 in (141 cm). She has no glandular breast tissue and has stage 4 pubic hair. There is no hirsutism or acne.

Laboratory test results:
Progesterone = 0.8 ng/mL (≤11.9 ng/mL) (SI: 2.5 nmol/L [≤37.8 nmol/L])
Estradiol = 8.2 pg/mL (≤283 pg/mL) (SI: 30.1 pmol/L [≤1038.9 pmol/L])
FSH = 102.5 mIU/mL (0.8-8.5 mIU/mL) (SI: 102.5 IU/L [0.8-8.5 IU/L])
LH = 38.3 mIU/mL (≤15.8 mIU/mL) (SI: 38.3 IU/L [≤38.3 IU/L])
Thyroid function, normal

Pelvic ultrasonography shows the presence of an echogenic structure behind the bladder measuring 5.2 × 1.2 × 1.8 cm not definitively identified as a uterus. Ovaries are not visualized.

Which of the following is the most likely underlying etiology?
- A. >200 CGG triplet repeats in the *FMR1* gene
- B. Excess ovarian androgen production
- C. Abnormal karyotype
- D. Ovarian failure due to follicle depletion
- E. Abnormally elevated prolactin levels

41 An overweight 15-year-old girl just returned from vacation in Mexico. A few days after taking some diet pills while on her trip, she developed a sore throat, palpitations, and a headache. She does not have the pills with her and cannot recall the name. Her parents brought her to the emergency department, where she was found to be tachycardic and hypertensive.

On physical examination, her blood pressure is 140/90 mm Hg and pulse rate is 124 beats/min. She has a fine tremor. She has no goiter and no thyroid gland tenderness.

Laboratory test results:
TSH = <0.03 mIU/L (0.35-5.00 mIU/L)
Free T_4 = 0.92 ng/dL (0.71-1.85 ng/dL) (SI: 11.8 pmol/L [9.1-23.8 pmol/L])
Total T_3 = 776 ng/dL (84-179 ng/dL) (SI: 12.0 nmol/L [1.3-2.8 nmol/L])
Erythrocyte sedimentation rate = 46 mm/h (0-20 mm/h)

Thyroid iodine uptake on a nuclear scan is low at 5.7% at 22 hours.

Which of the following assessment(s) should be ordered to determine whether she has subacute thyroiditis or exogenous intoxication?
   A. Complete blood cell count with differential
   B. Thyroglobulin measurement and assessment of thyroglobulin antibodies
   C. Calcitonin measurement
   D. Procalcitonin measurement
   E. Thyroid ultrasonography

42 A 6-month-old infant is seen by his pediatrician for surgical clearance for circumcision revision. He was born at 36 weeks' gestation and was discharged home with his parents after birth. He has since been lost to follow-up, but his mother reports exclusively breastfeeding him until he was 4 months old. At that time, his parents switched his diet to pureed table foods. They follow a vegan lifestyle. His birth weight was 6 lb, 5.1 oz (2865 g), and his current weight is 11 lb, 1.8 oz (5040 g).

On physical examination, he is alert but cachectic in appearance with palpable rachitic rosary, widened wrists, and frontal bossing. His blood pressure is normal, and he is breathing comfortably on room air.

Laboratory test results:
   Calcium = 5.1 mg/dL (8.0-10.5 mg/dL) (SI: 1.3 mmol/L [2.0-2.6 mmol/L])
   Phosphate = 3.3 mg/dL (4.2-8.0 mg/dL) (SI: 1.1 mmol/L [1.4-2.6 mmol/L])
   Magnesium = 1.7 mg/dL (1.7-2.5 mg/dL) (SI: 0.7 mmol/L [0.7-1.0 mmol/L])
   Albumin = 3.9 g/dL (2.6-4.7 g/dL) (SI: 39 g/L [26-47 g/L])
   Alkaline phosphatase = 434 U/L (124-383 U/L) (SI: 7.2 μkat/L [2.1-6.4 μkat/L])
   25-Hydroxyvitamin D = <4.0 ng/mL (20.0-60.0 ng/mL) (SI: 10.0 nmol/L [49.9-149.8 nmol/L])
   1,25-Dihydroxyvitamin D = 17.8 pg/mL (19.9-79.3 pg/mL) (SI: 46.3 pmol/L [51.7-206.2 pmol/L])
   PTH (1-84) = 312 pg/mL (15-87 pg/mL) (SI: 312 ng/L [15-87 ng/L])

Electrocardiography shows a borderline prolonged QTc interval of 430 ms.

In addition to inpatient admission for cardiac telemetry and monitoring weight gain on formula feeds, which of the following is the best next step in this patient's management?
   A. Vitamin D supplementation, 400 IU daily for 3 months, and enteral calcium, at least 50 mg/kg per day
   B. Calcitriol, 0.125 mcg twice daily; enteral calcium, at least 50 mg/kg per day; and enteral phosphorus, 30 mg/kg per day
   C. Calcitriol, 0.125 mcg twice daily, and intravenous calcium gluconate
   D. Reintroduction of breastfeeding; maternal high-dosage vitamin D supplementation; and enteral calcium, at least 50 mg/kg per day
   E. Vitamin D supplementation, 2000 IU daily; enteral calcium, 50 mg/kg per day; and intravenous calcium gluconate as needed

43 Liraglutide injection for subcutaneous use was approved in June 2019 for pediatric patients (10 years and older) with type 2 diabetes mellitus.

Which of the following is a "black box" warning for the product that must be discussed with patients and families?

A. Pancreatitis: postmarketing reports, including fatal and nonfatal hemorrhagic or necrotizing pancreatitis

B. Renal impairment: postmarketing reports, usually in association with nausea, vomiting, diarrhea, or dehydration, which may sometimes require hemodialysis

C. Thyroid C-cell tumors: contraindicated in patients with a personal or family history of medullary thyroid cancer or in patients with multiple endocrine neoplasia type 2

D. Serious hypoglycemia: risk of hypoglycemia is higher in pediatric patients aged 10 years and older regardless of concomitant antidiabetes therapies

E. Hypersensitivity: postmarketing reports of serious hypersensitivity reactions (eg, anaphylactic reactions and angioedema)

44 A 14-year-old boy with Klinefelter syndrome diagnosed by amniocentesis presents for evaluation. He is a freshman in a therapeutic day school. He has attention-deficit/hyperactivity disorder and aggressive behaviors. He has regular follow-up visits with his psychiatrist. He is not yet shaving.

On physical examination, his blood pressure is 115/74 mm Hg and pulse rate is 74 beats/min. His height is 71 in (180.3 cm) (>95th percentile), and weight is 194 lb (88.2 kg) (99th percentile) (BMI = 27.1 kg/m²). He is tall with long legs. He has cystic acne and a few facial hairs. His genitals are Tanner stage 5, pubic hair is Tanner stage 4, and testicular volume is 4 mL bilaterally.

Which of the following are the most likely expected laboratory findings for this boy?

Answer	LH	FSH	Testosterone	Inhibin B
A.	↑	↑	Normal or ↓	Normal
B.	Normal	↑	Normal	↑
C.	↑	↑	Normal or ↓	↑
D.	↑	↑	Normal or ↓	Undetectable
E.	↑	Normal	↓	Undetectable

45 A 15-year-old girl with a history of acute lymphocytic leukemia treated with chemotherapy and bone marrow transplant (including total body irradiation) has been diagnosed with stage I, multifocal, tall variant papillary thyroid carcinoma. Both thyroid lobes are involved, with the largest dimension of 3.5 cm, and there is extrathyroidal extension into adipose tissue and soft-tissue margin, as well as lymphatic, vascular, and perineural invasion. She has metastasis to bilateral cervical lymph nodes in the central neck and lateral neck, involving level VI and levels II and IV (17/32 lymph nodes, size of metastasis >1 cm without extracapsular invasion) (T3, N1b, MX). A ¹²³I whole-body scan following levothyroxine withdrawal and low-iodine diet demonstrates minimal thyroid bed uptake with no evidence of distal metastases. Stimulated thyroglobulin measurement is pending.

In addition to planning to optimize levothyroxine to maintain TSH <0.1 mIU/L, which of the following is the best next step in this patient's management?
  A. Reassure the family regarding ^{123}I uptake and arrange for follow-up in 6 months with neck ultrasonography and nonstimulated thyroglobulin measurement
  B. Reassure the family regarding ^{123}I uptake and arrange for follow-up in 12 months with neck ultrasonography and nonstimulated thyroglobulin measurement
  C. Reassure the family regarding ^{123}I uptake and arrange for follow-up with nonstimulated thyroglobulin measurement in 3 months
  D. Treat with ^{131}I 30 mCi (1110 MBq) and perform posttreatment scan 4 to 7 days later
  E. Treat with ^{131}I 120 mCi (4440 MBq) and perform posttreatment scan 4 to 7 days later

46 A 7-year-old girl is referred after a standard lipid assessment documented the following results:
Total cholesterol = 279 mg/dL (<170 mg/dL) (SI: 7.23 mmol/L [<4.40 mmol/L])
HDL cholesterol = 51 mg/dL (30-65 mg/dL) (SI: 1.32 mmol/L [0.78-1.68 mmol/L])
LDL cholesterol = 190 mg/dL (<130 mg/dL) (SI: 4.92 mmol/L [<3.37 mmol/L])
Triglycerides = 190 mg/dL (30-140 mg/dL) (SI: 2.15 mmol/L [0.34-1.58 mmol/L])

The blood draw was performed after she had eaten breakfast. The patient's mother reports that they have reduced sugary drinks and increased physical activity for the past 6 months because of her daughter's rising BMI. There is no family history of early cardiovascular disease. The patient's maternal grandmother has high cholesterol that was diagnosed in her 50s and she is doing well on medication. The patient's father is in his 40s and has a normal cholesterol level. The patient's mother has not had her cholesterol checked but plans to do so at her next check-up.

Which of the following is the best next step in this patient's management?
  A. Redraw a fasting lipid panel in 3 months
  B. Initiate the Cardiovascular Health Integrated Lifestyle Diet (CHILD-2 diet)
  C. Start a fibrate
  D. Start a statin
  E. Start fish oil

47 A 2-year-old boy with achondroplasia is referred to you by his primary care physician at the request of his parents for possible management of short stature. The patient was born via cesarean delivery at 38 weeks' gestation with a birth weight of 6 lb 0 oz (2730 g) and a birth length of 18.7 in (47.5 cm). The pregnancy was uneventful. The patient's father has achondroplasia and has the typical features of this condition. His father's height is 54.3 in (138 cm) (−5.26 SD). His mother is healthy, and her height is 59.8 in (152 cm) (−1.73 SD).

Physical examination reveals dysmorphic features consistent with achondroplasia, including short stature, macrocephaly, prominent forehead, midface hypoplasia, and short extremities. His height is 31.1 in (79 cm) (−2.35 SDS), and weight is 26.4 lb (12 kg) (−0.51 SDS). His arm span is 28.7 in (73 cm), and head circumference is 20 in (50.8 cm) (+2.5 SDS).

Laboratory tests show normal levels of IGF-1 and IGFBP-3, normal thyroid function, normal liver and kidney function, negative celiac screen, and normal inflammatory markers.

The parents inquire about potential therapeutic interventions for the management of their son's short stature to avoid the father's final height outcome, and they are eager to participate in a clinical study, if necessary.

Which of the following pharmacologic interventions appears promising for this condition?
  A. Recombinant human IGF-1
  B. C-type natriuretic peptide analogue
  C. GnRH analogues
  D. Recombinant human GH
  E. Aromatase inhibitors

48 A 6-and-6/12-year-old girl is being followed up in endocrine clinic. She has a diagnosis of classic congenital adrenal hyperplasia (CAH) secondary to 21-hydroxylase deficiency. She was born with ambiguous genitalia and has a family history of CAH. Her parents report that she is well with no episodes of illness necessitating increasing her hydrocortisone dosage. The patient's regimen consists of hydrocortisone, 11.3 mg/m^2 per day, and fludrocortisone, 100 mg daily.

On physical examination, her height is 37.8 in (96.1 cm) (–1.46 SDS), and weight is 30 lb (13.6 kg) (–1.56 SDS) (BMI = 14.7 kg/m^2 [–0.77 SDS]). Body surface area is 0.62 m^2. Her height velocity is 9.6 cm/y. Her blood pressure is 94/50 mm Hg.

Which of the following is the best next step in this patient's care?
  A. Perform a pubertal examination
  B. Determine bone age
  C. Measure 17-hydroxyprogesterone
  D. Increase the hydrocortisone dosage
  E. Reduce the fludrocortisone dosage

49 An 11-and-3/12-year-old girl was diagnosed with Graves disease 6 weeks ago. She had a moderately diffuse goiter, a fine tremor, and the following laboratory test results:
TSH = <0.03 mIU/L (0.35-5.00 mIU/L)
Total T$_4$ = 14.1 µg/dL (4.5-12.5 µg/dL) (SI: 181.5 nmol/L [57.9-160.9 nmol/L])
Total T$_3$ = 345 ng/dL (84-179 ng/dL) (SI: 5.3 nmol/L [1.3-2.38 nmol/L])
Thyroid-stimulating immunoglobulin = 480% (<140%)

At diagnosis, her weight was 72.2 lb (32.8 kg). Methimazole, 7.5 mg twice daily, and propranolol were prescribed. Propranolol was stopped less than 3 weeks later because her pulse rate was 96 beats/min. Six weeks after starting methimazole, the patient comes for a follow-up visit.

On physical examination today, her pulse rate is 84 beats/min. Goiter is unchanged and there is no tremor.

Laboratory test results:
TSH = <0.03 mIU/L
Total T$_4$ = 7.2 µg/dL (SI: 92.7 nmol/L)
Total T$_3$, pending
Complete blood cell count with differential, normal
Liver enzymes, normal

Which of the following is the best next step in this patient's management?
  A. Wait for the result of the T$_3$ measurement before adjusting the methimazole dosage
  B. Ask the laboratory to assess T$_3$ uptake on the sample from that day
  C. Reduce the methimazole dosage to 10 mg once daily
  D. Measure thyroid-stimulating immunoglobulin again
  E. Increase the methimazole dosage to 10 mg twice daily

50 A 16-and-8/12-year-old boy is referred to your clinic for concerns of low bone density. He is an avid cross-country runner and lacrosse player. Over the last 18 months, he has sustained 2 stress fractures and 1 growth plate fracture that have sidelined him from participating in sports. His orthopedic surgeon ordered a DXA scan and laboratory tests, which were done at an outside hospital. Osteopenia was diagnosed with a lumbar spine Z-score of –1.7. Serum 25-hydroxyvitamin D was in the insufficient range at 20.1 ng/mL (50.2 nmol/L), and alkaline phosphatase was reported as high at 280 U/L (4.68 µkat/L). Calcium, phosphate, magnesium, and PTH levels were normal.

He has no other history of fractures and no relevant medical history. Family history is notable for postmenopausal osteoporosis in his maternal grandmother. He follows a healthy diet with 3 servings of dairy each day. His parents are concerned that he will continue to be injured during physical activity and that his bone disease will impair his ability to join the military upon high school graduation.

On physical examination, he is a well-appearing young man. His height is at the 65th percentile and weight is at the 35th percentile. BMI is 19.5 kg/m². In the last year, he has grown 5 in (12.7 cm). His pubertal examination shows 15-mL testes bilaterally.

Which of the following is the most appropriate recommendation for this patient?
  A. Refer to sports medicine for evaluation of running mechanics
  B. Perform DXA of the total body and total hip to assess bone mineral density at cortical and weight-bearing skeletal sites
  C. Start vitamin D supplementation to address low vitamin D and elevated alkaline phosphatase
  D. Start prophylactic oral bisphosphonate therapy to increase bone mineral density
  E. Recommend avoidance of contact sports and suggest golf for weight-bearing exercise instead of running

51 An 11-year-old boy presents for evaluation of breast development. His parents report that for the past several months he has had swelling under the nipples bilaterally without discharge. This has caused him significant distress and he has started wearing large sweatshirts to hide the appearance of breasts. He reports no exposure to lavender or tea tree oil. He and his parents express a strong desire for treatment.

On physical examination, the patient's height is 60.6 in (154 cm) (91st percentile) and weight is 103.6 lb (47.1 kg) (88th percentile). He appears well. Examination findings are notable for 2 cm of glandular breast tissue bilaterally, Tanner stage 2 pubic hair development, and testicular volume of 6 mL bilaterally.

Laboratory test results:
  LH = 1.7 mIU/mL (0.03-3.70 mIU/mL [Tanner stage 2]) (SI: 1.7 IU/L [0.03-3.70 IU/L])
  Total testosterone (liquid chromatography–tandem mass spectrometry) = 58 ng/dL (18-150 ng/dL [Tanner stage 2]) (SI: 2.01 nmol/L [0.63-5.20 nmol/L])
  Estradiol (sensitive) = <2.5 pg/mL (5.0-16.0 pg/mL [Tanner stage 2]) (SI: <9.2 pmol/L [18.4-58.7 pmol/L])

Results from assessment of liver, kidney, and thyroid function are normal. Bone age is 11 years. Midparental target height is 66 in (167.6 cm).

Which of the following is the best next step in the management of this patient's condition?
  A. Order karyotype analysis
  B. Order testing for serum tumor markers
  C. Prescribe an aromatase inhibitor
  D. Refer to surgery for mastectomy
  E. Offer reassurance and follow-up in 6 months

52 A 1-year-old girl presents to clinic as a new patient regarding concern for excess weight gain. Her mother states that the patient was born full term after an uncomplicated pregnancy. Birth weight was 6 lb 6 oz (3000 g). Review of her growth charts demonstrates that her weight was already greater than the 97th percentile by 2 months of age and that it has continued to increase significantly over time. Her length has plotted consistently just above the 97th percentile since early infancy.

On physical examination, you observe a tall-for-age toddler with no obvious dysmorphic features. According to her mother, she always seems hungry and this has been true since she was a young infant. Developmental milestones have all been met appropriately thus far. She has generally been in good health with no history of frequent infections. Her mother comments that she herself has struggled with her weight all of her life and underwent sleeve gastrectomy in the past. There is a strong family history of significant obesity in multiple family members spanning generations.

Given the clinical phenotype, genetic testing is being considered. Which of the following is the most likely genetic finding?
   A. Pathogenic variant in the *BBS1* gene
   B. Pathogenic variant in the *LEP* gene
   C. Deletion in 15q11.2-q13 region on the paternal chromosome
   D. Pathogenic variant in the *MC4R* gene
   E. Pathogenic variants in the *ALMS1* gene

53 At 37 weeks' gestation, a male baby is born to a 28-year-old woman who had minimal prenatal care. The delivery is uncomplicated, and the baby's Apgar scores are 9 and 9. Birth weight is 5 lb 3 oz (2360 g). Physical examination is significant for bilateral cleft lip, partial cleft palate, and marked hypotelorism. Brain MRI reveals lobar holoprosencephaly with absence of cleavage of the inferior frontal lobe with characteristic fading away of the genu of the corpus callosum. The baby is initially given intravenous fluids on the first day of life, but he is subsequently transitioned to enteral feedings by 4 days of age, which he is tolerating well. The neonatal intensive care unit has asked for an endocrinology consult.

Which of the following is the most likely laboratory finding in this newborn?
   A. Low free T_4
   B. Elevated serum sodium
   C. Low GH
   D. Low glucose
   E. Low serum sodium

54 A 16-year-old girl presents for outpatient evaluation of thyroid nodules. Two weeks ago, she saw her primary care physician for evaluation of 9 months of secondary amenorrhea and increasing acne. Laboratory testing revealed an elevated serum testosterone concentration (355 ng/dL [9-58 ng/dL] [SI: 12.3 nmol/L (0.3-2.0 nmol/L)]), and pelvic ultrasonography demonstrated a 5.9-cm solid left ovarian mass. Preoperative staging CT demonstrated cysts in both lungs (1 to 2 cm in diameter) and multiple hypoattenuating lesions in the thyroid measuring up to 1.1 cm in diameter.

The patient was born preterm at 31 weeks' gestation. She underwent resection of a benign right lung cyst at age 22 months. She has never received external irradiation or chemotherapy. Her family history includes a maternal aunt diagnosed with breast cancer in her 40s.

The patient reports no symptoms of hypothyroidism or thyrotoxicosis, dysphagia, or voice changes. Her height is at the 11th percentile, weight is at the 82nd percentile, BMI is at the 92nd percentile (27 kg/m²), and head circumference is at the 88th percentile. Vital signs are normal. Thyroid examination reveals a mildly enlarged right lobe that is irregular in texture without discrete nodules. There is no lymphadenopathy. No abnormal skin pigmentation is present. The rest of the examination findings are normal.

Her serum TSH concentration is 2.63 mIU/L (0.7-5.7 mIU/L). Thyroid ultrasonography demonstrates multiple bilateral thyroid nodules measuring 1.0 to 1.7 cm in diameter (*see image*).

In addition to appropriate further evaluation of the patient's thyroid nodules, germline genetic testing should be performed for which of the following conditions?
   A. Carney complex
   B. *DICER1* syndrome
   C. Familial adenomatous polyposis
   D. McCune-Albright syndrome
   E. *PTEN* hamartoma tumor syndrome

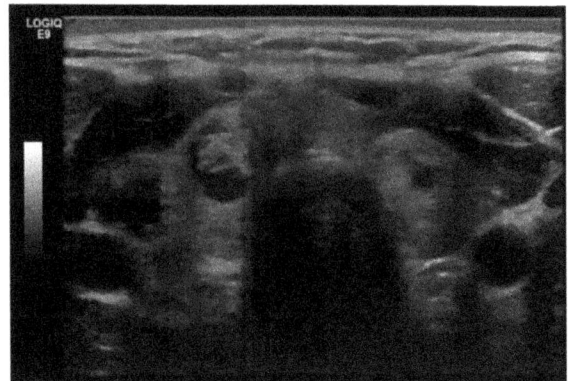

55 A 4-year-old boy is diagnosed with GH deficiency via an arginine-L-dopa stimulation test (peak GH = 0.8 ng/mL [0.8 μg/L]). Recombinant human GH replacement therapy is started at a dosage of 0.18 mg/kg per week. Several weeks after treatment initiation, the child presents to the emergency department with hypotension and hypoglycemia. In light of the recent initiation of recombinant human GH therapy and based on current symptoms, the patient is suspected to have adrenal insufficiency.

Which of the following mechanisms best explains the patient's presentation? GH-induced:
- A. Inhibition of 21-hydroxylase
- B. Stimulation of 11β-hydroxysteroid dehydrogenase 2
- C. Inhibition of 11β-hydroxysteroid dehydrogenase 2
- D. Stimulation of 11β-hydroxysteroid dehydrogenase 1
- E. Inhibition of 11β-hydroxysteroid dehydrogenase 1

56 A postpubertal 15-year-old boy presents with a healing right clavicle fracture diagnosed 4 weeks ago after he fell from standing height and was treated appropriately by the orthopedic team. This is his first-ever bone fracture.

Type 1 diabetes mellitus was diagnosed at age 2 and 9/12 years. His diabetes is managed by multiple daily insulin injections. His glycemic control is not optimal, and he has wide glycemic variation with weekly episodes of hypoglycemia followed by significant hyperglycemia. A hemoglobin A_{1c} measurement 3 months ago was 10.6% (92 mmol/mol). His point-of-care hemoglobin A_{1c} level today is 10.8% (95 mmol/mol). His mother believes he had elevated blood glucose values due to fracture-related pain.

He has celiac disease but is not adherent to a gluten-free diet. His current height is 67 in (170.2 cm) with a growth velocity less than 0.5 in/y. He is shorter than expected considering the calculated midparental height.

He has no family history of bone disease. Neither of his 2 older siblings has a history of frequent bone fractures.

Which of the following is the best next step in the assessment of this patient's bone health?
- A. Measurement of osteocalcin, bone-specific alkaline phosphatase, and C-terminal telopeptide of type I collagen
- B. Measurement of IGF-1, calcium, and 25-hydroxyvitamin D
- C. DXA scan
- D. Skeletal survey
- E. No further study (unless he has a second fracture)

57 A pediatric gastroenterologist asks for an opinion regarding a 9-year-old girl with a history of ulcerative colitis, which was diagnosed at age 8 years. Her condition has been refractory to treatment, and she has required intermittent steroid therapy. She underwent colectomy and ileostomy 2 months ago and was taking prednisolone, 20 mg once daily, which has since been reduced to 10 mg daily. Her physician would like to stop prednisolone therapy and is seeking an opinion.

Which of the following is the best course of action?
- A. Stop treatment now
- B. Measure 8-AM cortisol
- C. Change to alternate day treatment, then stop in 2 weeks
- D. Wean treatment and measure 8-AM serum cortisol
- E. Wean treatment and perform a standard cosyntropin-stimulation test

58 During a follow-up appointment for type 1 diabetes mellitus, an 18-year-old girl reports she is 16 weeks pregnant. Prenatal ultrasonography at 12-weeks' gestation was normal. Results from a first-trimester quadruple marker blood screen were normal. Cell-free DNA screening was negative for trisomy 21, 18, and 13 but showed monosomy X. She searched online and read about Turner syndrome. She is considering the option of medical termination of pregnancy and asks for an opinion.

In addition to encouraging the patient to have further discussions with her obstetrician, which of the following is the best next step?

A. Reassurance and follow-up in 3 months
B. Another cell-free DNA screen
C. Fetal karyotyping by amniocentesis
D. Fetal karyotyping by chorionic villus sampling
E. Referral for counseling about options regarding medical termination of pregnancy

59 A 6-week-old male infant presents to his primary care physician with recent-onset jaundice. On physical examination, he is found to have hemangiomas on his skin and an enlarged liver. Newborn screening results were normal, but his current TSH concentration is 42 mIU/L (0.35-5.0 mIU/L). He is referred for further evaluation.

On physical examination, his weight is 11 lb (5000 g) (50th percentile) and length is 21.7 in (55 cm) (25th percentile). He has a normal heart rate of 140 beats/min with low blood pressure for age (76/33 mm Hg). He has mild jaundice. On skin examination, there is a 3- to 4-second capillary refill and 3 hemangiomas on his trunk (the largest is 2 cm). The liver is enlarged, 4 cm below the costal margin. The spleen is not enlarged. Findings on heart examination are remarkable for a 2-3/6 systolic murmur radiating to the axilla.

Abdominal ultrasonography confirms an enlarged liver. He has multiple well-circumscribed lesions throughout the liver, predominantly hypoechoic, measuring up to 3.2 cm in diameter. Doppler ultrasonography reveals internal vascular flow. The lesions are compatible with multiple hepatic hemangiomas.

Echocardiography documents an enlarged heart with systolic dysfunction and mitral valve failure.

Another TSH measurement is 38.2 mIU/L (0.35-5.0 mIU/L).

Which of the following additional findings are likely in this infant?

Answer	Free T$_4$	Total T$_3$	Reverse T$_3$	Heart failure
A.	Normal	Low	High	Low-output
B.	Low	Normal	Low	Low-output
C.	Normal	Low	High	High-output
D.	Low	High	High	Low-output
E.	Low	Normal	Low	High-output

60 A 9-year-old girl presents for a follow-up visit. She has a history of craniopharyngioma, resected 1 year ago, that required subsequent radiation treatment. Her grandparents, who are her legal guardians, think that she has gained a lot of weight since her last visit 6 months ago. They have made a number of lifestyle modifications at home, including cutting back on portion sizes and increasing her physical activity, but they do not think these measures have impacted her weight gain. Review of her growth charts reveals that she has gained 17.5 lb (8 kg) since the last clinic visit. In addition to evaluating for pituitary deficiencies, further hormonal assessments are ordered.

Which of the following patterns is characteristic of this patient's condition?

Answer	Leptin	Insulin	Ghrelin
A.	Increased leptin	Increased insulin	Suppressed ghrelin
B.	Decreased leptin	Insulin resistance	Elevated ghrelin
C.	Increased leptin	Insulin resistance	Suppressed ghrelin
D.	Decreased leptin	Insulin sensitive	Elevated ghrelin
E.	Increased leptin	Increased insulin	Elevated ghrelin

61 A 2-week-old newborn presents for follow-up to her pediatrician. She was born full term to a G3 now P3 mother. Birth weight was 7 lb 11 oz (3500 g). Upon discharge at 36 hours of life, she weighed 7 lb 9 oz (3200 g). On examination today, her weight is 6 lb 9 oz (3000 g). The mother is breastfeeding and providing supplemental formula (1 oz every 3 hours, waking the baby overnight to feed). She has normal wet diapers, but bowel movements occur only once every 3 days.

On physical examination, the baby appears lethargic but is afebrile. She has no unusual facial features and no heart murmur. No bony abnormalities or signs of subcutaneous fat necrosis are noted.

Pertinent laboratory test results:
Calcium = 16.5 mg/dL (7.4-11.0 mg/dL) (SI: 4.1 mmol/L [1.9-2.8 mmol/L])
Phosphate = 6.6 mg/dL (4.6-8.5 mg/dL) (SI: 2.1 mmol/L [1.5-2.7 mmol/L])
Magnesium = 3.0 mg/dL (1.6-2.6 mg/dL) (SI: 1.2 mmol/L [0.7-1.1 mmol/L])
25-Hydroxyvitamin D = 32.8 ng/dL (20.0-60.0 ng/dL) (SI: 81.9 nmol/L [49.9-149.8 nmol/L])
1,25-Dihydroxyvitamin D = 43.4 pg/mL (19.9-79.3 pg/mL) (SI: 112.8 pmol/L [51.7-206.2 pmol/L])
Alkaline phosphatase = 161 U/L (90-273 U/L) (SI: 2.69 μkat/L [1.50-4.56 μkat/L])
PTH = 63 pg/mL (15-65 pg/mL) (SI: 63 ng/L [15-65 ng/L])

Family history is pertinent for mild hypercalcemia in the father, but he has no history of kidney stones. A maternal great aunt had a parathyroid adenoma removed at age 33 years. There is otherwise no family history of endocrine disorders.

Which of the following is the most likely pathogenic variant causing this infant's hypercalcemia?
A. Activating variant in *PTH1R*
B. Inactivating variant in *CASR*
C. Inactivating variant in *MEN1*
D. Inactivating variant in *CYP24A1*
E. Deletion of the *ELN* gene on chromosome 7

62 A 14-and-10/12-year-old boy with Down syndrome (trisomy 21), obesity, and history of acute lymphoblastic leukemia diagnosed at age 7 years is referred for evaluation. Results of annual thyroid function testing were normal, and there is no history of goiter. He has lost 4 lb (1.8 kg) in the past 2 months without trying to lose weight. He has no nocturia or other signs of diabetes mellitus.

His primary care physician ordered repeated thyroid function tests:
TSH = 0.01 mIU/L (0.5-4.3 mIU/L)
Total T_4 = 9.0 μg/dL (4.5-12.0 μg/dL) (SI: 115.8 nmol/L [57.9-154.4 nmol/L])

Leukemia has been in remission for more than 5 years. There is no history of asthma. He does not have palpitations, heat intolerance, or diarrhea, but he has been having sleep difficulties for 3 months, waking up at 3 AM and being unable to fall back asleep.

On physical examination, his height is 61.3 in (155.7 cm) (92nd percentile based on Down syndrome charts) and weight is 155.8 lb (70.7 kg) (85th percentile based on Down syndrome charts) (BMI = 29.1 kg/m² [97th percentile]). His blood pressure is 123/73 mm Hg, and pulse rate is 80 beats/min. He has typical Down syndrome facies. There is no lymphadenopathy. He has mild proptosis and no lid lag. His neck is short, and there is no goiter and no bruit. He has normal patellar reflexes and no tremor.

Laboratory tests repeated 1 month after the initial low TSH measurement demonstrate he is mildly hyperthyroid, and his antibodies confirm Graves disease.
TSH = <0.01 mIU/L (0.5-4.30 mIU/L)
Total T_4 = 11.5 μg/dL (4.5-12.0 μg/dL) (SI: 148.0 nmol/L [57.9-154.4 nmol/L])
Free T_4 = 2.2 ng/dL (0.9-1.4 ng/dL) (SI: 28.3 pmol/L [11.6-18.9 pmol/L])

Total T$_3$ = 244 ng/dL (84-179 ng/dL) (SI: 3.8 nmol/L [1.3-2.8 nmol/L])
TPO antibodies = 441 IU/mL (<9 IU/mL) (SI: 441 kIU/L [<9 kIU/L])
Thyroid-stimulating immunoglobulin = 361% (<140%)

Which of the following is the best next step in this child's management?
A. Perform total thyroidectomy
B. Start oral propranolol
C. Start oral methimazole
D. Observe and repeat thyroid function tests in 1 month
E. Perform radioactive iodine (^{131}I) ablation

63 A 6-and-6/12-year-old girl of African American descent is evaluated in the pediatric endocrinology clinic because of a 12-month history of body odor and acne. Over the last 6 months, her mother has noticed that she has developed pubic hair and had a growth spurt. She is the child of nonconsanguineous parents. She was born full term with a birth weight of 7 lb 13 oz (3550 g). She has been well with no hospital admissions. Her current height is at the 75th percentile. At her last check-up, her height was at the 50th percentile. Her bone age is advanced by 1.8 years compared with her chronologic age. There is no family history of early puberty. Her mother had menarche at age 10 years. Her 4-year-old brother is prepubertal.

On physical examination, breast development is Tanner stage 1, pubic hair is Tanner stage 2, and she has axillary hair development.

Which of the following diagnostic investigations should be ordered next?
A. Adrenal ultrasonography
B. LH measurement
C. Baseline 17-hydroxyprogesterone measurement
D. TSH measurement
E. Urinary steroid profile

64 A 17-year-old girl is referred for evaluation of secondary amenorrhea. Breast development started at age 10 years, and menarche occurred at age 12 years. She had menses monthly until approximately 8 months ago at which time menstrual periods ceased. She states that pregnancy is not a possibility and that she has otherwise been well. She has had no recent weight loss, vision problems, headaches, or breast discharge and takes no medications on a daily basis. Midparental target height is 65.5 in (166.4 cm).

On physical examination, her height is 64.2 in (163.1 cm) (50th percentile), weight is 142.6 lb (64.8 kg) (80th percentile) (BMI = 24.3 kg/m^2 [80th percentile]). She appears well. Examination findings are notable for Tanner stage 5 breast development with no nipple discharge. She does not have hirsutism. Peripheral vision is intact.

Laboratory test results:
Qualitative hCG, negative
TSH = 1.16 mIU/L (0.45-4.50 mIU/L)
Free T$_4$ = 1.1 ng/dL (0.8-1.8 ng/dL) (SI: 14.2 pmol/L [10.3-23.2 pmol/L])
LH = 1.2 mIU/mL (0.4-11.7 mIU/mL) (SI: 1.2 IU/L [0.4-11.7 IU/L])
FSH = 7.8 mIU/mL (0.8-8.5 mIU/mL) (SI: 7.8 IU/L [0.8-8.5 IU/L])
Estradiol = 12.2 pg/mL (12.5-211 pg/mL) (SI: 44.9 pmol/L [45.9-774.6 pmol/L])
Prolactin = 78.2 ng/mL (3.2-20.0 ng/mL) (SI: 3.4 nmol/L [0.14-0.87 nmol/L])

On brain MRI, her pituitary gland measures 5.2 mm with a normal neurohypophysis and infundibulum and no suprasellar mass. There is a 0.3 × 0.4 × 0.3-cm area of hypoenhancement in the left side of the pituitary gland.

Which of the following is recommended for this patient's management?
- A. Dynamic testing of prolactin secretion to confirm the diagnosis
- B. Neuro-ophthalmology examination for visual field deficits
- C. Monitoring with follow-up prolactin measurement and brain MRI in 3 to 6 months
- D. Initiation of once-daily bromocriptine and monitoring with annual echocardiography
- E. Initiation of twice-weekly cabergoline and counseling for psychiatric disturbance

65 An 11-month-old boy is admitted to the hospital for failure to thrive. His mother had gestational diabetes mellitus that was well controlled with dietary modifications. Prenatal course was normal. His birth weight and birth length were appropriate for age. He had normal weight gain and growth until 4 months of age, after which his weight gain declined drastically and growth slowed slightly. He has had intermittent vomiting for the last 1 month. He is otherwise a healthy child with normal development, appetite, and activity. Review of his growth chart documents length at the 11th percentile (–1.17 SDS) and weight at less than the 1st percentile (–3.89 SDS) (weight for length, –3.95 SDS). Head circumference is at 1.9 SDS.

On physical examination, he has a very thin build with a prominent forehead and very little subcutaneous fat on his chest and extremities. He is happy and interactive. The rest of the examination findings, including those from an ophthalmologic examination, are normal.

Laboratory test results:
    Complete blood cell count, normal
    Basic metabolic panel, normal
    Liver function, normal
    Free T_4, normal
    TSH, normal
    Random GH = 12.7 ng/mL (SI: 12.7 µg/L)
    IGF-1 = 110 ng/mL (17-248 ng/mL) (SI: 14.4 nmol/L [2.2-32.5 nmol/L])

Which of the following should be recommended as the best next step to confirm this patient's diagnosis?
- A. Brain MRI
- B. Cortisol level and cosyntropin-stimulation test
- C. Skeletal survey
- D. Bone age x-ray
- E. Refer to gastroenterology

66 A 6-week-old boy presents for outpatient evaluation of poor feeding and abdominal distention over the preceding 7 days. He was born full term following an uncomplicated singleton pregnancy. He was of normal weight and length at birth. He had mild neonatal jaundice that resolved without therapy. Results of newborn screening (sample obtained at 60 hours of life) were normal. The state newborn thyroid screen is TSH-based. Before the onset of symptoms, he had been healthy since birth and had been breastfeeding and gaining weight normally. His mother has no history of thyroid disease.

On physical examination, his length is at the 3rd percentile, weight is at the 10th percentile, weight for length is at the 67th percentile, and head circumference is at the 24th percentile. Pulse rate is 130 beats/min, respiratory rate is 24 breaths/min, and blood pressure is 92/55 mm Hg. The infant is sleeping comfortably and wakes easily. Fontanelles are open, soft, and normal in size. The thyroid gland is not palpable. Findings on pulmonary examination are normal, and there is a 2/6 systolic murmur. The abdomen is distended and nontender, and a firm liver edge is palpable 5 cm below the costal margin. The spleen is not palpable. A 5-mm cutaneous hemangioma is present on the left chest. The rest of the examination findings are normal.

Laboratory test results:

TSH = 94.5 mIU/L (0.7-5.7 mIU/L)

Free T_4 = 1.34 ng/dL (0.9-2.3 ng/dL) (SI: 17.2 pmol/L [11.6-29.6 pmol/L])

Which of the following additional laboratory findings is most likely to be present?

A. Elevated serum reverse T_3

B. Low serum thyroglobulin

C. Elevated serum T_3

D. Elevated serum TSH-receptor antibodies

E. Elevated urinary iodine

67 A 2-year-old boy with recently diagnosed acute lymphoblastic leukemia is hospitalized for fever with neutropenia and is found to have *Escherichia coli* bacteremia. Endocrinology is consulted for persistent hyponatremia. He is receiving tobramycin and piperacillin/tazobactam for the bacteremia and intravenous fluids (0.9% normal saline plus KCl [20 mmol/L]) at a maintenance rate. In addition to dexamethasone, he is currently on the following chemotherapy medications: daunorubicin, methotrexate, and vincristine.

On physical examination, his blood pressure is 90/52 mm Hg, pulse rate is 128 beats/min, respiratory rate is 24 breaths/min, and temperature is 98.6°F (37°C). His height is 36.5 in (92.7 cm), and weight is 29.7 lb (13.5 kg) (BMI = 15.78 kg/m²). He has moist mucous membranes. There is no thyromegaly. Findings on cardiac examination are normal. He is fussy, but his neurologic examination findings are otherwise normal. His extremities are well perfused. There is no edema.

Laboratory test results:

Sodium = 124 mEq/L (136-149 mEq/L) (SI: 124 mmol/L [136-149 mmol/L])

Potassium = 3.9 mEq/L (3.9-5.7 mEq/L) (SI: 3.9 mmol/L [3.9-5.7 mmol/L])

Chloride = 90 mEq/L (98-108 mEq/L) (SI: 90 mmol/L [98-108 mmol/L])

Carbon dioxide = 19.3 mEq/L (23.0-30.0 mEq/L) (SI: 19.3 mmol/L [23.0-30.0 mmol/L])

Glucose = 120 mg/dL (70-110 mg/dL) (SI: 6.7 mmol/L [3.9-6.1 mmol/L])

Serum urea nitrogen = 17 mg/dL (7-18 mg/dL) (SI: 6.1 mmol/L [2.5-6.4 mmol/L])

Creatinine = 0.16 mg/dL (0.25-0.74 mg/dL) (SI: 14.1 μmol/L [22.1-64.4 μmol/L])

Uric acid = 1.6 mg/dL (2.0-7.0 mg/dL) (SI: 95.2 μmol/L [119.0-416.4 μmol/L])

Triglycerides = 92 mg/dL (30-74 mg/dL) (SI: 1.04 mmol/L [0.34-0.74 mmol/L])

Free T_4 = 0.96 ng/dL (0.96-1.77 ng/dL) (SI: 12.4 pmol/L [12.4-22.8 pmol/L])

TSH = 0.9 mIU/L (0.70-5.97 mIU/L)

Serum cortisol (8 AM) = 0.3 μg/dL (2.3-15.0 μg/dL) (SI: 8.3 nmol/L [63.5-413.8 nmol/L])

Plasma osmolality = 264 mOsm/kg (285-295 mOsm/kg) (SI: 264 mmol/kg [285-295 mmol/kg])

Urine osmolality = 554 mOsm/kg (50-1400 mOsm/kg) (SI: 554 mmol/kg [50-1400 mmol/kg])

Urinary sodium (random) = 83 mEq/L (SI: 83 mmol/L)

Which of the following is the most likely primary cause of this patient's hyponatremia?

A. Hypertriglyceridemia

B. Cerebral/renal salt wasting

C. Excessive fluid administration

D. Syndrome of inappropriate antidiuresis

E. Cortisol insufficiency

68 A 9-and-10/12-year-old girl with Turner syndrome is being seen for follow-up evaluation of growth. Turner syndrome was diagnosed at age 15 months, and karyotype analysis documented a 45,X karyotype with no mosaicism. She has been receiving recombinant human GH since age 4 years after slowed growth was documented. Her response to GH therapy had been good (*see growth chart*): the red lines are the 5th, 50th, and 95th percentiles of the Centers for Disease Control chart for normal girls, and the green lines are the 5th, 10th, 25th, 50th, 75th, 90th, and 95th percentiles for girls with untreated Turner syndrome). Over the last 1.5 to 2 years, her linear growth has decelerated. Her growth velocity over the last 10 months was poor at 3.4 cm/y.

On physical examination, there is no evidence of pubertal development with Tanner stage 1 breast development and pubic hair. At previous appointments, her IGF-1 values have been in the upper reference range or slightly above. For this reason, she has been maintained on a relatively low GH dosage. Her current dosage is 0.9 mg subcutaneously 7 days a week, which translates into a total dose of 0.19 mg/kg per week. A bone age obtained at this visit is interpreted to be 8 years, 10 months at a chronologic age of 9 years, 10 months. Her IGF-1 concentration is 476 ng/mL (62.4 nmol/L) (Z-score, +2.1).

Midparental target height is 61.8 in (157 cm), which falls between the 10th and 25th percentile for women in the standard Centers for Disease Control growth charts.

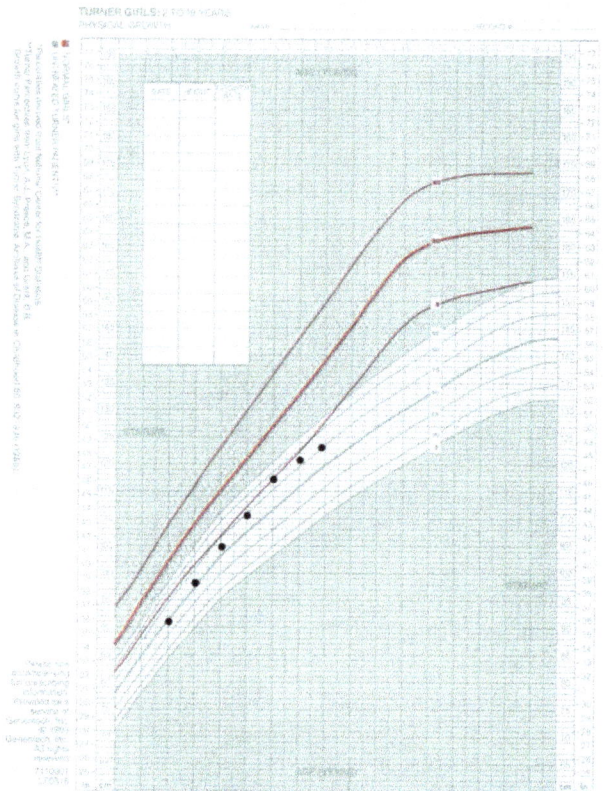

Which of the following is the most appropriate intervention to improve final height outcome?
   A. Increase the GH dosage to 0.35 mg/kg per week
   B. Start oral estradiol and maintain the current GH dosage
   C. Start oxandrolone at a dosage of 0.03 mg/kg daily and maintain the current GH dosage
   D. Start an aromatase inhibitor (anastrozole) at a dosage of 1 mg orally daily and maintain the current GH dosage
   E. Continue the current GH dosage and consider starting estradiol at age 14 to 16 years

69 A 13-year-old boy presents for evaluation of obesity. His BMI has consistently plotted at greater than the 95th percentile for weight since he was a young child. His family is very concerned about his risk for medical problems due to obesity. His pediatrician has screened him for glucose abnormalities and also ordered a fasting lipid panel, all of which had normal results. The family asks about screening him for liver problems because his mother, who also has obesity, states that she has "fatty liver."

Which of the following is the best next step in this patient's evaluation?
   A. Abdominal ultrasonography
   B. Measurement of AST
   C. Measurement of ALT
   D. Referral to gastroenterology
   E. Abdominal MRI

70 A 10-year-old girl was recently diagnosed with high-risk acute lymphocytic leukemia. Part of her induction chemotherapy included high-dosage prednisone, 20 mg twice daily, for the last month. She now frequently experiences back pain, but her parents cannot identify a preceding traumatic event. Since being diagnosed with acute lymphocytic leukemia, she has gained 6.6 lb (3 kg). She has not yet started puberty.

Which of the following is the best next step regarding the assessment and treatment of this patient's vertebral compression fractures?
   A. Strict bed rest until pain resolves
   B. Lumbar spine DXA; if results are normal, no further imaging is indicated
   C. Lumbar spine DXA and vertebral fracture analysis by DXA
   D. Lumbar spine DXA and dedicated spine x-rays
   E. Bisphosphonate therapy for treatment of vertebral compression fractures

71 A 16-year-old girl has been aware of a lump in the left side of her neck for the past few months. At her annual well-child visit, her pediatrician orders ultrasonography, which shows a thyroid nodule in the left lobe measuring 5 cm with features suspicious for thyroid cancer. It is solid and hypoechoic and has a few microcalcifications. There is no evidence of the nodule invading the capsule and no cervical lymphadenopathy. Thyroid cancer is suspected, and she is referred to pediatric endocrinology for ultrasound-guided FNA and laboratory tests.

The FNA is interpreted to be papillary thyroid cancer. Given the large nodule, neck CT is performed before total thyroidectomy, and it shows no cervical lymph nodes. Her preoperative thyroid function is normal and TPO and thyroglobulin antibodies are negative. Total thyroidectomy is uneventful. No neck dissection is performed based on her CT and ultrasonography staging. Pathologic examination confirms the diagnosis of papillary thyroid cancer in the left lobe, and no evidence of thyroid cancer is noted in the right lobe. The tumor does not invade the capsule and there is no evidence of lymphovascular invasion.

Levothyroxine, 150 mcg once daily, is initiated and the patient returns for her first visit 1 month after surgery.

On the basis of the 2015 Pediatric Guidelines for Children with Thyroid Nodules and Differentiated Thyroid Cancer, which of the following is the best strategy?
   A. Recommend ^{131}I radioablation in 1 month; measure thyroglobulin 2 months later while on levothyroxine
   B. Assess thyroid function now and aim for a TSH concentration <0.1 mIU/L; measure thyroglobulin in 2 to 3 months while on levothyroxine
   C. Assess thyroid function now and aim for a TSH concentration 0.1-0.5 mIU/L; measure thyroglobulin in 2 to 3 months while on levothyroxine
   D. Assess thyroid function now and aim for a TSH concentration 0.5-1.0 mIU/L; measure thyroglobulin in 2 to 3 months while on levothyroxine
   E. Stop levothyroxine; order a stimulated thyroglobulin measurement and whole-body scan to be done 2 weeks later when her TSH concentration is >30 mIU/L

72 A 3-year-old boy presents with lower-extremity bowing. He was born at 28 weeks' gestation, and the neonatal course was complicated by prolonged use of total parenteral nutrition due to necrotizing enterocolitis. He has been on full enteral feeds since approximately 4 months of age and now consumes 24 oz of milk daily. He also takes a chewable multivitamin.

He did not start walking until 18 months of age, which the family attributes to his prematurity. His parents initially noted the bowing deformity at that time and report that it appears to have worsened over the last year. The child is now in preschool and his parents note that compared with other children in his class, he seems to rest more often on the playground. Growth parameters, adjusted for prematurity, have been normal. Dentition is normal. Family history is relevant for recurrent stress fractures in the mother who is a marathon runner.

Laboratory test results:

Calcium = 9.8 mg/dL (8.3-10.6 mg/dL) (SI: 2.5 mmol/L [2.1-2.7 mmol/L])

Phosphate = 7.7 mg/dL (4.0-6.8 mg/dL) (SI: 2.5 mmol/L [1.3-2.2 mmol/L])

25-Hydroxyvitamin D = 73 ng/dL (20-60 ng/dL) (SI: 182.2 nmol/L [49.9-149.8 nmol/L])

Alkaline phosphatase = 76 U/L (78-300 U/L) (SI: 1.27 μkat/L [1.22-5.01 μkat/L])

PTH = 16 pg/mL (15-87 pg/mL) (SI: 16 ng/L [15-87 ng/L])

Which of the following is this child's most likely diagnosis?

A. Vitamin D intoxication
B. Hypoparathyroidism
C. Physiologic bowing
D. Hypophosphatasia
E. Rickets of prematurity

73 A 15-year-old boy is referred for evaluation of pubertal delay. His history is notable for cryptorchidism and orchiopexy at age 11 years. The only signs of puberty have been recent onset of pubic hair growth. He was followed by his pediatrician from birth until 2 years of age for poor growth, but he has grown well since then. He has no vision problems, headaches, or fatigue, but he does report a poor sense of smell.

His mother underwent menarche at age 13 years, and the timing of puberty in his father is unknown. His 18-year-old brother started puberty at 13 to 14 years of age. His midparental target height is 69.5 in (176.5 cm).

On physical examination, his height is 63.2 in (160.5 cm) (5th percentile) and weight is 117 lb (53.2 kg) (22nd percentile). He appears well. Pubic hair is Tanner stage 3 and testicular volume is 2 mL bilaterally.

Which of the following sets of laboratory test results would be most likely in this patient?

Answer	Inhibin B	Antimullerian hormone	FSH
A.	17.7 pg/mL (SI: 17.7 ng/L)	41 ng/mL (SI: 293 pmol/L)	0.33 mIU/mL (SI: 0.33 IU/L)
B.	186 pg/mL (SI: 186 ng/L)	114 ng/mL (SI: 814 pmol/L)	1.2 mIU/mL (SI: 1.2 IU/L)
C.	186 pg/mL (SI: 186 ng/L)	114 pg/mL (SI: 814 pmol/L)	34.6 mIU/mL (SI: 34.6 IU/L)
D.	17.7 pg/mL (SI: 17.7 ng/L)	41 ng/mL (SI: 293 pmol/L)	34.6 mIU/mL (SI: 34.6 IU/L)
E.	17.7 pg/mL (SI: 17.7 ng/L)	96 ng/mL (SI: 686 pmol/L)	0.33 mIU/mL (SI: 0.33 IU/L)

Reference Ranges:

Inhibin B

5-9.9 years	21-166 pg/mL (SI: 21-166 ng/L)
10-13.9 years	41-328 pg/mL (SI: 41-328 ng/L)
14-17.9 years	54-295 pg/mL (SI: 54-295 ng/L)
≥18 years	47-308 pg/mL (SI: 47-308 ng/L)

Source: Quest Diagnostics

Antimullerian hormone

<24 months	14.0-466.0 ng/mL (SI: 100-3329 pmol/L)
24 months-12 years	7.4-243.0 ng/mL (SI: 53-1736 pmol/L)
>12 years	0.7-19.0 ng/mL (SI: 5-136 pmol/L)

Source: Mayo Clinic Laboratories

74 A 6-and-2/12-year-old boy with Prader-Willi syndrome presents to the clinic for follow-up. He was born at full term. Birth weight and length were adequate for gestational age. He was noted to have significant hypotonia at birth and had dysmorphic features, including narrow biparietal diameter and undescended testes. He had issues with feeding and required a nasogastric tube and, later, a gastrostomy tube. The suspicion of Prader-Willi syndrome was confirmed with fluorescence in situ hybridization analysis.

At age 14 months, his length was below the 3rd percentile for age (SDS, –2.2) and weight was at the 4th percentile for age (SDS, –1.75). Given the reported benefits of GH therapy started early in children with Prader-Willi syndrome, he underwent a sleep study to rule out significant obstructive sleep apnea. The sleep study showed mild obstructive sleep apnea, as well as a component of central apnea. GH therapy was started at age 16 months when his length was 28.9 in (73.4 cm) (<3rd percentile; SDS, –2.18), weight was 20.9 lb (9.5 kg) (5th percentile; SDS, –1.64), and body surface area was 0.422 m². The initial GH dosage was 0.2 mg subcutaneously once daily (0.47 mg/m² daily or 0.15 mg/kg per week). Close surveillance with overnight pulse oximetry was recommended.

Now, at age 6-and-2/12 years, his height is 42.9 in (109 cm) (7th percentile; SDS, –1.46), weight is 44.7 lb (20.3 kg) (39th percentile; SDS, –0.27), and BMI is 17.1 kg/m² (85th percentile; SDS, +1.05). His body surface area is 0.775 m². He grew 1.5 in (3.8 cm) in the last 6 months, rendering a growth velocity of 7.6 cm/y. He has been doing well with the GH injections without evidence of adverse effects or worrisome signs or symptoms such as polyuria, polydipsia, nocturia, enuresis, headaches, or vision changes. His mother reports that since the initiation of GH therapy, the frequency of oxygen desaturations has decreased. She has also noticed continued improvement in his muscle tone, a finding that was corroborated in a recent follow-up appointment in neurology. His GH dosage is 0.7 mg subcutaneously once daily (0.24 mg/kg per week).

Laboratory test results:
    IGFBP-3 = 3.7 mg/L (1.5-3.4 mg/L)
    IGF-1 = 215 ng/mL (60-228 ng/mL) (SI: 28.2 nmol/L [7.86-29.9 nmol/L])
    IGF-1 Z-score = +2.49
    Random glucose = 128 mg/dL (70-100 mg/dL) (SI: 7.1 mmol/L [3.9-5.56 mmol/L])
    Hemoglobin A$_{1c}$ = 5.5% (4.3%-5.7%) (SI: 37 mmol/mol [23-39 mmol/mol])
    TSH = 6.2 mIU/L (0.8-8.2 mIU/L)
    Free T$_4$ = 1.35 ng/dL (0.8-1.8 ng/dL) (SI: 17.4 pmol/L [10.3-23.2 pmol/L])
    25-Hydroxyvitamin D = 30 ng/mL (25-100 ng/mL) (SI: 74.9 nmol/L [62.4-249.6 nmol/L])

On the basis of these results and clinical guidelines, which of the following is the best next step in this patient's management?
    A.   Continue the current dosage of GH
    B.   Start thyroid hormone replacement therapy
    C.   Decrease the GH dosage
    D.   Perform an oral glucose tolerance test
    E.   Start vitamin D therapy

75   A 15-year-old boy has recently been diagnosed with a pheochromocytoma. The 24-hour urine metanephrine results at the time of diagnosis were as follows:
    Urine volume = 961 mL (0-4440 mL)
    Urinary normetanephrine = 1765 µg/24 h (0-366 µg/24 h) (SI: 9637 nmol/d [0-2000 nmol/d])
    Urinary metanephrine = 114 µg/24 h (0-493 µg/24 h) (SI: 622 nmol/d [0-2692 nmol/d])

He undergoes unilateral adrenalectomy and has genetic testing.

A pathogenic variant in which of the following genes is most likely?
    A.   *RET* (ret proto-oncogene)
    B.   *VHL* (von Hippel-Lindau tumor suppressor)
    C.   *TMEM127* (transmembrane protein 127)
    D.   *NF1* (neurofibromin 1)
    E.   *SDHC* (succinate dehydrogenase complex subunit C)

76 A postpubertal 15-year-old boy is evaluated for suboptimally controlled type 1 diabetes mellitus diagnosed 7 years ago. He is treated with multiple daily insulin injections with long- and rapid-acting insulin pens.

His last 3 hemoglobin A_{1c} measurements have fluctuated between 8.2% and 9.7% (66-83 mmol/mol). He currently uses a glucose meter and does not want to switch to a continuous glucose monitoring device because he thinks it would "annoy" him. His blood glucose values vary widely from 54 mg/dL (3.0 mmol/L) to greater than 500 mg/dL (>27.8 mmol/L). His current 30-day glucose average is 229 mg/dL (12.7 mmol/L) with 1 standard deviation of 102 mg/dL (5.7 mmol/L).

He describes normal daily function without any symptoms. He is an avid soccer player and is physically active. He does not report any sleep disruption and has no nocturia. He is dismissive when asked about his vision.

His most recent set of laboratory results reveal normal thyroid function, undetectable tissue transglutaminase antibodies, elevated total cholesterol and triglycerides, normal LDL cholesterol, and normal-range urine albumin.

Which of the following subspecialists should this patient be referred to first to address concerns of microvascular complications?
- A. Cardiologist
- B. Nephrologist
- C. Neurologist
- D. Ophthalmologist
- E. Podiatrist

77 A 7-year-old girl is referred for evaluation of short stature. She was born at term but was small-for-gestational-age. She has a history of microcephaly, midface hypoplasia, hypoplastic optic nerves, mega cisterna magna, autism spectrum disorder, and mild global developmental delay. She has normal appetite, thirst, bowel movements, and urination. Whole-exome sequencing done at 6 months of age (ordered by a geneticist) identified a heterozygous pathogenic variant in the *IGF1R* gene (Arg739Trp). She has not had any hospital admissions since birth. Review of her growth chart shows that since infancy, her length and height have been at less than the first percentile and her weight has been at the third percentile.

Laboratory test results:
Erythrocyte sedimentation rate = 10 mm/h (0-32 mm/h)
IGF-1 = 278 ng/mL (49-267 ng/mL) (SI: 36.4 nmol/L [6.4-35.0 nmol/L])
TSH = 1.37 mIU/L (0.5-5.0 mIU/L)
Free T_4 = 1.46 ng/dL (0.90-1.67 ng/dL) (SI: 18.8 pmol/L [11.6-21.5 pmol/L])
Tissue transglutaminase antibodies IgA = <2 U/mL (0-3 U/mL)
IgA = 157 mg/dL (51-220 mg/dL)

Bone age is reported to be 8 years and 10 months at the chronologic age of 7 years and 5 months.

A problem with the function of which of the following proteins best explains the underlying pathology of this patient's poor growth?
- A. Cytokine receptor that activates the JAK-STAT signaling pathway
- B. Cell-surface receptor with intrinsic tyrosine kinase activity
- C. Nuclear receptor that regulates gene transcription
- D. Cytosolic receptor that regulates gene transcription
- E. Transmembrane G-protein–coupled receptor

78 A 5-week-old girl presents for outpatient evaluation of jaundice and decreasing oral intake over the preceding 4 days. The pregnancy was uncomplicated until the third trimester, when intrauterine growth restriction was observed. Delivery was induced at 38 weeks' gestation and was uncomplicated, and birth weight was 5 lb 8 oz (2500 g) (11th percentile). Her postnatal course was unremarkable, and results of newborn screening were normal (sample collected at 50 hours of life). She is exclusively breastfeeding and her weight has been increasing by 30 g daily. Her mother has no history of thyroid disease, takes a prenatal vitamin, and consumes 2 daily servings of a traditional Korean soup to stimulate lactation.

On physical examination, the infant's length is at the 10th percentile, weight is at the 15th percentile, and head circumference is at the 18th percentile. Her pulse rate is 120 beats/min, respiratory rate is 22 breaths/min, and blood pressure is 84/52 mm Hg. The infant appears calm, comfortable, and sleepy. She has jaundice and scleral icterus. Fontanelles are open, soft, and normal in size. The thyroid gland is not palpable. The abdomen is normal with no organomegaly. There are no skin lesions. The rest of the examination findings are normal.

Laboratory test results:
Total bilirubin = 7.2 mg/dL (0-7.0 mg/dL) (SI: 123.1 µmol/L [0-119.7 µmol/L])
Direct bilirubin = 0.6 mg/dL (0-0.6 mg/dL) (SI: 10.3 µmol/L [0-10.3 µmol/L])
Hematocrit = 36.2% (34.1%-41.8%) (SI: 0.362 [0.341-0.418])
TSH = 108 mIU/L (1.7-9.1 mIU/L)
Free T$_4$ = 0.39 ng/dL (0.9-2.3 ng/dL) (SI: 5.0 pmol/L [11.6-29.6 pmol/L])

Ultrasonography reveals a thyroid gland that is normal in size and appearance.

Measurement of which of the following is most likely to confirm the etiology of this patient's hypothyroidism?
   A.   Serum reverse T$_3$
   B.   Serum TPO antibodies
   C.   Serum T$_3$
   D.   Serum TSH-receptor antibodies
   E.   Urinary iodine

79   A 13-year-old girl with autoimmune polyglandular syndrome type 1 presents for routine follow-up. Her current diagnoses include hypoparathyroidism and malabsorption secondary to chronic diarrhea. She had the onset of thelarche approximately 3 years ago but has not yet had menses. Approximately 1 year ago, she required significant alteration in management of hypocalcemia with increasing dosages of calcium and calcitriol supplementation. Because of her malabsorption, she was eventually transitioned to recombinant PTH given once every evening with calcium carbonate supplementation continued once daily in the early afternoon. With this approach, her serum calcium levels have been stable.

On physical examination, the patient is thin. She has lost 6.6 lb (3 kg) since her last visit 6 months ago. She appears mildly dehydrated and reports fatigue, nausea, and vomiting. She has Tanner stage 4 breast development. Her pulse rate is 88 beats/min, blood pressure is 92/56 mm Hg, and respiratory rate is 16 breaths/min.

Current laboratory test results (8-AM specimen draw):
Calcium = 10.6 mg/dL (8.4-10.2 mg/dL) (SI: 2.7 mmol/L [2.1-2.6 mmol/L])
Phosphate = 4.8 mg/dL (3.7-6.5 mg/dL) (SI: 1.6 mmol/L [1.2-2.1 mmol/L])
Magnesium = 1.8 mg/dL (1.7-2.4 mg/dL) (SI: 0.7 mmol/L [0.7-1.0 mmol/L])
Albumin = 3.7 g/dL (3.3-4.8 g/dL) (SI: 37 g/L [33-48 g/L])
PTH (1-84) = <3 pg/mL (15-87 pg/mL) (SI: <3 ng/L [15-87 ng/L])
Urinary calcium-to-creatinine ratio = 0.14 (<0.2)

Which of the following is the most important next step in this patient's management?
   A.   Screen for adrenal insufficiency
   B.   Screen for primary ovarian insufficiency
   C.   Screen for thyroid disease
   D.   Reduce the dosage of recombinant PTH
   E.   Discontinue calcium carbonate supplementation

80 A family has recently moved to the United States. Their now 20-month-old son received the diagnosis of Prader-Willi syndrome (PWS) several months before their move to the United States, and they would like to establish care. The parents express frustration that the diagnosis was delayed since their son exhibited features soon after birth that they now recognize as being common in infants with this condition. They have been trying to learn more about PWS to ensure the best care. They are very worried about possible comorbidities associated with PWS, particularly the risks for overweight/obesity, and would like to know what they might expect in the upcoming months.

Which of the following is the most accurate description of what to expect regarding their child's weight status over the next 9 months?
A. Hyperphagia and lack of satiety leading to rapid weight gain
B. Increase in weight percentile without appreciable changes in appetite or calories
C. Increase in weight percentile associated with an increased interest in food
D. Maintenance of weight along the same percentile
E. Failure to thrive with difficulty gaining weight

81 A 6-year-old girl presents for evaluation of short stature. GH deficiency is being considered, and the next planned step is provocative GH-stimulation testing. The patient's mother asks how the testing works.

Which of the following best describes the mechanism of GH release?
A. Arginine inhibits somatostatin
B. Glucagon stimulates $\alpha2$ adrenergic receptors
C. Propranolol causes hypoglycemia
D. Clonidine inhibits $\alpha2$ adrenergic receptors
E. Levodopa leads to a $\beta2$ adrenergic antagonist effect on somatostatin

82 A 6-month-old girl presents to her pediatrician with failure to thrive, vomiting, and seizures. Biochemical analysis reveals hypoglycemia and primary adrenal insufficiency. She receives treatment, and her management regimen subsequently consists of glucocorticoid and mineralocorticoid replacement with regular monitoring.

Over the next 2 years, she is noted to have mild neurodevelopmental delay and develops ichthyosis and persistent lymphopenia. Primary hypothyroidism is diagnosed, and levothyroxine is initiated. At age 3 years, she develops nephrotic syndrome with proteinuria and hypoalbuminemia. Renal biopsy documents focal segmental glomerulosclerosis.

Pathogenic variants in which of the following genes are the most likely cause of her condition?
A. *SGPL1* (sphingosine-1-phosphate lyase 1)
B. *MRAP* (melanocortin 2 receptor accessory protein)
C. *POR* (cytochrome P450 oxidoreductase)
D. *AIRE* (autoimmune regulator)
E. *AAAS* (aladin WD repeat nucleoporin)

83 An otherwise healthy 4-year-old boy is referred for evaluation of short stature. He was born at 39 weeks' gestation via natural vaginal delivery. Birth weight was 3 lb 15 oz (1800 g) (<3rd percentile; SDS, –3.14) and birth length was 16.5 in (42 cm) (<3rd percentile; SDS, –4.4). He had a few episodes of hypoglycemia in the immediate neonatal period that resolved after 3 days, at which time he was discharged home with his mother.

Family history is negative for disorders of growth and puberty. Midparental target height is 68 ± 4 in (172.7 ± 10 cm). The patient has no siblings.

On physical examination, his height is 33.5 in (85 cm) (<3rd percentile; SDS, –4.16) and his weight is 29.7 lb (13.5 kg) (4th percentile; SDS, –1.68). He has a prominent forehead with relative macrocephaly and a small pointy chin. His right leg is 1 in (2.5 cm) longer than his left leg. He has clinodactyly of the fifth digits bilaterally. He has 2 café-au-lait spots on the right side of his lumbar area measuring 4 × 3 cm and 2 × 1.5 cm.

Initial laboratory test results:

IGF-1 = 115 ng/mL (54-178 ng/mL) (SI: 15.1 nmol/L [7.1-23.3 nmol/L])

IGFBP-3 = 2.8 mg/L (1.4-3.0 mg/L)

Thyroid function, normal

Erythrocyte sedimentation rate, normal

Screen for celiac disease, negative

Which of the following tests is most likely to reveal the etiology of this child's short stature?

A. Arginine-insulin tolerance test

B. *NF1* gene sequencing and deletion/duplication analysis

C. Uniparental disomy analysis of chromosome 7

D. Sequencing of the gene encoding the IGF-1 receptor

E. Methylation analysis of chromosome 11p15

84 A 17-year-old girl presents with classic symptoms of polyuria and polydipsia, and diabetes mellitus is diagnosed. Her urinalysis indicates no ketones. Her BMI is at the 65th percentile; the family reports no recent weight loss. She wears bilateral hearing aids. Her medical history is notable for bilateral sensory neural hearing loss and a learning disability. Her family history is relevant for insulin-requiring diabetes in her mother. Her older brother was diagnosed with diabetes at age 19 years and he is currently on oral therapy.

The patient is started on a basal-bolus insulin regimen. She responds well but requires much less insulin than initially prescribed due to frequent hypoglycemia episodes. At her 2-week follow-up visit, the following laboratory results are reviewed:

Hemoglobin A_{1c} = 8.5% (4.0%-5.6%) (69 mmol/mol [mmol/mol]) (it was 9.8% [84 mmol/mol] at diagnosis)

Glutamic acid decarboxylase 65 antibodies = <5 IU/mL (<5 IU/mL)

Insulin autoantibodies = <0.4 U/mL (<0.4 U/mL)

Islet-cell antibodies = <1.25 JDF units (<1.25 JDF units)

Electrolytes, normal

Liver enzymes, normal

Which of the following diagnostic approaches would reveal the etiology of this patient's diabetes mellitus?

A. Assessment for zinc transporter-8 [ZnT8] antibodies

B. HLA typing

C. *HNF1A* and *HNF4A* genetic testing

D. *WFS1* genetic testing

E. *MT-TL1* genetic testing

85 A 16-year-old girl is noted to have a thyroid nodule on examination, and ultrasonography confirms a right-sided 3-cm nodule with features suspicious for thyroid cancer. Furthermore, ultrasonography demonstrates a few lymph nodes in the right mid-cervical chain, anterior to the sternocleidomastoid muscle, that show a loss of the hilum and/or peripheral vascularity. She is euthyroid, and TPO and thyroglobulin antibodies are negative. Results of ultrasound-guided FNA of the nodule are interpreted as suspicious for papillary thyroid carcinoma. She undergoes total thyroidectomy, and based on the preoperative ultrasonography findings, the surgeon also performs a bilateral central neck dissection and a lateral right-sided neck dissection.

Histopathologic examination confirms the right nodule to be papillary thyroid carcinoma, measuring 3.2 cm in largest diameter with lymphovascular invasion. She has 2 smaller foci of papillary thyroid carcinoma in the left lobe. She has locoregional spread: 5/7 level 6 lymph nodes and 8/10 level 3 and 4 lymph nodes are malignant on the right side.

Which of the following is the best next step in this patient's management?
- A. Perform chest CT to search for pulmonary metastases; decide whether she needs ^{131}I radioablation
- B. Initiate levothyroxine to maintain TSH <0.1 mIU/L; 2 to 3 months after surgery, measure thyroglobulin
- C. Initiate levothyroxine to maintain TSH <0.1 mIU/L; 2 to 3 months after surgery, measure TSH-stimulated thyroglobulin and perform diagnostic whole-body ^{123}I scan
- D. Hold off on initiating levothyroxine postoperatively; administer ^{131}I once TSH is >30 mIU/L
- E. Initiate levothyroxine to maintain TSH between 0.1 and 0.5 mIU/L; perform postoperative ^{123}I whole-body scan

86 A 5-year-old boy is followed up in endocrine clinic for short stature. He was the product of a nonconsanguineous union and was born at 34.5 weeks gestational age with normal birth length (18.5 in [47 cm]) and weight (6 lb 5 oz [2865 g]). In the last year, he had 4 episodes of abdominal pain, vomiting, hypoglycemia, and ketosis requiring intravenous glucose infusions. His growth chart demonstrates postnatal growth delay with a current height at –3.0 SD. His BMI is at the 3rd percentile. He consumes approximately 2000 calories daily (normal, 1700-1800 calories daily).

His parents and 2 younger siblings have a normal phenotype. His mother's height is 61.4 in (156 cm) (–1.3 SD), and his father's height is 67.3 in (171 cm) (–0.6 SD). His father is overweight and had delayed puberty. His mother had normal puberty. The patient's father has a female first cousin who is very short (adult height 55.1 in [140 cm]), but she has never been evaluated for short stature.

The patient has proportional short stature and no dysmorphic features on examination. His current growth velocity is 4 cm/y. Bone age assessment at age 4 years and 8 months was interpreted to be 1 year and 6 months.

Laboratory test results (6 months ago):
    IGF-1 = 44 ng/mL (37-192 ng/mL) (SI: 5.8 nmol/L [4.8-25.2 nmol/L])
    Free T$_4$ = 1.1 ng/dL (0.9-1.7 ng/dL) (SI: 14.2 pmol/L [11.6-21.9 pmol/L])
    TSH = 3.5 mIU/L (0.6-5.5 mIU/L)
    Cortisol (8 AM) = 15.0 µg/dL (3.0-21.0 µg/dL) (SI: 413.8 nmol/L [82.8-579.4 nmol/L])

A dual-agent GH-stimulation test performed 2 months ago documented a peak GH concentration of 4.0 ng/mL (4.0 µg/L).
Findings on brain MRI are normal.

Which of the following is the best next step in this patient's management?
- A. Reassure and schedule follow-up in clinic in 6 months
- B. Refer to gastrointestinal clinic for evaluation and return to endocrine clinic once BMI has improved
- C. Start GH replacement therapy at 0.2 mg/kg per week
- D. Start GH replacement therapy at 0.35 mg/kg per week
- E. Repeat endocrine laboratory tests, including IGF-1, free T$_4$, TSH, and 8-AM cortisol

87 A 3-year-old girl presents for evaluation of precocious puberty. She was born at 31 weeks' gestation (birth weight 3 lb 3 oz [1446 g]) and spent time in the neonatal intensive care unit because of mild respiratory distress, anemia, and jaundice. She has reportedly had breast tissue since infancy and it has recently increased. She has developed some long, thick hairs in the pubic area. She has also started outgrowing her twin sister. Development has been normal, and she does not take any medications. She is otherwise healthy. Her mother is concerned that her daughter has episodes of unprovoked laughter lasting 30 to 45 seconds. Although she is able to speak during these episodes, she is unable to stop the laughter.

On physical examination, her height is 38.2 in (97 cm) (75th percentile). She appears well and findings on neurologic examination are normal. She has approximately 5 cm of glandular breast tissue bilaterally, several long, coarse pubic hairs along the labia, and dull pink vaginal mucosa. There are several café-au-lait macules measuring less than 5 cm each.

Laboratory test results:

    Thyroid function, normal

    Complete blood cell count, normal

    Complete metabolic panel, normal

    Estradiol = 25.2 pg/mL (<16 pg/mL) (SI: 92.5 pmol/L [<58.7 pmol/L])

    LH = 9.5 mIU/mL (<0.02-0.30 mIU/mL) (SI: 9.5 IU/L [<0.02-0.30 IU/L])

    FSH = 7.1 mIU/mL (0.5-6.0 mIU/mL) (SI: 7.1 IU/L [0.5-6.0 IU/L])

Which of the following is the most likely etiology of her precocious puberty?

    A. *MKRN3* gene variant

    B. *GNAS* gene variant

    C. Idiopathic

    D. Craniopharyngioma

    E. Hypothalamic hamartoma

88 A 2-and-11/12-year-old girl is referred for evaluation of short stature.

On physical examination, her length is below the 3rd percentile for age (SDS, –3.42), her weight is at the 8th percentile for age (SDS, –1.38), and her head circumference is at the 4th percentile for age (SDS, –1.74). She is a petite, nondysmorphic girl in no acute distress. Examination findings are unremarkable. There is no asymmetry or bowing of the lower extremities and no evidence of scoliosis. Her teeth are in good condition with no signs of decay. She is at Tanner stage 1 for breast development and pubic hair, and the appearance of her external genitalia is normal for a prepubertal girl. The growth chart available from her pediatrician is shown (*see image*), and it includes measurements obtained at the present visit.

She was born via cesarean delivery at a gestational age of 38 weeks' based on obstetric ultrasonography performed in early pregnancy. Birth length was 16.5 in (42 cm) (<3rd percentile; SDS, –3.55), birth weight was 4 lb 3 oz (1900 g) (<3rd percentile; SDS, –2.72), and head circumference was 11.8 in (30 cm) (<3rd percentile; SDS, –3.42). The obstetrician described the placenta as small.

She is the second child of otherwise healthy parents. Her father's height is 68 in (172.7 cm). He had normal timing of puberty and has no history of medical issues. Her mother's height is 62 in (157.5 cm). She experienced menarche at age 12 years and has had no health issues. Neither parent smokes cigarettes.

Laboratory test results:

    IGF-1 = 98 ng/mL (74-202 ng/mL) (SI: 12.8 nmol/L [9.7-26.5 nmol/L])

    IGFBP-3 = 1.7 mg/L (1.4-3.0 mg/L)

    TSH = 5.7 mIU/L (0.6-5.5 mIU/L)

    Free T_4 = 1.95 ng/dL (0.8-2.2 ng/dL) (SI: 25.1 pmol/L [10.3-28.3 pmol/L])

    Erythrocyte sedimentation rate = 12 mm/h (0-20 mm/h)

    Complete blood cell count, no anemia and normal differential

    Comprehensive chemistry panel, normal

    25-Hydroxyvitamin D = 33 ng/mL (30-100 ng/mL) (SI: 82.4 nmol/L [74.9-249.6 nmol/L])

    Karyotype = 46,XX

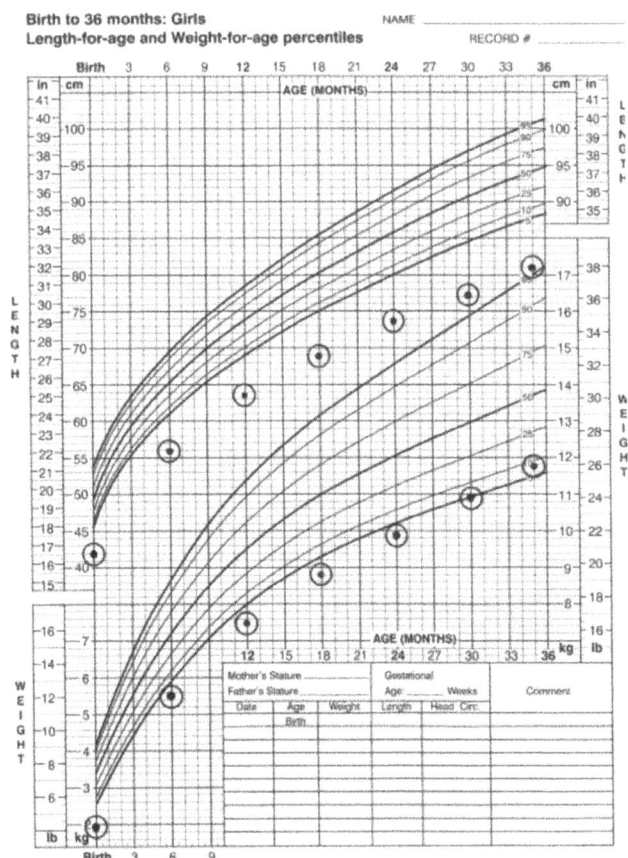

Birth to 36 months: Girls
Length-for-age and Weight-for-age percentiles

Which of the following is the most reasonable course of action?
- A. Start GH therapy
- B. Measure TPO and thyroglobulin antibodies
- C. Perform a GH-stimulation test
- D. Request a consultation with gastroenterology
- E. Follow clinically until age 5 years

89 A 4-year-old boy is being seen in the outpatient setting for ongoing care of congenital hypothyroidism. At this visit, his parents express concern that he does not speak as clearly as their older child did at the same age. He sometimes does not respond if they speak to him while he is watching television. They have no concerns about his vision or social development.

The patient was diagnosed with congenital hypothyroidism at 4 weeks of age after presenting with prolonged jaundice. He was born at home, and no newborn screening was performed. At diagnosis, his serum TSH concentration was 308 mIU/L and his free T_4 concentration was 0.5 ng/dL (6.4 pmol/L). Levothyroxine, 50 mcg daily (12 mcg/kg), was initiated, and 2 weeks after beginning treatment his serum TSH concentration had decreased to 46 mIU/L and his free T_4 concentration was 2.1 ng/dL (27.0 pmol/L). TSH normalized 1 month after treatment initiation. During the first 3 years of life, he had 5 episodes of elevated TSH (>10 mIU/L) due to variable adherence to treatment. His current levothyroxine dosage is 75 mcg daily.

On physical examination, his length is at the 23rd percentile and weight is at the 60th percentile. Vital signs are normal. He is alert and energetic. He makes good eye contact and responds to direct questions. His speech is 50% to 75% intelligible. Fontanelles are closed. Findings on external ear and otoscopic examination are normal. The thyroid gland is not palpable. The rest of the examination findings are normal.

Laboratory test results:
TSH = 4.4 mIU/L (0.7-5.7 mIU/L)
Free T_4 = 1.6 ng/dL (1.0-2.6 ng/dL) (SI: 20.6 pmol/L [12.9-33.5 pmol/L])

A possible hearing deficit may be contributing to the patient's speech delay.

Which of the following factors is most closely associated with the risk of hearing impairment in this patient?
- A. Delayed initiation of levothyroxine treatment
- B. Delayed normalization of TSH levels after initiation of treatment
- C. Severity of hypothyroidism at diagnosis
- D. Inadequate treatment of hypothyroidism during early childhood
- E. Male sex

90 A 16-year-old girl presents with weight loss, irritability, heat intolerance, difficulty sleeping, and a decline in school performance over the past several years. She is taking an oral contraceptive pill daily. Her medical history is unremarkable and she has no history of hearing problems. Her mother has a history of Graves disease, which was treated with radioactive iodine at age 36 years. Her mother now takes levothyroxine and has normal thyroid function. Her father's thyroid function was checked last year due to fatigue and results were normal. The patient's midparental height is 61 in (155 cm).

On physical examination, her pulse rate is 140 beats/min and blood pressure is 126/52 mm Hg. Her height is 68 in (172.7 cm) (90th percentile), and weight is 110 lb (50 kg) (25th percentile). Her skin is moist, and there is no exophthalmos or lid lag. She has a tremor of the outstretched hands, and the thyroid gland is diffusely enlarged without nodules or thyroid bruit. There is a hyperactive precordium with tachycardia and hyperactive reflexes.

Laboratory test results:

Free T$_4$ = 4.1 ng/dL (0.98-1.63 ng/dL) (SI: 52.8 pmol/L [12.6-21.0 pmol/L])

Total T$_3$ = 445 ng/dL (91-218 ng/dL) (SI: 6.9 nmol/L [1.4-3.3 nmol/L])

TSH = 14.0 mIU/L (0.51-4.3 mIU/L)

Which of the following is this patient's most likely diagnosis?
A. Medication interference causing abnormal laboratory findings
B. Resistance to thyroid hormone β
C. Familial dysalbuminemic hyperthyroxinemia
D. Graves disease
E. TSH-producing adenoma

91 A 3-year-old girl with new-onset diabetes mellitus is admitted to the hospital. Discharge is planned after her condition is stable for 24 hours following resolution of diabetic ketoacidosis. She is responding well to the basal-bolus insulin regimen and has cleared her ketosis. The family is interested in pursuing continuous glucose monitoring since they are fearful of nocturnal hypoglycemia. Insulin dosing and all safety precautions related to preventing hypoglycemia are reviewed. The patient weighs 33 lb (15 kg).

Which of the following prescriptions is most appropriate to use for emergency glucagon treatment in this patient?
A. Prefilled syringe, ready-to-inject glucagon, 0.5 mg
B. Prefilled syringe, ready-to-inject glucagon, 1 mg
C. Glucagon nasal powder, 3 mg
D. Glucagon nasal powder, 1.5 mg (half dose)
E. Glucagon reconstitution powder, 1 mg

92 A 10-year-old girl with myelomeningocele is referred to endocrinology for assessment of bone health due to a fracture of her right humerus that occurred when she fell during a school field trip. She had a prior low-trauma tibial fracture at 2 years of age.

The patient ambulates with the assistance of lower-extremity braces and a wheelchair for longer distances. She has a regular diet and consumes milk at breakfast and cheese at lunch. She also has a history of epilepsy that is well controlled with levetiracetam (she has been seizure-free for the last 2 years).

DXA of her total body less head shows a height-adjusted Z-score of –2.1. Metabolic bone workup reveals normal calcium, phosphate, and magnesium; mildly elevated alkaline phosphatase for age; and a 25-hydroxyvitamin D concentration of 15.8 ng/mL (39.4 nmol/L).

Which of the following interventions is the best next step to reduce this child's risk for subsequent fractures?
A. Start supplemental vitamin D
B. Start supplemental vitamin D and calcium
C. Start bisphosphonate therapy
D. Induce puberty
E. Consult with the neurologist about changing seizure treatment

93 A 13-year-old boy is seen for follow-up of congenital adrenal hyperplasia due to 21-hydroxylase deficiency. Over the last 2 years, his control has become suboptimal on hydrocortisone replacement therapy (14 mg/m² per day in 3 divided dosages), with persistently high 17-hydroxyprogesterone, androstenedione, and ACTH levels. He was receiving vitamin D supplementation and was treated with erythromycin for a chest infection. He has been growing along the same percentiles for height and weight. His current height is 55.5 in (149 cm) (50th percentile), and weight is 108 lb (49 kg) (75th percentile). Pubertal assessment reveals Tanner stage 4 genital development and pubic hair. Testicular volumes are 10 mL bilaterally. He has some mild symptoms of gastritis. Pharmacokinetic studies performed after administering 15 mg/m² of intravenous hydrocortisone document increased cortisol clearance with reduced half-life.

Which of the following is the most likely cause of suboptimally controlled congenital adrenal hyperplasia in this patient?
   A. Poor regimen adherence
   B. Puberty
   C. Gastritis
   D. Obesity
   E. Drug interaction

94 A 16-year-old boy presents to his pediatrician with a neck mass. On palpation, the pediatrician notes a 3-cm, firm nodule and 2 palpable lymph nodes on the right side and lateral to the thyroid gland. He is referred to a pediatric endocrinologist who orders thyroid and neck ultrasonography and laboratory tests. The patient is euthyroid and has negative thyroid antibodies. Calcitonin and calcium levels are normal. There is no family history of thyroid cancer.

Ultrasonography reveals a 2.8-cm, right-sided, hypoechoic, solid nodule with microcalcifications and a smaller 1.2-cm nodule on the left lower pole of the thyroid. Ultrasonography also identifies a number of right-sided lymph nodes that are suspicious for malignancy. Findings from FNA biopsy of both nodules are suspicious for malignancy. He undergoes total thyroidectomy, with bilateral central neck dissection and right lateral neck dissection. Histopathologic examination reveals classic papillary thyroid cancer involving both lobes, with spread to the central and lateral neck compartments (T2N1bMx).

Which of the following is the most likely pathogenic genetic alteration expected in this patient?
   A. *RET* proto-oncogene pathogenic variant
   B. *RET/PTC* fusion
   C. *PAX8/PPARG* fusion
   D. *NTRK3/ETV6* fusion
   E. *BRAF* V600E pathogenic variant

95 A 4-and-6/12-year-old girl is followed in clinic for short stature. Her height is −3.5 SDS with target height at −3.0 SDS. She was born full term with normal birth weight and length. She has no developmental delay. In addition to short stature in her father and 2 paternal first cousins, her family history is notable for multiple lumbar disk herniations and osteoarthritis of the knees in the third decade of life.

On physical examination, she is overweight and has brachydactyly and midface hypoplasia. She has no signs of puberty. Her sitting height to standing height ratio is 0.54, and her arm span is 1 cm more than her height. Her bone age is interpreted to be 6 years.

Which of the following is the most likely cause of this patient's short stature?
   A. Familial short stature
   B. *GNAS* pathogenic variant
   C. 45,X karyotype
   D. *FGFR3* pathogenic variant
   E. *ACAN* pathogenic variant

96 A 14-year-old boy presents for follow-up of obesity as part of the hospital's weight management program. He has a longstanding history of progressive weight gain. His current BMI is greater than 140% of the 95th percentile for age and sex (class III obesity). His parents report that they have made radical changes to their lifestyle as a family, including cutting out sugar-sweetened beverages, increasing fruit and vegetable intake, and cutting out fast food. His older brother takes him to the gym at least 3 days per week, where he uses the treadmill and stationary bike. Despite all of these efforts, his weight has increased by 6.6 lb (3 kg) in the last 4 months. His hemoglobin A_{1c} value is normal at today's visit today.

The patient and his parents would like to discuss potential pharmacotherapeutic options to help him lose weight.

After discussing the risks and benefits of starting a weight-loss medication, which of the following would be the most appropriate choice for this patient?
A. Phentermine
B. Octreotide
C. Metformin
D. Liraglutide
E. Orlistat

97 A 10-year-old girl with a large craniopharyngioma is followed for panhypopituitarism. She has diabetes insipidus and hypothalamic obesity with impaired glucose tolerance. In addition to pituitary hormone replacement with GH, levothyroxine, hydrocortisone, and desmopressin, she also takes metformin. She has tried to adhere to a strict low-carbohydrate diet, but she finds it very difficult to maintain and she has not been successful with weight loss. Through social media, her mother has heard of patients with hypothalamic obesity using inhaled oxytocin as a treatment for weight loss and she asks you about this. You inform her that use of oxytocin in this setting is experimental.

Which of the following is a proposed mechanism of action of oxytocin for weight loss in this setting?
A. Decreased energy consumption
B. Increased leptin resistance
C. Decreased fatty liver
D. Increased energy expenditure
E. Reduced insulin secretion

98 A 17-year-old girl is seen in the outpatient setting for follow-up of Graves disease. Graves disease was diagnosed 3 years ago and has been treated with methimazole, which she takes consistently. After a recent decrease in the methimazole dosage, hyperthyroidism recurred, and her prior methimazole dosage was resumed. Having not achieved remission of Graves disease, she wishes to pursue definitive therapy for hyperthyroidism. She reports no symptoms of hypothyroidism or hyperthyroidism. She has no eye or vision symptoms.

On physical examination, her height is at the 56th percentile, weight is at the 25th percentile, and BMI is at the 20th percentile (19.3 kg/m²). Her pulse rate is 74 beats/min, and blood pressure is 107/63 mm Hg. She is alert and oriented. She has normal extraocular movements, no proptosis, and no edema or erythema of the eyelids or conjunctivae. There is no cervical lymphadenopathy. Palpation of the thyroid reveals a firm, asymmetric gland, with the right lobe normal in size and the left lobe twice normal size, and no palpable discrete nodule. This represents a change from her examination 1 year ago, at which time the left thyroid lobe was only slightly larger than the right lobe. The rest of the examination findings are normal.

Her current TSH concentration is 1.3 mIU/L (0.7-5.7 mIU/L).

Based on the thyroid examination, thyroid ultrasonography is performed, which reveals a 3.5-cm, solid, hypoechoic nodule in the left thyroid lobe. The nodule contains echogenic foci consistent with possible calcifications.

Which of the following is the most appropriate next step in this patient's management?
  A. Continuation of methimazole and follow-up with ultrasonography in 3 months
  B. Radioactive iodine (^{131}I) therapy
  C. Thyroid scintigraphy
  D. FNA of the thyroid nodule
  E. Thyroidectomy

99 An 11-year-old child assigned male sex at birth who identifies as female is referred by a pediatrician. The parents state that their child has always identified as a girl. Starting in first grade, she would become distressed whenever she was referred to as a boy. She started seeing a therapist with experience in gender disorders and was diagnosed with gender dysphoria. She socially transitioned at age 7 years and has been well supported by her family.

Her parents are concerned that she has started showing signs of puberty, which is causing distress. They are worried about worsening gender dysphoria as puberty progresses. The patient is requesting intervention to prevent developing a male body. Stage 2 testicular development is noted on physical examination. Laboratory testing is notable for pubertal LH and testosterone levels.

Which of the following is the best advice for this patient?
  A. Start gender-affirming hormone treatment with low-dosage estradiol
  B. Start a GnRH analogue to prevent further pubertal changes
  C. Start medroxyprogesterone acetate to block testosterone production
  D. Refer for counseling to discuss the impact of treatment on fertility before starting medication
  E. Recommend allowing puberty to further progress to determine whether her gender identity is permanent before pursuing intervention

100 A 6-year-old boy diagnosed with acute lymphoblastic leukemia starts an induction chemotherapy protocol. Therapy includes prednisolone, vincristine, cyclophosphamide, daunorubicin, triple intrathecal injection, and pegylated L-asparaginase.

The treatment protocol is shown (*see figure*).

On day 18 of therapy, he develops fasting hypoglycemia (glucose = 51 mg/dL [2.8 mmol/L]) with severe hunger but no other signs or symptoms such as tremor, palpitation, anxiety, or sweating. On day 27 of therapy, he has another episode and critical blood sampling documents the following:

Fasting serum glucose = 45 mg/dL (70-99 mg/dL)
  (SI: 2.5 mmol/L [3.9-5.5 mmol/L])
Insulin = 14 µIU/mL (<17 µIU/mL) (SI: 97.2 pmol/L
  [<118.1 pmol/L])
Free fatty acids = 13.2 mg/dL (16.9-42.3 mg/dL)
  (SI: 0.47 mmol/L [0.6-1.5 mmol/L])
β-Hydroxybutyrate = 1.25 mg/dL (<2.91 mg/dL)
  (SI: 120 µmol/L [<280 µmol/L])

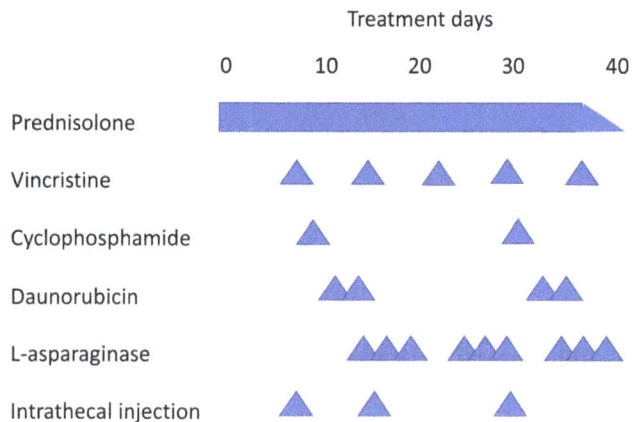

He repeatedly develops fasting hypoglycemia without serious complications (glucose ranging from 35-51 mg/dL [1.9-2.8 mmol/L]) until day 37.

His medical history is unremarkable. He was a full-term baby (size appropriate for gestational age) with no medical complications. His mother did not have gestational diabetes. No previous blood glucose problems are reported. His linear growth has always been steady. There is no family history of diabetes or hypoglycemia.

Which of the following is the most likely etiology of this patient's hypoglycemia?
- A. Iatrogenic adrenal insufficiency
- B. L-asparaginase–induced hypoglycemia
- C. Inadequate nutritional intake
- D. Intrathecal injection–induced GH deficiency
- E. Normal hypoglycemic response during chemotherapy

PEDIATRIC ENDOCRINE SELF-ASSESSMENT PROGRAM 2021-2022

Part II

1 ANSWER: B) Familial glucocorticoid deficiency

Familial glucocorticoid deficiency (Answer B) is the most likely diagnosis in view of this patient's extremely high plasma ACTH levels. He lacks biochemistry suggestive of congenital adrenal hyperplasia (Answer D), and mineralocorticoid deficiency and adrenal antibodies that would point towards congenital adrenal hypoplasia (Answer C) or Addison disease (Answer A), respectively. Very long-chain fatty acid levels were normal, thus excluding X-linked adrenoleukodystrophy (Answer E). This child was found to have a homozygous pathogenic variant in the gene encoding the ACTH receptor (*MC2R*; S74I [serine to isoleucine at amino acid position 74]), also known as the melanocortin 2 receptor. Many patients with this pathogenic variant are of Scottish descent. Familial glucocorticoid deficiency is an autosomal recessive disorder that typically manifests during early childhood or the neonatal period with symptoms of hypocortisolemia, the absence of mineralocorticoid deficiency, and very high plasma ACTH, which leads to intense hyperpigmentation. Tall stature, which normalizes after glucocorticoid replacement, is also a feature of *MC2R* pathogenic variants, probably through the action of ACTH on other melanocortin receptors expressed in bone. The diagnosis in this case is relatively late and demonstrates the phenotypic variability of this condition, even in those with the same pathogenic variant.

Seven other genes associated with familial glucocorticoid deficiency have been identified to date, including *MRAP* (melanocortin 2 receptor accessory protein), *STAR* (steroidogenic acute regulatory protein), *MCM4* (minichromosome maintenance complex component 4), *NNT* (nicotinamide nucleotide transhydrogenase), *TXNRD2* (thioredoxin reductase 2), *CYP11A1* (cytochrome P450 family 11 subfamily A member 1), and *SGPL1* (sphingosine-1-phosphate lyase 1). These genes are involved in diverse pathways, and the resulting phenotypes are caused by defective ACTH signaling, cholesterol transport, steroidogenesis, cellular redox homeostasis, DNA replication, or sphingolipid metabolism. There is increasing awareness of the variable phenotypes and associated conditions seen within the familial glucocorticoid deficiency umbrella of conditions. For example, evidence of mineralocorticoid deficiency (transient or permanent) has been described in those with severe pathogenic variants in *MC2R* and *MRAP*, as well as in patients with pathogenic variants in *NNT*. Later onset of symptoms has been observed in some persons with pathogenic variants in *NNT* and missense mutations in *MRAP* and *CYP11A1*. Furthermore, *MCM4* and *SGPL1* are associated with other disorders such as natural killer cell deficiency and progressive renal dysfunction, respectively.

The other causes of primary adrenal insufficiency (Addison disease [Answer A], congenital adrenal hypoplasia [Answer C], congenital adrenal hyperplasia [Answer D], and X-linked adrenoleukodystrophy [Answer E]) should certainly be considered in the differential diagnosis. Overall, autoimmune causes (Addison disease and polyglandular syndromes) account for 80% to 90% of primary adrenal insufficiency, and most individuals are adrenal antibody positive. Autoimmune destruction is usually associated with mineralocorticoid deficiency; hence, in the absence of both features, an autoimmune cause is unlikely. Because this is a male patient, *NR0B1* (formerly *DAX1*) pathogenic variants as a cause of congenital adrenal hypoplasia are also a possibility, but the late onset plus the lack of mineralocorticoid deficiency make this a less likely diagnosis. X-linked adrenoleukodystrophy should always be considered and excluded by measuring very long-chain fatty acid levels. Late-onset congenital adrenal hyperplasia is another consideration, especially in view of the unexplained tall stature. However, in this case, normal androgens and prepubertal findings on examination do not support this diagnosis.

Educational Objective

Explain the pathophysiology and phenotype variability of familial glucocorticoid deficiency.

Reference(s)

Maharaj A, Maudhoo A, Chan LF, et al. Isolated glucocorticoid deficiency: Genetic causes and animal models. *J Steroid Biochem Mol Biol.* 2019;189:73-80. PMID: 30817990

Bornstein SR, Allolio B, Arlt W, et al. Diagnosis and treatment of primary adrenal insufficiency: an Endocrine Society clinical practice guideline. *J Clin Endocrinol Metab.* 2016;101(2):364-389. PMID: 26760044

2 ANSWER: A) X-linked hypophosphatemic rickets

While many features of these skeletal conditions overlap, X-linked hypophosphatemic rickets (Answer A) (XLH) is frequently associated with progressive bowing of the lower extremities that appears when young children learn to stand and walk, a waddling gait, short stature, and craniosynostosis (particularly with premature fusion of the sagittal sutures, resulting in the elongation of the skull or dolichocephalic malformation). While the exact incidence is unknown, a recent retrospective study suggests that craniosynostosis may occur in more than 50% of affected patients. Dental abscesses may develop as children get older.

Craniosynostosis can result in increased intracranial hypertension and Chiari malformation type 1 with herniation of the cerebellar tonsils. In some cases, craniosynostosis does not occur until later in skull development, resulting in little morphologic changes and sufficient room for brain growth. However, craniosynostosis can be the presenting feature of XLH and can occur in children as young as 3 months. When cranial sutures fuse at a young age, surgical intervention may be required to prevent complications.

Craniosynostosis syndromes can be due to pathogenic variants in the fibroblast growth factor (FGF) receptors. FGF receptor 1 (*FGFR1*) and FGF receptor 2 (*FGFR2*) are involved in intramembranous osteogenesis, whereas FGF receptor 3 (*FGFR3*) has a primary role as an inhibitor of endochondral ossification. The primary receptor for FGF-23 is *FGFR1*, and thus this may explain the association of craniosynostosis with this disorder.

Pathogenic variants in *FGFR3* are associated with hypochondroplasia (Answer C). Patients with this condition also have short stature, macrocephaly, and bowed legs, but frequently have short, broad hands and feet. However, these individuals rarely present with craniosynostosis or radiographic signs of rickets, so hypochondroplasia is an unlikely diagnosis in this case. One-third to two-thirds of patients with infantile hypophosphatasia (Answer B) also have craniosynostosis, frequently by 6 months of age. Affected children generally have other manifestations such as bell-shaped chest deformity, respiratory compromise, seizures, and characteristic x-ray findings of metaphyseal tongues.

While severe vitamin D deficiency (Answer D) could explain the radiographic findings in this patient, craniotabes is a rare skull manifestation of this condition, not craniosynostosis. There have been case reports of vitamin D excess causing craniosynostosis.

Apert syndrome (Answer E) is due to pathogenic variants in the *FGFR2* gene and is associated with short stature and bicoronal synostosis with resultant widely spaced eyes, exophthalmos, and midface hypoplasia. Affected patients also have characteristic changes of the hands including syndactyly, most commonly of the second through fourth fingers with a single common nail.

Educational Objective
Identify craniosynostosis as an initial presentation of X-linked hypophosphatemic rickets.

Reference(s)
Rothenbuhler A, Fadel N, Debza Y, et al. High incidence of cranial synostosis and Chiari I malformation in children with X-linked hypophosphatemic rickets (XLHR). *J Bone Miner Res.* 2019;34(3):490-496. PMID: 30352126

Wang J, Liu S, Li J, Yi Z. The role of the fibroblast growth factor family in bone-related diseases. *Chem Biol Drug Des.* 2019;94(4):1740-1749. PMID: 31260189

Vakharia JD, Matlock K, Taylor HO, Backeljauw PF, Topor LS. Craniosynostosis as the presenting feature of X-linked hypophosphatemic rickets. *Pediatrics.* 2018;141(Suppl 5):S515-S519. PMID: 29610183

Whyte MP, Leung E, Wilcox WR, et al; Study 011-10 Investigators. Natural history of perinatal and infantile hypophosphatasia: a retrospective study. *J Pediatr.* 2019;209:116-124. PMID: 30979546

3   ANSWER: C) 8 units
Calculating the needs for mixed-meal insulin in children with type 1 diabetes is challenging. Both the type and the amount of carbohydrate found in foods influence postprandial glucose levels and can also affect overall glycemic control in individuals with diabetes. Added sugars such as sucrose and high-fructose corn syrup are digested, absorbed, and fully metabolized in a similar fashion to naturally occurring monosaccharides and disaccharides. Only about half of the carbohydrate grams from sugar alcohols and half or less from dietary fiber are metabolized to glucose, whereas almost all "other carbohydrate" (mainly starch such as amylose and amylopectin) becomes blood glucose.

All food labels indicate the amount of dietary fiber in the serving size, and newer labels provide further details about soluble and insoluble amounts. If the total fiber amount is greater than 5 g, half of the total amount, which usually corresponds to the insoluble portion, should be subtracted from the total carbohydrate amount to calculate the insulin dose. If insoluble fiber amount is listed, then it can be used to calculate directly.

In this vignette, the patient plans to consume 54 g (27 g × 2 servings) of total carbohydrates. The insoluble fiber amount is 3 g per serving, totaling 6 g. The amount of carbohydrate that needs to be considered for an insulin bolus is 54 minus 6, which equals 48 g. The correct insulin dose should be calculated by dividing 48 g by 6, which equals 8 units (Answer C).

Ignoring the fiber content and calculating the insulin amount on the basis of the total carbohydrate of 54 g divided by 6, which equals 9 units (Answer B), would be incorrect.

Subtracting all of the fiber content from the total carbohydrate amount (54 minus 10, which equals 44 → divided by 6, which equals 7.3 → rounded to 7 units [Answer D]) is also incorrect.

Ten units (Answer A) provide extra insulin beyond the carbohydrate calculation. This may be valid in some practices that account for the fat and the protein content of the consumed food when determining the insulin calculation. There are data to suggest that 25% to 50% extra insulin may be needed to cover the fat and protein load of meals and snacks, delivered in an extended fashion that can be achieved by insulin pumps. However, in this vignette, there is no additional information to prompt one to consider extra insulin.

Eating her snack and monitoring her glucose to decide on the amount of insulin (Answer E) is also wrong and goes against the concept that all "meal" insulin should be received before food consumption. This idea may be valid in special circumstances such as pending severe hypoglycemia if the patient's continuous glucose monitoring indicated such scenario.

Educational Objective
Incorporate dietary fiber into the insulin calculation for meals and snacks in patients with type 1 diabetes mellitus.

Reference(s)
van der Hoogt M, van Dyk JC, Dolman RC, Pieters M. Protein and fat meal content increase insulin requirement in children with type 1 diabetes - role of duration of diabetes. *J Clin Transl Endocrinol.* 2017;10:15-21. PMID: 29204367

Matteucci E, Giampietro O. Dietary strategies for adult type 1 diabetes in light of outcome evidence. *Eur J Clin Nutr.* 2015;69(3):285-290. PMID: 25293432

Wheeler ML, Pi-Sunyer FX. Carbohydrate issues: type and amount. *J Am Diet Assoc.* 2008;108(4 Suppl 1):S34-S39. PMID: 18358253

4 **ANSWER: B) Optimize levothyroxine treatment to maintain TSH between 0.5 and 1.0 mIU/L and follow-up with thyroglobulin measurement (while on levothyroxine) 12 weeks after surgery**

Postoperative systems have not been validated in children with papillary thyroid carcinoma (PTC). However, the American Joint Committee on Cancer TNM classification system can describe the extent of the disease. The inaugural management guidelines for children with thyroid nodules and differentiated thyroid cancer (DTC), published in 2015, use the TNM system to categorize pediatric patients into 1 of 3 risk group categories to determine which patients are at higher risk for persistent cervical disease or distant metastasis.

- **American Thyroid Association (ATA) pediatric low-risk category** is defined as disease confined to the thyroid, with no nodal metastasis, unknown nodal metastasis, or incidental finding of microscopic metastasis in a small number of central lymph nodes. This group of patients is at low risk for distant metastasis, but may still be at risk for residual local disease.
- **ATA pediatric intermediate-risk category** is defined as extensive central nodal disease (N1a) or minimal nodal disease in other neck compartments (N1b). These patients have increased risk of persistent local disease, although they are still considered to be at low risk for distant metastasis.
- **ATA pediatric high-risk category** is defined as extensive N1b disease or locally invasive tumors (T4 tumors that extend beyond the thyroid capsule to invade extrathyroidal soft tissue, fascia, carotid artery, or mediastinal vessels).

The patient in this vignette belongs in the ATA low-risk category. She has a classic papillary thyroid microcarcinoma (tumor less than 1 cm) confined to the thyroid, without nodal disease.

Assuming that the patient had adequate preoperative staging and that surgery was performed by a high-volume thyroid cancer surgeon, the current guidelines for pediatric ATA low-risk thyroid cancer recommend (1) postoperative staging by measuring a TSH-suppressed (on levothyroxine) thyroglobulin concentration 12 weeks after surgery, (2) treatment with levothyroxine to maintain TSH between 0.5 and 1.0 mIU/L (Answer B), and (3) follow-up with measurement of TSH-suppressed thyroglobulin every 3 to 6 months for 2 years and then annually and neck ultrasonography 6 months after surgery and then annually.

For patients in the intermediate- and high-risk categories, TSH-stimulated thyroglobulin measurement and whole-body scan (Answer A) are recommended to assess for residual disease and to determine whether the patient may benefit from ^{131}I treatment. This patient, however, is in the low-risk category.

For patients in the high-risk category, radioactive iodine is generally recommended.

Universal ^{131}I treatment for DTC (Answer C) is not recommended for children and adolescents, as the goal for radioactive iodine treatment is to decrease the recurrence risk and to improve mortality, while minimizing unnecessary exposure to radioactive iodine to prevent permanent adverse effects (lifelong xerostomia, increased risk for salivary gland malignancy, gonadal damage, suppression of the bone marrow, possible risk of secondary malignancies). Interestingly, Jin et al recently described how radioactive iodine uptake and stimulated thyroglobulin measurement may also be useful in deciding the dose of radioactive iodine treatment in adults with DTC. This study confirms the value of a TSH-stimulated thyroglobulin level less than 2 ng/mL (<2 µg/L) as a predictor of the absence of DTC.

The TSH goal of 0.1 to 0.5 mIU/L (Answer D) has been recommended for patients at intermediate risk, and less than 0.1 mIU/L has been recommended for patients at high risk. Maintaining TSH in the normal range (Answer E) is not recommended for patients with a history of DTC.

Of note, although this patient does not currently have thyroglobulin antibodies, it is important to always measure thyroglobulin antibodies when obtaining thyroglobulin levels, as the presence of thyroglobulin antibodies makes the thyroglobulin measurement unreliable. Presence of thyroglobulin antibodies in a patient previously negative for antibodies is nonreassuring. In the presence of antibodies, monitoring the antibodies using the same assay is recommended.

Educational Objective
Explain the indications for use of ^{131}I in treating differentiated thyroid carcinoma and the role of levothyroxine for TSH suppression in its management.

Reference(s)
Francis GL, Waguespack SG, Bauer AJ, et al; American Thyroid Association Guidelines Task Force. Management guidelines for children with thyroid nodules and differentiated thyroid cancer. *Thyroid.* 25(7):716-759. PMID: 25900731

Jin Y, Ruan M, Cheng L, et al. Radioiodine uptake and thyroglobulin-guided radioiodine remnant ablation in patients with differentiated thyroid cancer: a prospective, randomized, open-label, controlled trial. *Thyroid.* 2019;29(1):101-110. PMID: 30560716

5 ANSWER: C) Measure prolactin again in 2 to 4 weeks
Breast tissue is commonly found in term infants, and some milk secretion is common as well. Transient neonatal gynecomastia is thought to be caused by placental conversion of weak androgens to estrogens, which enter the fetal circulation and stimulate glandular proliferation in the breast. The patient in this case was referred because of the unusually large amount of breast tissue.

There are few reports of hyperprolactinemia in children younger than 5 years and most are associated with other signs of pituitary/hypothalamic dysfunction. Defining the normal range for prolactin levels in the newborn is challenging; laboratory reference ranges do not identify separate ranges for infants and indicate a normal range of less than 10 ng/mL (<0.4 nmol/L) for prepubertal males. One study of prolactin levels in infants and children suggests that the normal range for prolactin levels in 1-week-old neonates may be as high as 496 ng/mL (21.6 nmol/L), but drops to 63 ng/mL (2.7 nmol/L) in infants 2 to 12 months of age. Data on the 1-week to 2-month age range are lacking. While it is difficult to determine whether the infant in this case has an elevated prolactin level for his age, his value of 108.5 ng/mL (4.7 nmol/L) should prompt another measurement (Answer C) to ensure that it is decreasing. While pathology in such a young patient would be rare, there have been some reports of persistently elevated prolactin levels in infants.

This infant's prolactin level will most likely decrease over time, and therefore performing MRI of the brain and the pituitary gland (Answer A) would be premature. Imaging would be indicated if the prolactin level does not decrease over time, as there would be a greater chance of finding a hypothalamic pituitary defect. Given that this infant most likely has an exaggerated form of nonpathologic neonatal breast hypertrophy, dopamine agonist therapy (Answer D) to decrease the prolactin level is not indicated. This treatment would only be considered if the prolactin level does not decrease, and only after CNS imaging and further evaluation of hypothalamic/pituitary function.

LH, FSH, and testosterone levels are most likely to be detectable due to the mini puberty of infancy and their measurement (Answer B) would not contribute to determining whether there is an underlying pathologic cause for this patient's breast hypertrophy.

Multiple endocrine neoplasia type 1 is associated with tumors of the pituitary gland. Individuals known or suspected to have multiple endocrine neoplasia type 1 are advised to have MRI of the brain and measurement of prolactin, IGF-1, fasting glucose, insulin, and proinsulin every 1 to 3 years starting as early as age 5 years. While prolactin-secreting pituitary adenomas are common in this syndrome, such manifestations would not be expected in an infant. Therefore, genetic testing (Answer E) is not warranted.

Educational Objective
Evaluate breast enlargement and galactorrhea in a neonate.

Reference(s)

Wiedermann G, Jonetz-Mentzel L. Establishment of reference ranges for prolactin in neonates, infants, children and adolescents. *Eur J Clin Chem Clin Biochem.* 1993;31(7):447-451. PMID: 8399785

Leung AKC, Leung AAC. Gynecomastia in infants, children, and adolescents. *Recent Pat Endocr Metab Immune Drug Discov.* 2017;10(2):127-137. PMID: 28260521

Amer A, Fischer H. Images in clinical medicine: neonatal breast enlargement. *N Engl J Med.* 2009;360(14):1445. PMID: 19339724

6 **ANSWER: D) Perform a glucagon-stimulation test; if abnormal, start GH therapy at a dosage of 1.0 mg daily and titrate based on IGF-1 levels**

This patient has completed her growth and showed good response to GH and levothyroxine treatment for GH and TSH deficiencies, respectively, after craniospinal radiation for a brain tumor. She also had appropriate pubertal development and regular menstrual cycles on hormone replacement therapy for primary ovarian insufficiency, which was most likely due to chemotherapy and spinal radiation. She has had tiredness and fatigue while off GH therapy for a year after achieving final adult height, despite maintaining a normal thyroid hormone level and having regular menstrual cycles on levothyroxine and estrogen/progesterone replacement therapy.

Unlike anterior pituitary hormone deficiencies, antidiuretic hormone deficiency has not been reported after cranial radiation. Thus, she is not at risk for diabetes insipidus. Antidiuretic hormone deficiency can be seen due to mass effect if the tumor (eg, germinoma) is anatomically close to the hypothalamus and/or pituitary. In this case, patient's fluid intake is not excessive, and her nocturia is therefore most likely habitual. She does not need to be screened with first-morning laboratory tests for diabetes insipidus (Answer A).

She has no notable symptoms or signs of cortisol insufficiency other than fatigue. Even though she is at risk for ACTH deficiency due to cranial radiation, an 8-AM cortisol value of 17 μg/dL (469 nmol/L) is robust and does not warrant cosyntropin-stimulation testing (Answer B).

Children receiving GH treatment for childhood GH deficiency should be evaluated for adult GH deficiency once growth is completed if they have a high likelihood of permanent GH deficiency (eg, history of cranial radiation, structural lesions causing panhypopituitarism, proven genetic causes). GH deficiency is the most common pituitary hormone deficiency in childhood cancer survivors. The IGF-1 level can generally be used as a surrogate marker for GH status; however, in childhood cancer survivors, IGF-1 performs poorly, making GH-stimulation testing necessary to diagnose GH deficiency in those patients at high risk. Although failure to respond to 2 different GH secretagogues is recommended to diagnose childhood GH deficiency, single-agent testing is acceptable to diagnose adult GH deficiency using 1 of the following 3 tests based on availability and patient eligibility: (1) GHRH-stimulation test, (2) insulin tolerance test, and (3) glucagon-stimulation test. Several different GH cutoff values have been proposed to diagnose adult GH deficiency based on the agent used for testing and the age and BMI of the patient tested. More recently, macimorelin, an orally active GH secretagogue, has been shown to be a potential alternative agent that could be used to diagnose adult GH deficiency.

Once a patient has been confirmed to have adult GH deficiency, GH therapy (at an appropriate dosage) should be restarted in adolescent and young adult patients. In patients with GH deficiency, long gaps in GH treatment should be avoided during the transition from childhood to adulthood to minimize the risk for compromised bone health, cardiovascular health, and poor quality of life. Adults younger than 30 years could be started at a GH dosage of 0.5 mg daily, although transition-age adolescents and young adults could be started at a slightly higher dosage such as 1.0 mg daily. Generally, patients with adult GH deficiency are started on low-dosage GH (0.5 to 1.0 mg daily), which can be up-titrated every 1 to 2 months based on IGF-1 levels, aiming to keep the IGF-1 level in the upper half of the reference range (thus, Answer D is correct and Answer C is incorrect). Reassuring a patient with a history of high-dosage cranial radiation who has symptoms such as tiredness and fatigue and not performing further workup for adult GH deficiency (Answer E) is incorrect.

Fleseriu M, Hashim IA, Karavitaki N, et al. Hormonal replacement in hypopituitarism in adults: an Endocrine Society clinical practice guideline. *J Clin Endocrinol Metab.* 2016;101(11):3888-3921. PMID: 27736313

Molitch ME, Clemmon DR, Malozowski S, Merriam GR, Vance ML; Endocrine Society. Evaluation and treatment of adult growth hormone deficiency: an Endocrine Society clinical practice guideline. *J Clin Endocrinol Metab.* 2011;96(6):1587-609. PMID: 21602453

Chemaitilly W, Li Z, Huang S, et al. Anterior hypopituitarism in adult survivors of childhood cancers treated with cranial radiotherapy: a report from the St Jude Lifetime Cohort study. *J Clin Oncol.* 2015;33(5):492-500. PMID: 25559807

Dichtel LE, Yuen KC, Bredella MA, et al. Overweight/obese adults with pituitary disorders require lower peak growth hormone cutoff values on glucagon stimulation testing to avoid overdiagnosis of growth hormone deficiency. *J Clin Endocrinol Metab.* 2014;99(12):4712-4719. PMID: 25210883

Garcia JM, Biller BMK, Korbonits M, et al. Macimorelin as a diagnostic test for adult GH deficiency. *J Clin Endocrinol Metab.* 2018;103(8):3083-3093. PMID: 29860473

7 ANSWER: A) Glycogen debrancher deficiency

This patient's presentation is consistent with glycogen storage disease (GSD). Hepatosplenomegaly, elevated triglycerides, and hypoglycemia are the hallmark findings of GSD that presents in infancy. GSD types I through IV are the most common forms that present in infancy and are associated with hepatosplenomegaly. However, GSD type I (known as von Gierke disease) and GSD type III (known as Cori disease, Forbes disease, and limit dextrinosis) are the 2 forms associated with ketotic hypoglycemia, hepatosplenomegaly, and hyperlipidemia as observed in this patient. Because of this patient's normal lactic acid level, the most likely diagnosis is GSD type III, or glycogen debrancher deficiency (Answer A). Lactic acid excess in GSD type I is due to buildup of glucose-6-phosphate, a condition not generally present in GSD type III.

GSD type I, or glucose-6-phosphatase deficiency (Answer C), is classically associated with ketotic hypoglycemia as a result of suppressed insulin secretion and increased secretion of counterregulatory hormones in response to hypoglycemia. Elevated glucose-6-phosphate is unable to be converted to glucose; therefore, it is converted to pyruvate. Excess pyruvate gets converted to lactate, especially in the presence of acidosis. These hormonal changes cause increased glycogenolysis and gluconeogenesis, with lactic acidosis representing increased formation and decreased use of lactate. The hormonal changes also promote exaggerated lipolysis. This leads to an influx of free fatty acids to the liver, where a substantial fraction is converted to triglycerides, and increasing secretion of VLDL.

In GSD type III, complete glycogenolysis is prevented by the lack of the glycogen debrancher enzyme, or amyloglucosidase, whose gene is located on chromosome 1p21. There are 4 subtypes of GSD type III as determined by variability in tissue expression of the debrancher enzyme:

- GSD IIIa represents about 85% of all GSD type III cases (liver and muscle involvement)
- GSD IIIb represents about 15% of all GSD type III cases (only liver involvement)
- GSD IIIc is very rare and is considered to be caused by a defect in glucosidase debranching activity
- GSD IIId is also very uncommon and is thought to be caused by a defect in transferase debranching activity

During glycogenolysis and prior to the presentation to the debrancher enzyme, phosphorylase breaks down glycogen to 2 to 4 linked glucose molecules or limit dextrins. Then, the debrancher enzyme works through 2 processes: cleavage of a dextrin branch from the remaining glycogen molecule (amylo-1,6-glucosidase activity), as well as through the transfer of the dextrin to the free end of a dextran polymer (oligo-1,4-1,4-glucanotransferase activity) to release free glucose molecules. The defects associated with this disorder, and thus their clinical manifestation in patients, are variable.

GSD type III, in contrast to GSD type I, can be associated with weakness, wasting of skeletal muscle, hypotonia, and cardiac defects. Cardiomyopathy can be found with or without left ventricular hypertrophy, and often presents in childhood. The skeletal findings and weakness are often manifested in adulthood. Osteopenia and osteoporosis commonly occur and appear to be due to lack of good metabolic control.

Hepatomegaly and elevated transaminase levels generally improve as patients become older and often normalize after puberty. Adenomas are rarely found, but they have been reported to progress to hepatocellular carcinoma.

GSD type VII (phosphofructokinase deficiency) (Answer B), GSD type VI (liver phosphorylase deficiency) (Answer D), and glucose transporter 2 deficiency (Answer E) do not present with the above findings.

Educational Objective

Differentiate among the various glycogen storage disorders on the basis of clinical findings.

Reference(s)

Kanungo S, Wells K, Tribett T, El-Gharbawy A. Glycogen metabolism and glycogen storage disorders. *Ann Transl Med.* 2018;6(24):474. PMID: 30740405

Kishnani PS, Austin SL, Arn P, et al. Glycogen storage disease type III diagnosis and management guidelines [published correction appears in *Genet Med.* 2010;12(9):566]. *Genet Med.* 2010;12(7):446-463. PMID: 20631546

8 ANSWER: E) Loss-of-function pathogenic variant in the *PAPPA2* gene (pappalysin 2)

Recently described pathogenic variants in the *PAPPA2* gene (pappalysin 2; pregnancy-associated plasma protein-A2) (Answer E) are associated with an autosomal recessive syndrome of postnatal growth failure and short stature. Individuals homozygous or compound heterozygous for pathogenic variants in this gene present with postnatal growth failure with varying degrees of proportionate short stature. No major dysmorphic features have been described other than mild microcephaly and long, thin bones on x-ray. This patient's parents are probably heterozygous and are unaffected. Given the presence of consanguinity in this family, the risk of autosomal recessive disorders is increased.

The IGF-1 half-life is increased by its binding to IGFBPs (IGF-binding proteins) in circulation. Only free IGF-1 can interact with the IGF-1 receptor to induce biologic activity. PAPP-A2 is a metalloproteinase that releases IGF-1 from the complexes it forms with the binding proteins (mainly IGFBP-3 and IGFBP-5). Inactivating pathogenic variants in *PAPPA2*, therefore, result in decreased levels of free IGF-1, leading to decreased linear growth. The absence of negative feedback of free IGF-1 on GH synthesis leads to an increase in GH production, which, in turn, induces an increase in the hepatic production of IGF-1, IGF-2, and IGFBP-3. Prenatal growth is dependent on IGF-1 and IGF-2. Fetal production of IGFs is largely independent from GH regulation except during the last few weeks of gestation. Normal maternal PAPP-A2 potentially maintains adequate free IGF levels in the fetus; therefore, no intrauterine growth failure occurs, which is consistent with this patient's history of intrauterine growth that was adequate for gestational age based on birth weight. She has proportionate short stature as suggested by very similar measurements of arm span and height. Measurements of free IGF-1 would show low levels in her case. However, this test is only available in research laboratories and not yet in clinical practice.

Loss-of-function pathogenic variants in the *GHR* gene (Answer A) are responsible for Laron-type dwarfism, also an autosomal recessive disorder characterized by severe postnatal growth failure. While GH levels may be elevated because of GH insensitivity, IGF-1 levels are low. Additionally, measurements of GH-binding protein, which represents the extracellular domain of the GH receptor, are low or undetectable. Gain-of-function pathogenic variants in the *GHR* gene (Answer B) have not been described, but they would theoretically result in an overgrowth syndrome.

Signal transducer and activator of transcription (STAT) 5b is one of the proteins in the GH postreceptor cascade. Inactivating pathogenic variants in the *STAT5B* gene (Answer D) lead to a Laron-like syndrome with postnatal growth failure, immune deficiency manifested by frequent respiratory infections, normal GH-binding protein, and elevated GH levels but low IGF-1 levels.

Inactivating pathogenic variants in the gene encoding the IGF-1 receptor (Answer C) are characterized by both prenatal and postnatal growth failure given that prenatal growth is dependent on IGF-1 and IGF-2 to which these individuals are unresponsive. Intrauterine growth is not dependent on GH, except for the last few weeks of gestation. GH therapy may induce a slight improvement in postnatal growth velocity, probably due to direct (ie, not mediated by IGF-1) action of GH on the growth plates.

Educational Objective

Explain the importance of IGF-1 bioavailability in the normal functioning of the GH-IGF-1 axis and identify pathogenic variants in the *PAPPA2* gene as a cause of postnatal growth failure and short stature.

Reference(s)

Rosenfeld R. Insulin-like growth factors and the basis of growth. *N Engl J Med.* 2003;349(23):2184-2186. PMID: 14657423

Dauber A, Muñoz-Calvo MT, Barrios V, et al. Mutations in pregnancy-associated plasma protein A2 cause short stature due to low IGF-I availability. *EMBO Mol Med.* 2016;8(4):363-374. PMID: 26902202

Argente J, Chowen JA, Pérez-Jurado LA, Frystyk J, Oxvig C. One level up: abnormal proteolytic regulation of IGF activity plays a role in human pathophysiology. *EMBO Mol Med.* 2017;9(10):1338-1345. PMID: 28801361

Kofoed EM, Hwa V, Little B, et al. Growth hormone insensitivity associated with STAT5b mutation. *N Engl J Med.* 2003;349(12):1139-1147. PMID: 13679528

Abuzzahab MJ, Schneider A, Goddard A, et al; Intrauterine Growth Retardation (IUGR) Study Group. IGF-1 receptor mutations resulting in intrauterine and postnatal growth retardation. *N Engl J Med.* 2003;349(23):2211-2222. PMID: 14657428

9 ANSWER: A) Measure TSH and T_4 in 1 week (off levothyroxine) and measure the mother's TSH and T_4

With a TSH value greater than 100 mIU/L due to congenital hypothyroidism, one would expect a much lower total T_4 or free T_4 level. Without a firm diagnosis of congenital hypothyroidism, starting levothyroxine (Answer C) would be incorrect and might prevent completion of the diagnostic evaluation, or in this case in which free and total T_4 are elevated, it may result in overtreatment. Guidelines in Europe (European Society for Paediatric Endocrinology) and the United States (American Academy of Pediatrics, American Thyroid Association) do not directly address a scenario whereby total or free T_4 is elevated. Further observation and testing is usually reserved for instances in which TSH is mildly elevated and T_4 is normal. At this patient's visit on day of life 8, he did not have jaundice, as might be expected in congenital hypothyroidism. Lower T_4 is also expected in resistance to TSH in those who are homozygous or compound heterozygous for pathogenic variants in *TSHR*, and TSH is often not as high as in this case, although there is a wide range. Resistance to TSH can also be observed in Albright hereditary osteodystrophy with PTH resistance, but TSH is only mildly elevated in affected patients. Therefore, measuring calcium and PTH (Answer B) is incorrect.

Mothers can transfer thyroid antibodies to the fetus, including TSH-receptor antibodies, which can block the TSH receptor and are expected to lead to high TSH and low or low-normal T_4. In the right clinical setting, it is recommended to measure the level of such blocking antibodies in the baby. Therefore, assessing the mother's thyroid antibodies (Answer D) is incorrect.

Thyroid ultrasonography (Answer E) is helpful in distinguishing between cases of congenital hypothyroidism due to an ectopic gland vs a gland located in the normal position, but this is not indicated here, as the technetium nuclear scanning showed a normal-sized thyroid gland in the correct location. This baby had normal TSH receptor–binding inhibiting immunoglobulins. This suggests the possibility of abnormal TSH or assay interference. Although much has been talked about regarding the effects of biotin, this is not relevant in this scenario on day of life 4 and onwards, even if the mother had been taking biotin during pregnancy. Repeated laboratory tests using different TSH assays and methodologies have shown normal T_4 levels associated with elevated TSH. On day of life 16, this baby's TSH value was 27.4 mIU/L, and the total T_4 value was 9.6 μg/dL (123.6 nmol/L) (same assay as the one used for testing on day of life 8).

Testing to assess for evidence of interfering heterophile antibodies was negative. HAMA wash yielded the same result.

Macro-TSH is a large circulating form of TSH composed of monomeric TSH complexed with autoimmune TSH antibodies. Macro-TSH can be detected on gel filtration chromatography with a prevalence ranging from 0.6% to 1.6%. Unlike TSH, which is a small bioactive hormone of 28 kDa easily filtered by the kidney, macro-TSH is a large molecule of at least 150 kDa that most likely accumulates in the circulation, resulting in measurements indicating falsely increased TSH levels. Currently, none of the available 2-site immunometric assays used for TSH testing can completely discriminate macro-TSH from bioactive free TSH, even if some platforms are more sensitive to its presence. Interference should be suspected in a patient with isolated TSH elevation (typically markedly elevated) with thyroid hormones in the upper half of the normal range and no signs or symptoms of thyroid dysfunction. An increased recovery of diluted samples showing nonlinearity may be indicative of macro-TSH. It should be noted, however, that the dilution procedure is neither specific nor sensitive. Lack of parallelism can be encountered with other interfering antibodies (eg, heterophilic antibodies). Gel filtration chromatography proved this patient had macro-TSH.

Transplacental transfer of macro-TSH has been documented in neonates as a cause of falsely elevated TSH, which is why it is important to recheck the TSH and T_4 levels a week later in the baby and in the mother (Answer A). Laboratory studies documented the following results in the patient's mother:

TSH = 16.42 mIU/L (0.5-4.30 mIU/L)
Total T_3 = 118 ng/dL (86-192 ng/dL) (SI: 1.8 nmol/L [1.3-3.0 nmol/L])
Total T_4 = 9.0 μg/dL (4.5-12.0 μg/dL) (SI: 115.8 nmol/L [57.9-154.4 nmol/L])

At 6 weeks of life, the infant's TSH concentration was still 21.4 mIU/L. Only at 7 months of life did it normalize, as the transplacental macro-TSH was washed out.

Diagnose macro-TSH as a confounder in newborns with elevated TSH and normal total or free T_4.

Reference(s)

Sunthornthepvarakul T, Gottschalk ME, Hayashi Y, Refetoff S. Brief report: resistance to thyrotropin caused by mutations in the thyrotropin-receptor gene. *N Engl J Med*. 1995;332(3):155-160. PMID: 7528344

Favresse J, Burlacu MC, Maiter D, Gruson D. Interferences with thyroid function immunoassays: clinical implications and detection algorithm. *Endocr Rev*. 2018;39(5):830-850. PMID: 29982406

American Academy of Pediatrics, Rose SR, Section on Endocrinology and Committee on Genetics, et al. Update of newborn screening and therapy for congenital hypothyroidism. *Pediatrics*. 2006;117(6):2290-2303. PMID: 16740880

Leger J, Olivieri A, Donaldson M, et al; ESPE-PSE-SLEP-JSPE-APEG-APPES-ISPAE; Congenital Hypothyroidism Consensus Conference Group. European Society for Paediatric Endocrinology consensus guidelines on screening, diagnosis, and management of congenital hypothyroidism. *Horm Res Paediatr*. 2014;81(2):80-103. PMID: 24662106

10 ANSWER: C) Measurement of urinary or plasma metanephrines

Urinary or plasma metanephrine measurement (Answer C) would be the most useful test to establish the presence of a pheochromocytoma and/or a catecholamine-secreting paraganglioma, which is the most likely diagnosis in view of the paroxysmal nature of the classic triad of symptoms (palpitations, diaphoresis, and headaches). Normal thyroid function test results and normal renal function exclude thyrotoxicosis and chronic renal disease as causes, which are on the list of differential diagnoses. Echocardiography (Answer A) could be useful to exclude a cardiac cause of hypertension such as aortic coarctation or to assess end-organ damage. Similarly, head MRI (Answer B) could be useful if Cushing disease were suspected or to assess the consequences of hypertension. However, neither of these options would be the next diagnostic investigation considering the symptomatology. MIBG scan (Answer D) and abdominal CT (Answer E) would be secondary investigations to locate the lesion following a biochemical diagnosis of pheochromocytoma and/or catecholamine-secreting paraganglioma.

The 24-hour urine metanephrine results in this case are shown (*see table*).

Analyte	Result	Reference Range
Urine volume	961 mL	0-4440 mL
Normetanephrine	1765 µg/24 h (SI: 9637 nmol/d)	0-366 µg/24 h (SI: 0-2000 nmol/d)
Metanephrine	114 µg/24 h (SI: 579 nmol/d)	0-493 µg/24 h (SI: 0-2500 nmol/d)

This patient had no phenotypic features of Cushing syndrome. MRI brain showed multifocal cortical deep white matter and basal ganglia edema predominantly within the basal ganglia, occipital lobes, and brain stem, findings consistent with posterior reversible encephalopathy syndrome. Findings on echocardiography were normal, with an ejection fraction of 60% and no evidence of cardiomyopathy. MIBG scan showed avid uptake within the left adrenal gland, while abdominal CT showed a 4.1-cm lesion anterior to the left renal pelvis displacing the renal vessels.

Phenoxybenzamine, 10 mg twice daily were initiated. He was discharged home on phenoxybenzamine, 20 mg 4 times daily, and propranolol, 4 times daily. He returned 2 weeks later for an elective left adrenalectomy and genetic testing.

Pheochromocytomas and catecholamine-secreting paragangliomas are neuroendocrine tumors derived from chromaffin cells of the adrenal medulla or tumors that originate from the paraganglia of the autonomic nervous system. Pheochromocytomas and catecholamine-secreting paragangliomas account for 0.1% to 0.6% of cases of hypertension in adults and 1% of cases in pediatric patients. The reported incidence is 2 to 5 cases per million per year, of which 10% occur in children. Pheochromocytomas and catecholamine-secreting paragangliomas secrete catecholamines and other peptides. They cause morbidity and mortality through their secretory effects, mass effect, and/or malignant potential. The complete classic symptom triad of palpitations, diaphoresis, and headaches occurs in only 4% of patients, making the diagnosis difficult. Affected individuals can present with a wide range of symptoms, including anxiety, fatigue, weight loss, heat intolerance, vision disturbance, pallor, tremors, abdominal or chest pain, nausea, dizziness, change in bowel habits, neurologic symptoms, and worsening or new-onset diabetes. The episodic nature of symptoms with complete resolution between episodes should trigger a high index of clinical suspicion, and the diagnosis should be considered in all patients with sustained hypertension (60%-90% of pediatric cases), difficult-to-control hypertension, symptomatic hypertension, or a positive family history.

Biochemical studies in the form of measuring 24-hour urinary metanephrines or plasma metanephrines are the first-line investigation to exclude pheochromocytomas and catecholamine-secreting paragangliomas. Careful evaluation is required in those with results in the upper-normal reference range. False-negative results are uncommon, except in cases of incomplete 24-hour urinary collection. Plasma metanephrines can be more reliable and convenient for this reason. However, false-positive results do occur. Medications including acetaminophen, α- and β-adrenergic blockers, tricyclic antidepressants, monoamine oxidase inhibitors, and sympathomimetic agents (nicotine, ephedrine, pseudoephedrine, cocaine) can all cause false-positive results. Circumstances of sample collection are also important. For plasma metanephrines, the patient should fast from midnight and be supine for 30 minutes before the blood test. The sample must be centrifuged within 2 hours. For urinary metanephrines, a complete 24-hour urine collection is required for accuracy. In both cases, patients should avoid common medications such as acetaminophen and pseudoephedrine on the day of the test.

Imaging and genetic testing are recommended once a diagnosis of pheochromocytoma or catecholamine-secreting paraganglioma is established. Currently, it is recognized that 40% to 50% of pheochromocytomas and catecholamine-secreting paragangliomas are due to underlying genetic pathogenic variants. These fall into 2 clusters of genes. Cluster 1 includes pathogenic variants in genes encoding the von Hippel-Lindau tumor suppressor (*VHL*), subunits of succinate dehydrogenase (*SDHA, SDHB, SDHC,* and *SDHD*), succinate dehydrogenase complex assembly factor 2 (*SDHAF2*), fumarate hydratase (*FH*), malate dehydrogenase 2 (*MDH2*), and egl-9 family hypoxia inducible factors (*EGLN1, EGLN2*), which result in activation of hypoxia signaling pathways. Cluster 2 includes pathogenic variants in genes encoding neurofibromatosis type 1 (*NF1*), ret proto-oncogene (*RET*), transmembrane protein 127 (*TMEM127*), MYC-associated factor X (*MAX*), HRas proto-oncogene GTPase (*HRAS*), and endothelial PAS domain protein 1 (*EPAS1*), which affect kinase receptor signaling pathways.

Educational Objective
Diagnose pheochromocytoma in a child and conduct the appropriate investigations.

Reference(s)
Pamporaki C, Hamplova B, Peitzsch M, et al. Characteristics of pediatric vs adult pheochromocytomas and paragangliomas. *J Clin Endocrinol Metab.* 2017;102(4):1122-1132. PMID: 28324046

Lenders JW, Duh QY, Eisenhofer G, et al; Endocrine Society. Pheochromocytoma and paraganglioma: an endocrine society clinical practice guideline. *J Clin Endocrinol Metab.* 2014;99(6):1915-1942. PMID: 24893135

Martucci VL, Pacak K. Pheochromocytoma and paraganglioma: diagnosis, genetics, management, and treatment. *Curr Probl Cancer.* 2014;38(1):7-41. PMID: 24636754

Bholah R, Bunchman TE, Review of pediatric pheochromocytoma and paraganglioma. *Front Pediatr.* 2017;5:155. PMID: 28752085

11 ANSWER: C) Effect of the somatostatin analogue
This patient presented with rapid growth, tall stature, galactorrhea, irregular menses, elevated prolactin, elevated GH, elevated IGF-1, failure of GH to suppress with oral glucose tolerance testing, and a sellar/suprasellar mass on MRI—findings consistent with a GH/prolactin-secreting pituitary adenoma. First-line therapy for a GH/prolactin-secreting macroadenoma is surgical resection. However, this patient continued to have evidence of GH excess postoperatively and was therefore treated with a somatostatin analogue.

Somatostatin is an inhibitory 14–amino acid peptide hormone present both in the hypothalamus and peripheral tissues. Somatostatin is involved in the inhibition of the release of GH and TSH, as well as gastrointestinal hormones, pancreatic enzymes, and neuropeptides. Somatostatin binds to receptors belonging to the 7 transmembrane G-protein–coupled receptor superfamily. Analogues of somatostatin, such as octreotide and lanreotide, were developed and initially used for the treatment of acromegaly and gastroenteropancreatic tumors and are highly effective for the treatment of GH excess. Because somatostatin inhibits TSH release, treatment with a somatostatin analogue (Answer C) is the most likely cause of this patient's low TSH level.

While destruction of thyrotrope cells can occur with a large mass (Answer A), this girl's thyroid function tests were normal at presentation. Surgical resection (Answer B) could result in central hypothyroidism, gonadotropin deficiency, ACTH deficiency, and even diabetes insipidus. However, her thyroid function tests were normal postoperatively. Hyperprolactinemia and GH excess were present initially, but prolactin levels (Answer D) normalized postoperatively. GH and IGF-1 levels (Answer E) normalized with medical therapy.

Educational Objective
Explain the effects of somatostatin and somatostatin analogues on TSH and GH secretion.

Reference(s)
Theodoropoulou M, Stalla GK. Somatostatin receptors: from signaling to clinical practice. *Front Neuroendocrinol.* 2013;34(3):228-252. PMID: 23872332

12 ANSWER: A) Measure uric acid, order a lipid panel, and refer to a metabolic nutritionist

Patients with hypoglycemia pose an interesting challenge to everyday clinical practice in endocrinology. GH deficiency, cortisol deficiency, and hyperinsulinemia could result in hypoglycemia. However, hepatomegaly (as evidenced by the protruding abdomen in this patient) and elevated lactate levels in the setting of hypoglycemia are seen in patients with glycogen storage disease (GSD). Elevated lactate levels and b-hydroxybutyrate with acidosis at the time of hypoglycemia in a patient with hepatomegaly are indications of possible GSD and warrant further metabolic workup and treatment. Patients with GSD type 1 also have hyperuricemia and hypertriglyceridemia. Therefore, measuring uric acid and performing a lipid panel (Answer A) is the best next step.

GSD type 1 occurs in patients with homozygous or compound heterozygous pathogenic variants in the genes encoding glucose-6-phosphatase (GSD type 1a) or glucose-6-phosphate translocase (GSD type 1b). Patients with GSD type 1 can present with hypoglycemia in the neonatal period, infancy, or early childhood, but more commonly present at 3 to 6 months of age. Clinical characteristics can mimic those of Cushing syndrome, including doll-like facies, poor growth, short stature, and a distended abdomen due to pronounced hepatomegaly and nephromegaly. Biochemical manifestations include hypoglycemia, hyperlipidemia, hypertriglyceridemia, hyperlactatemia, and hyperuricemia. Patients with GSD type 1b also have neutropenia and impaired neutrophil function, resulting in recurrent bacterial infections and oral and intestinal mucosa ulceration. Patients with GSD type 1 do not have skeletal myopathy or increased creatine kinase levels, which are characteristic of GSD type 3a.

Frequent feeds with complex carbohydrates and cornstarch every 3 to 5 hours, as well as close monitoring of blood glucose levels, are essential in patients with GSD type 1. Long-acting cornstarch is approved for overnight use in children older than 5 years. In 2018, the US FDA approved the first gene therapy trial for patients with GSD type 1, which, if successful, could ultimately obviate the lifelong dependence on cornstarch for survival in these patients.

GH and cortisol measured at the time of hypoglycemia may not be high enough to exclude GH deficiency and cortisol deficiency. Thus, in a patient with clinical and laboratory findings suggestive of a metabolic disorder such as GSD type 1, proceeding to expensive diagnostic testing such as MRI that could be also be invasive if it requires sedation given the patient's age (Answer C) is incorrect. Proceeding with cosyntropin-stimulation testing (Answer B) or GH-simulation testing (Answer E) could delay the correct diagnosis or potentially result in wrong diagnosis and neither is the best next step. Follow-up in 6 months without further investigation and in-depth counseling on diet (Answer D) could be life-threatening in patients with GSD type 1 and is thus is not acceptable.

Educational Objective
Diagnose glycogen storage disease in a patient with hypoglycemia based on their concurrent clinical and laboratory findings.

Reference(s)
Kishnani PS, Austin SL, Abdenur JE, et al. Diagnosis and management of glycogen storage disease type I: a practice guideline of the American College of Medical Genetics and Genomics. *Genet Med.* 2014;16(11):e1. PMID: 25356975

Heller S, Worona L, Consuelo A. Nutritional therapy for glycogen storage diseases. *J Pediatr Gastroenterol Nutr.* 2008;47(Suppl 1):S15-S21. PMID: 18667910

Kelly A, Tang R, Becker S, Stanley CA. Poor specificity of low growth hormone and cortisol levels during fasting hypoglycemia for the diagnoses of growth hormone deficiency and adrenal insufficiency. *Pediatrics.* 2008;122(3):e522-e528. PMID: 18694902

13 ANSWER: D) High risk for aggressive medullary thyroid carcinoma; total thyroidectomy is recommended now

The *RET* proto-oncogene encodes a transmembrane receptor of the tyrosine kinase family. It has a fundamental role in the development of sporadic or familial aggressive medullary thyroid carcinoma (MTC) and other malignant and nonmalignant diseases. Genetic counseling and genetic testing for germline pathogenic variants in *RET* should be offered to first-degree relatives of patients with proven MTC or known *RET* pathogenic variants.

In 2015, the American Thyroid Association published revised guidelines and changed the risk categories for MTC. Detailed information on risk classification of patients based on their *RET* pathogenic variant can be found in these guidelines. The highest-risk category includes patients with multiple endocrine neoplasia (MEN) type 2B and the *RET* codon M918T pathogenic variant. The high-risk category includes patients with *RET* pathogenic variants in codon 634 and the codon A883F pathogenic variant. Other common pathogenic variants, previously labeled as A and B categories, are now referred to as moderate-risk pathogenic variants.

Patients with MEN 2B have marfanoid body habitus, narrow, long facies, generalized ganglioneuromatosis, skeletal malformations (usually pes cavus, although other skeletal malformations can be seen), and ophthalmologic abnormalities (ie, alacrima, prominent corneal nerve fibers across corneas, plexiform subconjunctival neuromas, conjunctival hyperemia with superficial peripheral corneal neovascularization, and blepharitis) (Answer E). The patient described in the vignette does not have the M918T pathogenic variant seen in 95% of patients with MEN 2B, and she also has a normal physical examination. Patients with a pathogenic variant in this codon require total thyroidectomy before the age of 1 year.

For patients with the *RET* C634R pathogenic variant, it is recommended to screen for MTC with annual physical examination, cervical ultrasonography, and measurement of calcitonin starting at age 3 years. Studies have shown no lymph node metastasis in children with MEN 2A when the calcitonin level is below 30 or 40 pg/mL (<8.8 or 11.7 pmol/L). However, all patients with MEN 2A require total thyroidectomy. For children in the high-risk category, total thyroidectomy is recommended at or before age 5 years. The patient in this vignette is at high risk to have aggressive MTC. She is 7 years old, and total thyroidectomy ideally should have been done sooner. Therefore, this procedure is recommended now (Answer D). Patients with *RET* pathogenic variants at moderate risk should have total thyroidectomy in childhood or young adulthood, with the timing of operation being dependent primarily on calcitonin levels.

Pheochromocytoma may develop before age 12 years in patients with MEN 2, although it has been reported as early as 8 years. Currently, it is recommended to start routine screening at age 11 years for patients in the high- and highest-risk categories and at the age of 16 years for patients in the moderate-risk category, although earlier screening could be done based on clinical judgment. However, pheochromocytoma screening (Answer B) is not the best answer.

Hyperparathyroidism has been reported to occur as early as 2, 6, 7, and 10 years of age in patients in the high- and moderate-risk categories. However, current guidelines recommend screening by age 11 years for patients at high risk and by age 16 years for patients at moderate risk. Thus, screening for hyperparathyroidism (Answer A) is not the best choice.

Patients with certain *RET* pathogenic variants are at risk for developing Hirschsprung disease and cutaneous lichen amyloidosis (Answer C). The *RET* C634R pathogenic variant is associated with cutaneous lichen amyloidosis. In patients with MEN 2A, this condition manifests as localized, interscapular amyloidosis, usually preceded by pruritus. Although she may develop this condition, her examination findings are not consistent with this diagnosis. Also, the *RET* C634R mutation is not associated with Hirschsprung disease.

This patient's calcitonin concentration was elevated at 109 pg/mL (31.8 pg/mL). She underwent total thyroidectomy and was found to have MTC with local invasion and angioinvasion, localized to the thyroid. Five lymph nodes were negative for carcinoma. Although she has a 20% probability of developing hyperparathyroidism and a 50% probability of developing pheochromocytoma, the priority now is to proceed with total thyroidectomy. Screening for pheochromocytoma and hyperparathyroidism is recommended by age 11 years, although one could consider screening sooner if a patient has symptoms or abnormal vital signs.

Educational Objective
Guide decision-making regarding prophylactic thyroidectomy in a family with multiple endocrine neoplasia type 2A.

Reference(s)
Wells SA Jr, Asa SL, Dralle H, et al; American Thyroid Association Guidelines Task Force on Medullary Thyroid Carcinoma. Revised American Thyroid Association guidelines for the management of medullary thyroid carcinoma. *Thyroid*. 2015;25(6):567-610. PMID: 25810047

Verga U, Fugazzola L, Cambiaghi S, et al. Frequent association between MEN 2A and cutaneous lichen amyloidosis. *Clin Endocrinol (Oxf)*. 2003;59(2):156-161. PMID: 12864791

Castinetti F, Moley J, Mulligan L, Waguespack SG. A comprehensive review on MEN2B. *Endocr Relat Cancer*. 2018;25(2):T29-T39. PMID: 28698189

14

ANSWER: B) LH, low; TSH, very high; hCG, normal

LH, FSH, TSH, and hCG are glycoprotein hormones consisting of 2 chains, the α- and β-subunits, which are noncovalently bound. The α-subunits of LH, FSH, hCG, and TSH are identical in amino acid sequence (92 amino acids), although each of their β chains is unique and is responsible for the biologic specificity of the intact hormones. However, approximately 80% of the first 115 amino acids of the β-subunit of hCG is homologous to the sequence of the β-subunit of LH.

This girl presented with early pubertal changes with rapid progression to vaginal bleeding but slow linear growth. Her examination findings are notable for short stature, normal weight, presence of secondary sexual characteristics, periorbital edema, and hypertrichosis. Her bone age is delayed. These findings are consistent with primary hypothyroidism leading to the so-called overlap or Van Wyk-Grumbach syndrome. In this scenario, TSH would be markedly elevated, LH would be low, and hCG would be normal (Answer B). FSH levels can be normal or elevated. One theory to explain the mechanism that occurs in Van Wyk-Grumbach syndrome is thought to be related to a markedly elevated TSH concentration exerting FSH-like effects at the FSH receptor, via the common α-subunit, leading to an increase in gonadal size and steroidogenesis. The isolated rise in FSH is postulated to be from slowing of the GnRH pulse frequency in primary hypothyroidism. The low LH may be due to hyperprolactinemia from increased thyrotropin-releasing hormone leading to decreased GnRH secretion. In girls, the increase in estrogen from the ovaries leads to breast development and uterine bleeding in the absence of pubic and axillary hair development. The patient in this vignette did have pubic hair development; however, this can be normal for age. In boys, testicular enlargement without other signs of virilization is seen.

Gonadotropin-dependent precocious puberty, in which LH and FSH would be increased for age and TSH and hCG would be normal (Answer A), would be expected to cause linear growth acceleration, tall stature, and advanced bone age. Granulosa-cell tumors of the ovary, in which estradiol levels would be high, with suppressed LH and FSH levels and normal TSH and hCG levels (Answer C), usually present with rapid onset of pubertal changes and vaginal bleeding but would not be expected to be associated with short stature, periorbital edema, or hypertrichosis. A germ-cell tumor of the central nervous system, in which hCG levels are elevated and LH levels are low, can manifest with early pubertal changes. However, this phenomenon is only seen in boys. hCG and LH share the same receptor, so elevations in hCG would be expected to result in secondary sexual characteristics in boys due to stimulation of Leydig cells, with subsequent testosterone production. However, in girls, both LH (or hCG) and FSH are needed for ovarian estradiol production. A germ-cell tumor of the central nervous system would also not be likely to have an elevated TSH level as in Answer D. Low LH, low FSH, low TSH, and normal hCG (Answer E) might be seen in a girl with McCune-Albright syndrome who has gonadotropin-independent precocious puberty and hyperthyroidism due to constitutive activation of the G-protein–stimulatory subunit. Linear growth acceleration with bone age advancement would be expected in this scenario. Also, this patient has no evidence of café-au-lait macules or fibrous dysplasia on examination.

Educational Objective
Explain that LH, FSH, TSH, and hCG are heterodimers composed of a common α-subunit and a hormone-specific β-subunit.

Reference(s)

Eugster EA. Update on precocious puberty in girls. *J Pediatr Adolesc Gynecol.* 2019;32(5):455-459. PMID: 31158483

Van Wyk JJ, Grumbach MM. Syndrome of precocious menstruation and galactorrhea in juvenile hypothyroidism: an example of hormonal overlap in pituitary feedback. *J Pediatr.* 1960;57:416-435.

Hachicha M, Maaloul I, Aissa K, Kamoun T, Aloulou H. Van Wyk-Grumbach syndrome: a rare cause of precocious puberty. *Presse Med.* 2018;47(5):483-486. PMID: 29555166

15

ANSWER: D) Magnesium deficiency secondary to inadequate supplementation

Magnesium is a divalent cation (as is calcium) essential for both the secretion and function of PTH. In this clinical scenario, the patient has symptoms of profound tetany despite a corrected calcium of 7.7 mg/dL (1.9 mmol/L). PTH is exquisitely sensitive to calcium changes. Thus, the value of 40 pg/mL (40 ng/L) is lower than expected. However, this is due to the profound hypomagnesemia impairing the function of the calcium-sensing receptor. Acquired hypoparathyroidism (Answer B) is theoretically possible, but it would require ongoing treatment with calcium and calcitriol and would not resolve with magnesium supplementation alone. In addition, hypoparathyroidism is associated with hyperphosphatemia and an increased fractional excretion of calcium in the urine, neither of which is present in this patient.

Rare autosomal recessive pathogenic variants in the *TRPM6* gene (Answer A) on chromosome 9q22 cause hypomagnesemia with impaired urinary magnesium excretion. Affected patients present with symptoms of seizures and tetany in the first few weeks of life. Despite having a congenital malabsorption syndrome, her bowel pattern has not changed, and calcium, magnesium, and phosphate levels have previously been normal.

Gitelman syndrome (Answer E) is due to a defect in the sodium-chloride channel causing impaired resorption of several electrolytes at the distal tubule of the kidney. Laboratory findings include hypokalemic metabolic alkalosis, hypocalciuria, and hypomagnesemia due to renal magnesium wasting. Affected patients generally present in later childhood with symptoms of muscle weakness, lethargy, muscle cramps, and tetany. Because most calcium reabsorption is mediated by the calcium-sensing receptor thick ascending loop of Henle, these patients have low urinary calcium excretion in contrast to patients with Bartter syndrome.

This patient's pathogenic variants in *SPINT2* cause intractable watery diarrhea and tufting of enterocytes, leading to malabsorption and metabolic acidosis with resultant intestinal failure. Affected patients also present with woolly hair, intrauterine growth restriction, short stature, immunodeficiency, skin abnormalities, and liver disease. While enteric magnesium losses are possible at diagnosis, she has not had any changes in her bowel habits, and prior electrolyte measurements have been normal. Shortages of various electrolytes and micronutrients have been known to cause significant clinical consequences if patients are not carefully monitored. Patients on total parenteral nutrition are at risk for hypothyroidism due to iodine deficiency, which has been a previous concern for this patient. Iodine deficiency (Answer C) can cause fatigue, weakness, dry brittle hair, and dry skin, but it would not be expected to cause hypomagnesemia. Her TSH level was also checked and was normal. At the time of this patient's episode, there was a national shortage of magnesium. Because she was receiving some nutrition enterally, she was not identified as an at-risk patient despite her history of malabsorption. This led to both calcium and magnesium mineral supplementation being removed from her parenteral nutrition 2 weeks before her presentation (Answer D).

Educational Objective
Diagnose magnesium deficiency, which can present similarly to hypocalcemia, and identify total parenteral nutrition as potentially placing a patient at risk.

Reference(s)
Walder RY, Landau D, Meyer P, et al. Mutation of TRPM6 causes familial hypomagnesemia with secondary hypocalcemia. *Nat Genet.* 2002;31(2):171-174. PMID: 12032570

Seyberth HW, Weber S, Komhoff M. Bartter's and Gitelman's syndrome. *Curr Opin Pediatr.* 2017;29(2):179-186. PMID: 27906863

Ikomi C, Cole CR, Vale E, et al. Hypothyroidism and iodine deficiency in children on chronic parenteral nutrition. *Pediatrics.* 2018;141(4). PMID: 29496904

Plogsted S, Adams SC, Allen K, et al; Clinical Practice Committee's Nutrition Product Shortage Subcommittee of the American Society for Parenteral and Enteral Nutrition. Parenteral nutrition electrolyte and mineral product shortage considerations. *Nutr Clin Pract.* 2016;31(1):132-134. PMID: 26703958

16   ANSWER: D) Apolipoprotein B
Polycystic ovary syndrome is a known metabolic disorder associated with insulin resistance and dyslipidemia. Women with this condition often have metabolic syndrome. Metabolic syndrome is characterized by a group of cardiovascular risk factors, including central obesity, high blood pressure, elevated triglycerides, low HDL cholesterol (thus, Answer E is incorrect), and elevated fasting glucose. In pediatric patients, metabolic syndrome is most often diagnosed according to criteria that are adapted from adult criteria, such as those developed by the National Cholesterol Education Program. The most commonly used criteria specify the following cutoff values:

- Fasting blood glucose = typically >100 mg/dL (SI: >5.5 mmol/L)
- HDL cholesterol = <40 mg/dL (SI: <1.04 mmol/L)
- Triglycerides = >110 mg/dL (SI: >1.24 mmol/L)
- Blood pressure greater than the 90th percentile for sex, age, and height
- Waist circumference greater than the 90th percentile for age and sex

To be classified as having metabolic syndrome, an adolescent must have abnormal values for at least 3 of these 5 criteria.

Polycystic ovary syndrome contributes to the metabolic derangements with hyperandrogenemia, which has been associated with enhanced lipogenesis. While patients with polycystic ovary syndrome often have insulin resistance (Answer A), recent studies support the idea that the presence of elevated apolipoprotein B (Answer D), such as intestinal apolipoprotein B_{48} and hepatic apolipoprotein B_{100}, are strong predictors of future cardiovascular disease. Increased lipid synthesis via increased activation of the nuclear transcription factor sterol regulatory-element binding protein-1c is also a strong predictor of future cardiovascular disease.

African American patients appear to manifest metabolic syndrome differently than white and Hispanic patients. Black patients with metabolic syndrome are much less likely to exhibit elevated triglycerides. In a survey of 2456 adolescents, Johnson et al documented that although 26% to 32% of white and Hispanic adolescents had triglyceride concentrations above 110 mg/dL (>1.24 mmol/L), only 10% of black adolescents exhibited triglyceride elevations (Answer C), potentially because of lower levels of lipoprotein lipase. LDL-cholesterol elevations (Answer B) are not significantly associated with metabolic syndrome. The mainstay of treatment for metabolic syndrome and related abnormalities is lifestyle modification with increased physical activity and decreased caloric intake. However, metformin therapy has been associated with improvements in a number of the metabolic derangements noted in polycystic ovary syndrome in adolescent and adult women.

Educational Objective
List the lipid characteristics associated with metabolic syndrome in the context of polycystic ovary syndrome in adolescent patients and explain the differences observed in the manifestation of this syndrome in various racial/ethnic groups.

Reference(s)

Vine DF, Beilin LJ, Burrows S, et al. ApoB48-lipoproteins are associated with cardiometabolic risk in adolescents with and without polycystic ovary syndrome, *J Endocr Soc.* 2020;4(8):bvaa061. PMID: 32803089

Vine DF, Wang Y, Jetha MM, Ball GD, Proctor SD. Impaired ApoB-lipoprotein and triglyceride metabolism in obese adolescents with polycystic ovary syndrome. *J Clin Endocrinol Metab.* 2017;102(3):970-982. PMID: 27997268

Johnson WD, Kroon JJ, Greenway FL, Bouchard C, Ryan D, Katzmarzyk PT. Prevalence of risk factors for metabolic syndrome in adolescents: National Health and Nutrition Examination Survey (NHANES), 2001-2006. *Arch Pediatr Adolesc Med.* 2009;163(4):371-377. PMID: 19349567

17 ANSWER: E) FNA biopsy of both nodules

The most common form of well-differentiated thyroid cancer is papillary thyroid cancer (PTC). Because PTC is usually multifocal, it is crucial to determine via FNA biopsy if a thyroid nodule represents PTC. While more adults than children have thyroid nodules, thyroid nodules in children are more likely to be malignant. In pediatric patients, all instances of FNA biopsy should be ultrasound-guided. In this case, although the 2 nodules are in the left thyroid lobe, removing the left lobe alone (Answer A) is incorrect. If this patient has PTC, she would need completion thyroidectomy surgery.

Although evaluating whether this patient has Hashimoto thyroiditis (Answer B) could be done, it is not the best next step. Even if she has autoimmune thyroiditis, one would still need to perform FNA biopsy to determine whether she has thyroid cancer.

The ultrasonography features of thyroid nodules can indicate whether a nodule is likely to be malignant. Performing FNA biopsy of only the largest nodule (Answer C) is incorrect, as the smaller nodule could be malignant as well. In this case, the smaller nodule has a few features that confer a higher risk of malignancy: solid and hypoechoic composition, taller-than-wide shape, increased blood flow, and a possible microcalcification. Ultrasonography images of various thyroid nodules, illustrating the features of very low, low, intermediate, and high suspicion for risk of malignancy in thyroid nodules are depicted well in the adult American Thyroid Association guidelines from 2015. The same features apply when evaluating nodules in pediatric patients. While the smaller lesion has some high-risk features, performing FNA biopsy on this lesion alone (Answer D) is incorrect, as this patient requires assessment for multifocal disease. Irregular margins—another high-risk feature—were not present. Having cervical adenopathy also raises the suspicion of thyroid cancer, but this was not noted on ultrasonography or physical examination in this patient. When performing FNA biopsy on the larger lesion in this adolescent, ultrasound guidance should aim to sample the solid areas of the lesion where malignancy is more likely. For a complete evaluation, this patient should undergo ultrasound-guided FNA biopsy of both lesions (Answer E).

Educational Objective

Identify the high-risk features for thyroid cancer on ultrasonography and evaluate for malignancy in an adolescent with thyroid nodules.

Reference(s)

Francis GL, Waguespack SG, Bauer AJ, et al; American Thyroid Association Guidelines Task Force. Management guidelines for children with thyroid nodules and differentiated thyroid cancer. *Thyroid*. 2015;25(7):716-759. PMID: 25900731

Creo A, Alahdab F, Al Nofal A, Thomas K, Kolbe A, Pittock ST. Ultrasonography and the American Thyroid Association ultrasound-based risk stratification tool: utility in pediatric and adolescent thyroid nodules. *Horm Res Paediatr*. 2018;90(2):93-101. PMID: 30021204

Haugen BR, Alexander EK, Bible KC, et al. 2015 American Thyroid Association management guidelines for adult patients with thyroid nodules and differentiated thyroid cancer: the American Thyroid Association Guidelines Task Force on Thyroid Nodules and Differentiated Thyroid Cancer. *Thyroid*. 2016;26(1):1-133. PMID: 26462967

18 ANSWER: E) Discuss switching from risperidone to another atypical antipsychotic with her psychiatrist

Secondary amenorrhea is defined as the absence of menses for 3 consecutive cycles after menarche. Physiologic causes of secondary amenorrhea include functional hypothalamic amenorrhea, pregnancy, and lactation. An elevated prolactin level in a patient with secondary amenorrhea raises concern for pathologic causes such as prolactin-secreting adenomas, sellar masses, pituitary stalk disruption, and primary hypothyroidism. Patients with psychiatric disorders are at higher risk of amenorrhea or menstrual irregularities, most likely related to hypothalamic-pituitary dysfunction.

First-generation antipsychotic agents and the atypical antipsychotic risperidone can increase prolactin levels via dopamine receptor antagonism. Compared with risperidone, other atypical antipsychotics (serotonin-dopamine antagonists) and partial dopamine antagonists (ie, aripiprazole) are associated with lower serum prolactin levels. Switching from risperidone to another atypical antipsychotic (Answer E) may help resolve amenorrhea without worsening psychiatric symptoms, but this should only be undertaken after discussion with the prescribing physician. If an elevated prolactin value is documented, current guidelines recommend discontinuing medications that are known to increase prolactin before performing additional testing.

While the cause of this patient's amenorrhea and hyperprolactinemia is most likely risperidone, this cannot be assumed without further assessment, so simply providing reassurance (Answer D) is incorrect. A pituitary MRI (Answer A) would be recommended only if the antipsychotic medication cannot be discontinued or if the prolactin level remains above 50 ng/mL (>2.2 nmol/L) after switching medications.

This patient also has findings of mild hirsutism and a mild elevation in free testosterone, which could be caused by polycystic ovary syndrome or nonclassic CAH. While further workup for these conditions should be considered (Answer B), the first priority is to assess the elevated prolactin level. It is expected that menses would resume if the prolactin level decreases below 50 ng/mL (<2.2 nmol/L). Thus, if menses do not resume, additional testing would be indicated. A progestin withdrawal challenge (Answer C) would not add useful diagnostic information at this point given that her estrogen level is normal.

Initial laboratory test results were reviewed with this patient's psychiatrist, who switched her medication from risperidone to aripiprazole. Testing 4 weeks later showed that her prolactin level decreased to 24.6 ng/mL (1.1 nmol/L). Her hyperprolactinemia was therefore attributed to risperidone.

Educational Objective

Differentiate among causes of secondary amenorrhea.

Reference(s)

Melmed S, Casanueva FF, Hoffman AR, et al; Endocrine Society. Diagnosis and treatment of hyperprolactinemia: an Endocrine Society clinical practice guideline. *J Clin Endocrinol Metab*. 2011;96(2):273-288. PMID: 21296991

Fourman LT, Fazeli PK. Neuroendocrine causes of amenorrhea--an update. *J Clin Endocrinol Metab*. 2015;100(3):812-824. PMID: 25581597

Pritts S. Secondary amenorrhea: don't dismiss it as 'normal'. *Curr Psychiatr*. 2004;3(10):57-70.

19

ANSWER: D) Recommend a small insulin bolus before lifting weights

Type 1 diabetes mellitus is a challenging condition to manage with various physiologic changes of the human body. Regular exercise is essential, but management of different forms of physical activity is particularly challenging for both the individual with type 1 diabetes and the health care provider. Daily exercise is highly encouraged for patients with type 1 diabetes, as it is the best practice to recommend for any patient. Patients with type 1 diabetes benefit from exercise by improving glycemic control, as well as body composition and general well-being. However, different types and intensities of exercise have various effects on blood glucose concentrations. Understanding the metabolic and neuroendocrine responses to various types of exercise is essential to offer proper advice to patients. During aerobic exercise, insulin secretion decreases and glucagon secretion increases in the portal vein to facilitate release of glucose from the liver to match the rate of glucose uptake into the working muscles. During predominantly anaerobic activities such as sprinting and during a high-intensity training session such as weight lifting, circulating insulin concentrations do not decrease as markedly as in purely aerobic activities, in part because the duration of activity is typically shorter. Insulin concentrations increase above baseline in early recovery from a high-intensity training session to offset the rise in glucose caused by the elevations in counterregulatory hormones and other metabolites.

Blood glucose levels tend to remain steady or drop precipitously in patients with diabetes during aerobic forms of exercise such as biking, hiking, walking, and rollerblading, depending on the amount of active insulin on board (basal and/or bolus). However, in most anaerobic forms of exercise such as weight lifting, blood glucose rises since the insulin dose is mostly adjusted for the resting state. This can be prevented by giving a small dose (30%-50% less) of a blood glucose correction bolus (or half of the hourly basal rate) before the anaerobic exercise (Answer D).

Not trusting a patient's reporting by suspecting erroneous glucose measurements and requesting another report in 1 week (Answer A) could alienate the patient. Increasing the basal insulin dose by 20% before and during exercise (temporary basal rate) would most likely provide a similar solution if the patient is managed via insulin pump therapy. However, increasing the daily basal insulin by 20% (Answer B) would increase the risk of hypoglycemia throughout the day. Increasing the insulin bolus for the meal before lifting weights (Answer C) may cause hypoglycemia depending on the timing of the meal and should not be recommended. Reassurance (Answer E) will send the wrong message to the patient in terms of tolerating hyperglycemia and would increase the risk of ketosis during anaerobic exercise.

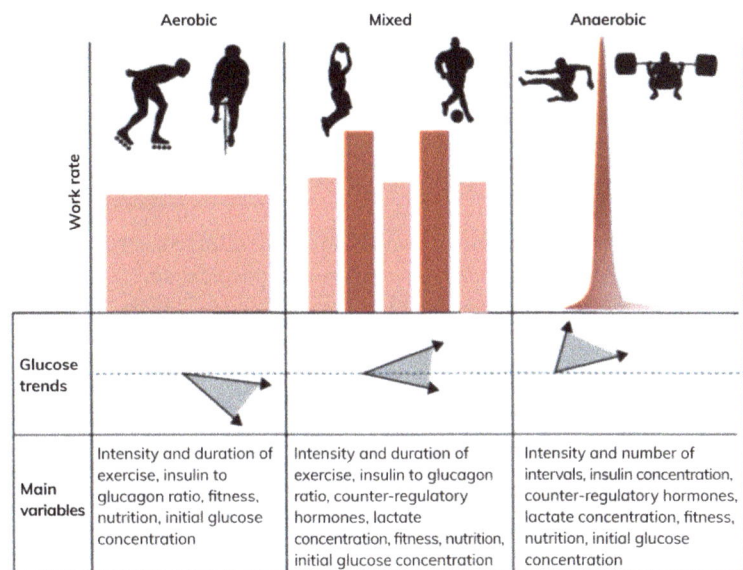

Image reprinted from Riddell MC, Gallen IW, Smart CE, et al. Exercise management in type 1 diabetes: a consensus statement. *Lancet Diabetes Endocrinol.* 2017;5(5):377-390.

Educational Objective
Advise patients on how to adjust their insulin regimen during anaerobic forms of exercise.

Reference(s)

Riddell MC, Gallen IW, Smart CE, et al. Exercise management in type 1 diabetes: a consensus statement. *Lancet Diabetes Endocrinol.* 2017;5(5):377-390. PMID: 28126459

Lukacs A, Barkai L. Effect of aerobic and anaerobic exercises on glycemic control in type 1 diabetic youths. *World J Diabetes.* 2015;6(3):534-542. PMID: 25897363

20

ANSWER: E) Shortened fourth metacarpals and metatarsals

The description of the child in this vignette most closely matches a diagnosis of pseudohypoparathyroidism type 1A (Albright hereditary osteodystrophy). Therefore, of the physical findings listed, the classic finding of shortened fourth metacarpals and metatarsals (Answer E) is the most likely to be observed. He has additional physical manifestations consistent with this disorder, including short stature, stocky build, obesity, and cognitive impairment/developmental delay. His workup shows mild hypocalcemia with slight hyperphosphatemia, as well as elevated PTH, which suggests the presence of PTH dysfunction. The history of seizures in infancy is most likely the result of hypocalcemia.

Manifestations of pseudohypoparathyroidism include a spectrum of abnormal physical features, neurocognitive deficiencies, and endocrine abnormalities that are most commonly caused by the defective hormonal signaling for those hormones that act through G protein–coupled receptors. Loss-of-function pathogenic variants in the gene encoding the α subunit of the stimulatory G protein ($G_s\alpha$) lead to lack of activation of the postreceptor cascade after interaction of the hormone (ligand) with the G protein–coupled receptor (receptor), thus leading to hormone resistance. As such, individuals with pseudohypoparathyroidism have primarily functional hypoparathyroidism with elevated PTH levels because of resistance to PTH leading to hypocalcemia and hyperphosphatemia. They may also present with hypothyroidism due to resistance to TSH, hypogonadism due to resistance to LH and FSH, and GH deficiency due to resistance to GHRH. Physical manifestations of pseudohypoparathyroidism include short stature, stocky build, early-onset obesity, skeletal deformities (most commonly brachydactyly), ectopic ossifications (not described in the vignette), premature closure of growth plates, and neurocognitive abnormalities (eg, developmental delay and loss of intellectual function).

Almond-shaped eyes (Answer A) are commonly associated with Prader-Willi syndrome. This condition is also associated with short stature but not commonly with thyroid dysfunction or PTH abnormalities.

Focal dysplasia of the distal radial physis (Answer B), or Madelung deformity, is often seen in patients with *SHOX* pathogenic variants. Affected patients uniformly have short stature, but they do not have associated thyroid or calcium disturbances.

Noonan syndrome is associated with widely-spaced eyes, eyelid ptosis, and low-set ears (Answer C). Patients with Noonan syndrome commonly present with a heart murmur or developmental delays. They do not have thyroid or calcium abnormalities.

Silver-Russell syndrome is associated with short stature and hemihypertrophy (Answer D). Affected patients commonly present with failure to thrive and poor feeding. Obesity and thyroid dysfunction are not typical findings in patients with this syndrome.

Educational Objective

Identify pseudohypoparathyroidism type 1A as a cause of short stature and list the clinical and laboratory abnormalities associated with this disorder.

Reference(s)

Mantovani G, Bastepe M, Monk D, et al. Diagnosis and management of pseudohypoparathyroidism and related disorders: first international consensus statement. *Nat Rev Endocrinol.* 2018;14(8):476-500. PMID: 29959430

Dauber A, Rosenfeld RG, Hirschhorn JN. Genetic evaluation of short stature. *J Clin Endocrinol Metab.* 2014;99(9):3080-3092. PMID: 24915122

21

ANSWER: D) Adrenal adenoma

An adrenal adenoma (Answer D) is the most likely diagnosis in this case, although glucocorticoid remediable aldosteronism (not given as an option) should be excluded. Glucocorticoid remediable aldosteronism is an autosomal dominant form of hyperaldosteronism due a genetic defect that gives rise to fusion of the promoter region of the *CYP11A1* gene with the coding sequences of the *CYP11B2* gene (encoding aldosterone synthase), resulting in a chimeric *CYP11A1/CYP11B2* gene. As a result, aldosterone synthase is expressed in cortisol-producing zona fasciculata cells, and excess aldosterone is secreted in response to endogenous plasma ACTH. Biochemically, this causes a picture of low-renin hypertension with aldosterone excess. Treatment with dexamethasone to suppress ACTH did not alter this patient's serum aldosterone levels, which rules out glucocorticoid remediable aldosteronism.

When this patient's CT images (which were initially reported as normal) were reviewed at a specialist center, a 10-mm nodule at the apex of the left adrenal gland was noted. A repeated scan demonstrated a stable lesion with no changes in size. Due to the washout characteristics of 40%, the lesion was thought to be a lipid-poor adenoma. The renal arteries were normal, as were the kidneys and left adrenal gland. The patient underwent a left-sided adrenalectomy. Macroscopically, a homogenous bright yellow nodule measuring approximately 14 × 12 × 4 mm was present without necrosis or hemorrhage, thus confirming a diagnosis of adrenal cortical adenoma. Postoperatively, the patient's blood pressure normalized and all medications were subsequently stopped. Genetic analysis did not reveal any germline pathogenic variants in known genes, but analysis of the adenoma itself revealed a heterozygous somatic gain-of-function pathogenic variant (T158A) in the *KCNJ5* gene. The *KCNJ5* gene encodes the potassium channel Kir 3.4 (potassium inwardly rectifying channel, subfamily J, member 5). Gain-of-function *KCNJ5* pathogenic variants, both somatic and germline, cluster in the selectivity filter of Kir3.4, and as such, lead to changes in ion selectivity, increased sodium conductance, and cell depolarization. This opens voltage-dependent calcium channels and influx of calcium in zona glomerulosa cells, resulting in constitutive secretion of aldosterone and cell proliferation.

Renal artery stenosis (Answer A) results in activation of the renin-angiotensin-aldosterone system, leading to elevated renin levels. In this case, renin is completely suppressed, which excludes renal artery stenosis as a diagnosis.

Hypertension is a feature of congenital adrenal hyperplasia (Answer B), in particular 11β-hydroxylase deficiency and 17α-hydroxylase deficiency. However, this is due to the excess production of 11-deoxycorticosterone acting on the mineralocorticoid receptor, leading to a low renin and low aldosterone state.

Liddle syndrome (Answer C) is an autosomal dominant condition caused by pathogenic variants in the sodium channel epithelial 1 β and γ subunit genes (*SCNN1B* and *SCNN1G*), which encode the subunits that make up the epithelial sodium channel. Pathogenic variants lead to constitutive activation of sodium reabsorption along with water retention and increased potassium excretion. Liddle syndrome is biochemically associated with low plasma renin activity, low blood potassium, and normal to low levels of aldosterone.

Licorice root ingestion (Answer E) mimics true hyperaldosteronism, but aldosterone levels are low, so this is an incorrect diagnosis in this case.

The prevalence of hypertension (primary and secondary) in children is reported to be between 4.5% and 13%. Secondary causes are more common in children than in adults. In one study, secondary causes account for 57% of all pediatric hypertension cases. Of these, more than 50% of hypertension cases are due to renal disease, while endocrine causes account for approximately 10%. Endocrine causes include primary aldosteronism, pheochromocytoma, Cushing syndrome, acromegaly, hyperparathyroidism, congenital adrenal hyperplasia, hypothyroidism, hyperthyroidism, and renin-secreting tumors.

The diagnosis of primary aldosteronism is made biochemically by documenting elevated aldosterone together with a low or undetectable plasma renin activity. The Endocrine Society guidelines suggest 2 separate measurements to confirm the diagnosis, except in cases where there is spontaneous hypokalemia, a plasma aldosterone concentration greater than 19.8 ng/dL (>550 pmol/L), and plasma renin activity below detectable limits. Adrenal venous sampling is recommended to distinguish between unilateral or bilateral disease. In this child, adrenal venous sampling was considered, but it was deemed unnecessary due to marked primary aldosteronism, his young age, and positive CT findings. Genetic testing is also recommended in patients with confirmed primary aldosteronism who are younger than 20 years, in those with a family history of primary aldosteronism, or in patients who experience stroke at an age younger than 40 years.

Unilateral laparoscopic adrenalectomy for patients with documented unilateral primary aldosteronism is the treatment of choice. Medical treatment with a mineralocorticoid receptor antagonist, usually spironolactone, should be considered if surgery is not possible or in cases of bilateral disease.

Educational Objective
Diagnose and manage primary aldosteronism due to an aldosterone-producing adenoma.

Reference(s)
Pons Fernandez N, Moreno F, Morata J, et al. Familial hyperaldosteronism type III a novel case and review of literature. *Rev Endocr Metab Disord*. 2019;20(1):27-36. PMID: 30569443

Williams TA, Reincke M. Management of endocrine disease: diagnosis and management of primary aldosteronism: the Endocrine Society guideline 2016 revisited. *Eur J Endocrinol*. 2018;179(1):R19-R29. PMID: 29674485

Funder JW, Carey RM, Mantero F, et al. The management of primary aldosteronism: case detection, diagnosis, and treatment: an Endocrine Society clinical practice guideline. *J Clin Endocrinol Metab*. 2016;101(5):1889-1916. PMID: 26934393

22

ANSWER: A) Discuss the adverse effects of her cancer therapy and have her return for follow-up in 6 months

Chronic myeloid leukemia (CML) is rare and accounts for less than 1% of all leukemias in children. Use of tyrosine kinase inhibitors (TKIs) in the treatment of CML has significantly improved the life expectancy of adults and children. Since the first-generation TKI imatinib was approved for CML therapy in 2003, several new TKI agents have emerged such as dasatinib, nilotinib, bosutinib, and ponatinib. These potent agents are taken orally and target the BCR-ABL1 fusion protein. Because children with CML require lifelong TKI therapy, there is concern for potential off-target inhibition of other kinases leading to long-term adverse effects.

TKIs may inhibit the GHRH signaling cascade, GH signaling cascade, and IGF-1 signal transduction, resulting in GH deficiency or resistance. TKIs may also inhibit chondrocyte activity in growth plates. Many patients have a significant decrease in their prepubertal growth, but experience catch-up growth during puberty. Thus, the best course of action is to discuss the adverse effects of her cancer therapy and have her return for follow-up in 6 months (Answer A). Use of GH during active malignancy is contraindicated because of concerns of neoplasia risks. Thus, further research is needed to assess whether GH therapy (Answer C) can be safely used in patients with CML on TKI therapy who have poor growth due to GH deficiency or GH resistance.

TKIs are associated with subclinical and overt primary hypothyroidism and hyperthyroidism. Mechanisms by which TKIs result in thyroid dysfunction are unclear, but they are thought to be related to increased clearance, decreased iodine uptake, thyroiditis, and TPO inhibition. Thus, it is important to ensure thyroid function is normal before starting TKIs and to periodically monitor thyroid function—usually twice a year—while on TKI therapy. This patient had normal free T_4 and TSH levels documented 1 week before the clinic visit. Thus, it is not necessary to prescribe levothyroxine at this time (Answer B). Because children on TKI therapy for CML tend to have catch-up growth during puberty, it is expected that this patient's growth will improve, as she is in early puberty now. She will not necessarily have short stature as an adult (Answer D).

TKIs lead to dysregulation in bone remodeling by inhibiting the activity of c-FMS, the macrophage colony-stimulating factor receptor, on osteoclasts and PDGF-R (platelet-derived growth factor receptor) and c-Abl1 on osteoblasts. TKIs may promote bone formation in adults, but they cause bone demineralization in children. TKIs also alter calcium and phosphate metabolism, resulting in hypocalcemia and hypophosphatemia. It is important to optimize bone health in these patients. However, DXA (Answer E) is not warranted unless the patient has an unprovoked fracture or is noted to have low bone mineral density on plain radiographs.

Educational Objective
Explain the endocrine adverse effects of tyrosine kinase inhibitor therapy in children.

Reference(s)
Samis J, Lee P, Zimmerman D, Arceci RJ, Suttorp M, Hijiya N. Recognizing endocrinopathies associated with tyrosine kinase inhibitor therapy in children with chronic myelogenous leukemia. *Pediatr Blood Cancer*. 2016;63(8):1332-1338. PMID: 27100618

Sabnis HS, Keenum C, Lewis RW, et al. Growth disturbances in children and adolescents receiving long-term tyrosine kinase inhibitor therapy for chronic myeloid leukaemia or Philadelphia chromosome-positive acute lymphoblastic leukaemia. *Br J Haematol*. 2019;185(4):795-799. PMID: 30407613

23

ANSWER: E) Start thyroid hormone replacement and measure TSH and free T_4 again in 2 weeks

The overall incidence of congenital hypothyroidism is 1 in 3000, although the incidence seems to be rising. Congenital hypothyroidism is one of the most preventable causes of intellectual disability. Therefore, newborn screening aims to identify children with this condition to initiate treatment as soon as possible. Usually, newborn screening identifies babies with congenital hypothyroidism based on elevated TSH in the first 24 to 48 hours of life, with or without a low T_4 level. However, in preterm babies, there is an atypical form of congenital hypothyroidism characterized by a delayed rise in TSH.

The fetal thyroid gland produces thyroid hormones around the end of the first trimester; however, the hypothalamic-pituitary-thyroid axis is not mature until after birth, and both TSH and thyroid hormone levels increase during gestation. Following delivery, there is a TSH surge in term infants, to about 60 to 80 mIU/L, which declines to about 20 mIU/L at 24 to 48 hours of life and to 6 to 10 mIU/L by 1 week of age.

In premature babies, this pattern also occurs, but the thyroid hormone levels reached are reduced compared with those of full-term newborns. In most preterm babies, the levels eventually improve over time, and a rise in

TSH and T$_4$ is seen as they recover from the several factors causing hypothyroxinemia of prematurity. However, in some babies with congenital hypothyroidism, extreme prematurity, and low birth weight, the TSH rise may not be seen before the age of 30 days (delayed TSH rise). These babies will not be diagnosed by routine TSH-based newborn screening.

Several studies have confirmed that preterm infants are at higher risk to have congenital hypothyroidism, which may be missed by routine newborn screening. Vigone et al found that in preterm infants with a birth weight of 640 to 1975 g, only 5 of 24 newborns with congenital hypothyroidism were identified by initial newborn screening, while the other 19 were detected by second or third screening performed between 15 and 30 days of life. This is similar to the study of Kaluarachchi et al, which showed that of 26 premature infants found to have thyroid dysfunction, only 3 were detected by newborn screening, while the others were detected when TSH and free T$_4$ were routinely obtained at 30 days of life. In a larger study, Hunter et al also documented that 63 infants were missed by initial newborn screening due to delayed TSH rise. A study by Tfayli et al confirmed similar data showing a late TSH surge in very low–birth weight infants (<1500 g) in Lebanon.

The ideal timing for second or third screening in this population is debated, and it has been generally thought that the delayed TSH rise can be captured at 30 days of life. Other areas of debate are the TSH cutoff at this time and whether to consider treatment vs follow-up—no data are available on whether lack of treatment of mildly elevated TSH levels on the second or third screening is harmful. Most experts agree with continuing treatment until age 2 or 3 years.

A recent systematic review of screening of congenital hypothyroidism in preterm, low–birth weight, and very low–birth weight neonates recommends careful interpretation of thyroid function studies in this population. The authors recommend screening with TSH and free T$_4$ levels in the second, sixth, and tenth weeks of life and treating if the TSH concentration is 20 mIU/L or greater. They also recommend treating if any TSH value is greater than 10 mIU/L with a free T$_4$ value below 0.7 ng/dL (<9.0 pmol/L) during the third to sixth weeks of life and any TSH value between 10 and 20 mIU/L with a normal free T$_4$ level on 2 occasions.

A recent study in Ireland found that if TSH measurement had been repeated at 2 weeks of life only, 48% of cases with congenital hypothyroidism would have been missed. If the final screen had occurred at 4 weeks of life, 26% cases would have been missed. The authors recommend screening on days 3 to 5, at 1 week, at 2 weeks, at 4 weeks, and at term-corrected gestational age. Although there is no consensus on when to screen premature and very low–birth weight newborns, it is important to be aware of this form of congenital hypothyroidism with delayed TSH surge and the importance of monitoring this fragile population to protect and maximize their brain development.

The patient in this vignette is a premature newborn with very low-birth weight and TSH concentration greater than 20 mIU/L at 4 weeks of life. This baby most likely has congenital hypothyroidism with delayed TSH surge and would benefit from treatment at this time, with close follow-up (Answer E). Although some clinicians may want to confirm results before starting treatment, waiting 4 weeks (Answer A) would most likely delay needed treatment in this infant. Assessing antibodies in the mother (Answer B) would not change management. In addition, there is no maternal history of thyroid dysfunction and determining whether the baby's hypothyroidism is transient could be reevaluated in the future. Measuring TSH, free T$_4$ by equilibrium dialysis, and total T$_3$ (Answer C) would be more appropriate when evaluating an infant for hypothyroxinemia with a normal TSH level to differentiate among central hypothyroidism, nonthyroidal illness, or low thyroxine-binding globulin. However, this would not change management in this setting. Although recovery from nonthyroidal illness is in the differential diagnosis for this patient, the TSH value above 20 mIU/L with a low-normal free T$_4$ concentration is more suggestive of congenital hypothyroidism with delayed TSH surge. Reassurance and no intervention and no follow-up with thyroid function studies (Answer E) would be incorrect. If no intervention is elected at this time, very close follow-up with repeated TSH and free T$_4$ measurements is recommended.

Educational Objective
Describe the clinical significance of the effect of prematurity on thyroid function in the neonate.

Reference(s)

Hunter MK, Mandel SH, Sesser DE, et al. Follow-up of newborns with low thyroxine and nonelevated thyroid-stimulating hormone-screening concentrations: results of the 20-year experience in the Northwest Regional Newborn Screening Program. *J Pediatr.* 1998;132(1):70-74. PMID: 9470003

Mandel SJ, Hermos RJ, Larson CA, Prigozhin AB, Rojas DA, Mitchell ML. Atypical hypothyroidism and the very low birthweight infant. *Thyroid.* 2000;10(8):693-695. PMID: 11014314

LaFranchi SH. Screening preterm infants for congenital hypothyroidism: better the second time around. *J Pediatr.* 2014;164(6):1259-1261. PMID: 24657124

Vigone MC, Caiulo S, Di Frenna M, et al. Evolution of thyroid function in preterm infants detected by screening for congenital hypothyroidism. *J Pediatr.* 2014;164(6):1296-1302. PMID: 24518164

Kaluarachchi DC, Colaizy TT, Pesce LM, Tansey M, Klein JM. Congenital hypothyroidism with delayed thyroid-stimulating hormone elevation in premature infants born at less than 30 weeks gestation. *J Perinatol.* 2017;37(3):277-282. PMID: 27906195

Tfayli H, Charafeddine L, Tamim H, Saade J, Daher RT, Yunis K. Higher incidence rates of hypothyroidism and late TSH rise in preterm very-low-birth-weight infants at a tertiary care center. *Horm Res Paediatr.* 2018;89(4):224-232. PMID: 29642061

Hashemipour M, Hovsepian S, Ansari A, Keikha M, Khalighinejad P, Niknam N. Screening of congenital hypothyroidism in preterm, low birth weight and very low birth weight neonates: a systematic review. *Pediatr Neonatol.* 2018;59(1):3-14. PMID: 28811156

McGrath N, Hawkes CP, Mayne P, Murphy NP. Optimal timing of repeat newborn screening for congenital hypothyroidism in preterm infants to detect delayed thyroid-stimulating hormone elevation. *J Pediatr.* 2019;205:77-82. PMID: 30529133

24 ANSWER: B) Adipsia

This patient presented with recurrent cystic growth of a craniopharyngioma. Although her pituitary function was initially normal, with subsequent surgeries she developed panhypopituitarism, central diabetes insipidus, and hypothalamic obesity. Patients with lesions of the pituitary gland or hypothalamus can present with hormone deficiencies preoperatively, during surgery, postoperatively, or following cranial irradiation. Central diabetes insipidus occurs due to dysfunction of the vasopressinergic neurons of the supraoptic and paraventricular nuclei. Arginine vasopressin (AVP) secretion is regulated by plasma and interstitial osmotic pressure sensed by osmoreceptors in the hypothalamus, as well as by circulating blood volume, sensed by baroreceptors. Plasma osmolality is normally maintained in a relatively narrow physiologic range by water intake and output regulated by AVP and thirst. Like AVP, thirst is stimulated by hyperosmolality. The osmoreceptors that regulate thirst are in close proximity to those regulating AVP. Adipsia (inappropriate lack of thirst) typically results from lesions that impair thirst and AVP secretion (eg, structural abnormalities of the hypothalamic-pituitary region due to congenital malformations such as optic nerve hypoplasia, septo-optic dysplasia, holoprosencephaly, tumors such as craniopharyngioma, trauma, and surgery). This patient initially had normal thirst. Postoperatively, her sodium was normal at first. However, when she was allowed to take fluids ad lib, she became hypernatremic. This patient most likely developed unrecognized adipsia (Answer B) as a result of the surgery.

Excess fluid administration (Answer A) is a common cause of postoperative polyuria, but it is unlikely to cause hypernatremia if there is normal kidney function and thirst. Her serum urea nitrogen and creatinine remained normal, so excess fluid administration is incorrect.

Symptoms of diabetes insipidus can be masked by glucocorticoid deficiency until cortisol replacement is administered. However, this patient already had a known diagnosis of ACTH deficiency and central diabetes insipidus, and her diabetes insipidus had been well controlled on her home desmopressin and hydrocortisone dosages. Additionally, if her thirst mechanism were intact, she would have been able to avoid hypernatremia by increasing her fluid intake. Therefore, stress doses of hydrocortisone worsening the diabetes insipidus (Answer C) is incorrect.

Hyperglycemia is a common cause of polyuria, but not hypernatremia (Answer D). She did have some mild postoperative hyperglycemia, but her glucose levels were not elevated enough to cause significant increases in urine output and subsequent dehydration.

At home she had good control on desmopressin. While her dosage certainly could have required adjustments postoperatively, she should have been able to maintain normal sodium levels by increasing her oral fluid intake in response to increases in plasma osmolality. Therefore, an insufficient desmopressin dosage (Answer E) is incorrect.

Educational Objective
Differentiate among the conditions responsible for pathologic loss of thirst.

Reference(s)
Di Iorgi N, Morana G, Napoli F, Allegri AE, Rossi A, Maghnie M. Management of diabetes insipidus and adipsia in the child. *Best Pract Res Clin Endocrinol Metab.* 2015;29(3):415-436. PMID: 26051300

25 **ANSWER: D) Increase all basal rates by 30% within 6 to 12 hours after initiating prednisone**
Insulin requirements to maintain normoglycemia during glucocorticoid therapy and stress are often difficult to estimate. The total daily insulin requirement may increase 30% to 100% within 6 to 12 hours after the first prednisone dose and return to baseline amounts 24 to 48 hours after therapy. Increasing the basal insulin rate by 30% within 6 to 12 hours after initiating prednisone (Answer D) is the best initial management strategy to prevent anticipated hyperglycemia.

High-dosage glucocorticoids are associated with insulin resistance and increased hepatic gluconeogenesis. These effects markedly increase insulin requirements in patients with type 1 diabetes and may even result in ketosis. The impact of glucocorticoid therapy on glycemic control is typically not seen immediately upon treatment initiation and the effects may persist for several days after discontinuing therapy. The longer the half-life of the glucocorticoid, the longer it will affect glycemic control. The effects of glucocorticoids on blood glucose values are influenced by the specific glucocorticoid chosen, the dosage, and the timing of the doses. Higher doses and more potent glucocorticoids are associated with higher insulin requirements.

Because glucocorticoids increase insulin requirements due to increased gluconeogenesis, these effects persist throughout the day. Increasing the insulin-to-carbohydrate ratios by 30%, which would be used only for mealtimes (Answer C), would not provide stable glycemic control beyond the mealtimes, especially overnight. Likewise, increasing the correction/sensitivity factors (Answer A) would be helpful for controlling blood glucose after hyperglycemia occurs, but would do little to prevent the development of hyperglycemia. The reactive approach of just monitoring blood glucose values and correcting the hyperglycemia (Answer E) with the existing correction factor will not be sufficient to maintain blood glucose in the target range because of insulin resistance.

Increasing basal rates within 6 to 12 hours after initiating prednisone (Answer D)—not immediately (Answer B) (which may cause hypoglycemia)—is a reasonable first step to ameliorate the anticipated deterioration of glycemic control. A 30% increase is a good place to begin, although some patients may require more aggressive increases in basal rates. If a patient continues to have significant glycemic excursions after meals, it is reasonable to also increase meal bolus insulin coverage by intensifying insulin-to-carbohydrate ratios and even the correction/ sensitivity factors.

The insulin management strategy highlighted in this vignette is specific to patients who are on insulin pump therapy. If the patient were on multiple daily injections of insulin, the concept of increasing basal insulin by 30% would still be a valid approach. Yet, depending on the timing of the "basal" insulin injection, there could be a delay in increasing the basal insulin amount. The delay could potentially result in interval hyperglycemia, which could be remedied by administering frequent (every 3 hours) "correction" bolus doses of rapid-acting insulin until the adjustment in basal insulin takes effect.

Educational Objective
Anticipate changes needed in the insulin regimen of a patient with diabetes mellitus to address hyperglycemia associated with glucocorticoid therapy.

Reference(s)
Tamez-Pérez HE, Quintanilla-Flores DL, Rodríguez-Gutiérrez R, González-González JG, Tamez-Peña AL. Steroid hyperglycemia: prevalence, early detection and therapeutic recommendations: a narrative review. *World J Diabetes.* 2015;6(8):1073-1081. PMID: 26240704

Bevier WC, Zisser HC, Jovanovič L, et al. Use of continuous glucose monitoring to estimate insulin requirements in patients with type 1 diabetes mellitus during a short course of prednisone. *J Diabetes Sci Technol.* 2008;2(4):578-583. PMID: 19885233

26 **ANSWER: C) Activating pathogenic variant in the *FGFR3* gene**
This patient has poor growth, short stature, obesity, macrocephaly, brachydactyly, and short limbs. She had normal onset and progression of puberty. These features are indicative of skeletal dysplasia. Achondroplasia is the most common form of dwarfism, occuring in 1 in 15,000 to 25,000 individuals. Autosomal dominant gain-of-function pathogenic variants in the *FGFR3* gene (Answer C), most of them sporadic but with 100% penetrance, are the most common cause of achondroplasia and related chondrodysplasia syndromes, including hypochondroplasia, severe achondroplasia with developmental delay and acanthosis nigricans (SADDAN), and the lethal form thanatophoric dysplasia.

Obstructive and central sleep apnea are common in individuals with achondroplasia, and a sleep study is recommended for all patients with this condition. Other common issues in individuals with achondroplasia include middle ear dysfunction, lower-extremity bowing, kyphosis, spinal stenosis, joint laxity, and arthritis. Thus, regular evaluation with otolaryngology and orthopedics is indicated for individuals with achondroplasia. Contact sports, joint hyperextension, trampoline use, diving, and hanging upside down from knees/feet should all be avoided due to risk of injury to the spinal cord at the craniocervical junction. References are available for anthropometric variables in achondroplasia such as sitting height, leg length, arm span, relative sitting height (sitting height/height), and foot length.

Short-term and long-term GH therapy in patients with achondroplasia has led to some height improvement, but a recent meta-analysis concluded that there are insufficient data on final adult height and changes in body proportion with GH therapy. C-type natriuretic peptide analogue has been proposed as a potential treatment option in clinical trials, as it antagonizes FGFR3 signaling by down-regulating the mitogen-activated protein kinase pathway, which is activated as a result of an *FGFR3* gain-of-function pathogenic variant in affected patients.

Maternal uniparental disomy of chromosome 15 (Answer A) results in Prader-Willi syndrome, which is associated with hypotonia, hyperphagia after infancy, morbid obesity, developmental delays, and hypogonadism. However, the patient in this vignette does not have any of these features.

Although patients with Turner syndrome (Answer B) are also at high risk for frequent ear infections, macrocephaly and short limbs are not characteristic of this condition.

Patients with an inactivating pathogenic variant in the maternal allele of the *GNAS* gene (Answer D) have Albright hereditary osteodystrophy with short stature, brachydactyly, and evidence of hormone resistance such as hypocalcemia due to PTH resistance and abnormal thyroid function tests. In this patient, the normal comprehensive metabolic panel, normal thyroid function, and presence of macrocephaly and short limbs make Albright hereditary osteodystrophy less likely to be the diagnosis.

Pathogenic variants in the *FMR1* gene (Answer E) result in fragile X syndrome, which is associated with developmental delay, learning disabilities, mental retardation, and some characteristic dysmorphic features. *FMR1* pathogenic variants are not associated with short stature and macrocephaly.

Educational Objective
List the physical characteristics of short stature in patients with achondroplasia and identify pathogenic variants in the *FGFR3* gene as the cause of achondroplasia.

Reference(s)
Ornitz DM, Legeai-Mallet L. Achondroplasia: development, pathogenesis, and therapy. *Dev Dyn.* 2017;246(4):291-309. PMID: 27987249

Merker A, Neumeyer L, Hertel NT, Grigelioniene G, Mohnike K, Hagenas L. Development of body proportions in achondroplasia: Sitting height, leg length, arm span, and foot length. *Am J Med Genet A.* 2018;176(9):1819-1829. PMID: 30152086

Miccoli M, Bertelloni S, Massart F. Height outcome of recombinant human growth hormone treatment in achondroplasia children: a meta-analysis. *Horm Res Paediatr.* 2016;86(1):27-34. PMID: 27355624

Trotter TL, Hall JG; American Academy of Pediatrics Committee on Genetics. Health supervision for children with achondroplasia [published correction appears in *Pediatrics.* 2005;116(6):1615]. *Pediatrics.* 2005;116(3):771-783. PMID: 16140722

27 ANSWER: D) Partial androgen insensitivity syndrome
Hypospadias is one of the most common congenital anomalies in newborn males, affecting up to 1 in 200 boys. While hypospadias has been described in more than 200 syndromes, a genetic cause is identified in only 30% of cases. When associated with other abnormalities such as cryptorchidism or micropenis, there is a higher likelihood of androgen deficiency. Heritability appears to vary with severity. Severe (proximal) hypospadias is also associated with intrauterine growth restriction, maternal hypertension, and oligohydramnios, suggesting that placental insufficiency can have a role, possibly through a decrease in the fetus's exposure to hCG.

The infant in this scenario has both environmental and genetic risk factors. Given that he also has microphallus (<2.5 cm), investigation for an underlying cause is warranted. Although he most likely has idiopathic hypospadias, of the options given, partial androgen insensitivity syndrome (PAIS) (Answer D) is most consistent with his presentation. PAIS is an X-linked recessive disorder characterized by ambiguous genitalia, with perineoscrotal hypospadias, microphallus, and bifid scrotum. Testes can be undescended, palpable, or anywhere in between.

Affected infants usually have a normal neonatal testosterone surge, although this may be reduced in the setting of complete androgen insensitivity syndrome. LH and testosterone levels are often, but not always, elevated. The ability to synthesize testosterone is intact, but there is loss of negative feedback inhibition of gonadotropins. The diagnosis is confirmed by molecular genetic testing of the androgen receptor gene (*AR*), which would be an appropriate next step for this infant. The frequency of detecting *AR* pathogenic variants ranges from 65% to 95% in individuals with complete androgen insensitivity and from 40% to 45% in those with PAIS.

Individuals with 5α-reductase deficiency (Answer A) have normal testosterone production but do not undergo normal virilization due to a defect in converting testosterone to dihydrotestosterone. While the phenotype ranges from normal female appearance to nearly normal male appearance of external genitalia, approximately 75% of affected individuals are identified as female at birth. A testosterone-to-dihydrotestosterone ratio greater than 10 is suggestive of this disorder; however, timing of laboratory studies is critical. Hormone levels should be assessed by gas or liquid chromatography–mass spectrometry (LC/MS) to avoid cross-reactivity. This assessment should be performed between 1 week and 6 months of age. In this vignette, LH and testosterone levels are consistent with the mini-puberty of infancy, so interpretation of hormone levels without hCG-stimulation testing can be considered reliable. While this infant's phenotype is consistent with possible 5α-reductase deficiency, the testosterone-to-dihydrotestosterone ratio of 3.6 makes this less likely.

Congenital adrenal hyperplasia due to 3β-hydroxysteroid dehydrogenase deficiency (Answer B) leads to undervirilization in 46,XY individuals due to testosterone deficiency. Undervirilization can range from a severe presentation, associated with salt-losing adrenal crises, to a mild presentation with hypospadias and microphallus. Characteristic laboratory findings include elevated pregnenolone, 17-hydroxypregnenolone, and DHEA concentrations. In this vignette, laboratory findings are not consistent with 3β-hydroxysteroid dehydrogenase deficiency.

Swyer syndrome (Answer C) is one form of partial XY gonadal dysgenesis, and it can be caused by pathogenic variants in one of several genes required for sexual differentiation of the fetus. Swyer syndrome is most often due to pathogenic variants in the *SRY* gene. Affected individuals typically have a female external appearance, thus Swyer syndrome would be an unlikely diagnosis in this vignette. Pelvic ultrasonography would demonstrate the presence of a uterus, which helps distinguish this condition from androgen insensitivity syndrome.

Individuals with pathogenic variants in the *LHCGR* gene (luteinizing hormone choriogonadotropin receptor) (Answer E) demonstrate a phenotype ranging from mild undervirilization to completely female external genitalia. Testes are typically inguinal or intraabdominal. While the phenotype in this vignette is consistent with an *LHCGR* pathogenic variant, laboratory testing would be expected to demonstrate a low testosterone level with elevated LH due to Leydig-cell hypoplasia.

Educational Objective
Evaluate the etiology of undervirilization in an infant with a 46,XY karyotype.

Reference(s)
Bouty A, Ayers KL, Pask A, Heloury Y, Sinclair AH. The genetic and environmental factors underlying hypospadias. *Sex Dev.* 2015;9(5):239-259. PMID: 26613581

---

28 **ANSWER: B) Stop atorvastatin; wait 2 weeks and then reintroduce atorvastatin and assess for symptoms**

Although statins are an effective way of lowering LDL-cholesterol levels, myopathy remains an important potential adverse effect. This has been reported predominantly in adults, but it has also been described in adolescents. This is a risk factor for rhabdomyolysis when creatine kinase levels are greater than 10 times the upper normal limit. The reasons for this boy's muscle soreness and creatine kinase elevations are unclear. However, his creatine kinase elevations are mild, which can be observed following vigorous physical activity. A practice guideline for pediatric statin treatment states, "Practitioners should be aware that recommended monitoring of creatine kinase levels is more likely to result in numerous mild to severe sporadic increases that may not be attributable to the statin. Vigorous exercise, particularly contact sports or weightlifting, may cause physiological increases, and it is important that not all increases are immediately attributed to the statin." This boy has clear reasons for being on a statin, with a high pretreatment LDL-cholesterol level and a family history of early death due to cardiovascular disease, so continuing adequate treatment for his dyslipidemia should be part of his care plan.

However, since this is the second event of myalgias, most experts would recommend stopping the statin, waiting for symptoms to resolve, and reintroducing either the same or different statin and assessing for symptoms (Answer B). Continuing atorvastatin and measuring creatine kinase in 2 days (Answer A) is incorrect. There are no guidelines for either adult or pediatric myopathies, so clinical judgment continues to be the best approach to caring for patients with this symptom. Since the statin was very effective in reducing this patient's LDL-cholesterol level and he is in the high-risk category for cardiovascular events in the future, an attempt should be made to remain on statin therapy.

This boy's creatine kinase elevations do not currently require hospitalization (Answer D) and are not concerning enough to recommend permanent discontinuation of statin treatment (Answer C).

MRI (Answer E) would not be expected to reveal any notable findings, even in the setting of a muscle reaction. Despite the mild nature of the patient's pain and degree of creatine kinase elevation, there remains the possibility that this is an early step in the process of myocyte damage.

While this boy's liver transaminase levels were normal, statin use in adults has been associated with a 0.5% rate of elevated transaminase levels (>3 times the upper normal limit. In studies of pediatric patients, there have been similar rates of elevated transaminase levels among patients taking statins and those taking placebo, potentially because of higher rates of underlying nonalcoholic steatohepatitis among treated patients.

Few nonstatin treatments have adequate safety data in children, and those that do are less effective than statins in reducing LDL-cholesterol levels. Therefore, they would not be warranted without adequate suspicion of statin-related myopathy. Nonstatin therapies include ezetimibe, bile acid sequestrants, PCSK9 inhibitors, and bempedoic acid.

Ezetimibe lowers LDL-cholesterol levels by inhibiting cholesterol absorption and up-regulating hepatic LDL receptors. While often used as an add-on therapy to statin treatment, recent studies using it as monotherapy in children showed promising results.

Bile acid sequestrants have long been known to reduce cholesterol levels. Their mechanism of action is to decrease the absorption of bile acids, which results in increased synthesis of bile acids from cholesterol leading to a decrease in hepatic cholesterol and an up-regulation of hepatic LDL receptors. They are not very well tolerated by children.

PCSK9 monoclonal antibodies lower LDL cholesterol by binding PCSK9 (regulator of LDL receptors), reducing the breakdown of LDL receptors, as well as by reducing lipoprotein (a) levels. Often used when statins are not tolerated, PCSK9 inhibitors are in phase 3 clinical trials in children.

Bempedoic acid lowers LDL cholesterol by inhibiting hepatic ATP citrate lyase activity, thereby reducing cholesterol synthesis in the liver and up-regulating LDL receptors. Bempedoic acid is also used in patients who do not tolerate statins. It has not been studied in children to date.

Educational Objective
Evaluate the possibility of statin-induced myopathy in an adolescent.

Reference(s)
Luirink IK, Wiegman A, Kusters DM, et al. 20-year follow-up of statins in children with familial hypercholesterolemia. *N Engl J Med.* 2019;381(16):1547-1556. PMID: 31618540

Selva-O'Callaghan A, Alvarado-Cardenas M, Pinal-Fernández I, et al. Statin-induced myalgia and myositis: an update on pathogenesis and clinical recommendations. *Expert Rev Clin Immunol.* 2018;14(3):215-224. PMID: 29473763

Avis HJ, Vissers MN, Stein EA, et al. A systematic review and meta-analysis of statin therapy in children with familial hypercholesterolemia. *Arterioscler Thromb Vasc Biol.* 2007;27(8):1803-1810. PMID: 17569881

29 ANSWER: C) Graves disease
A hot nodule (Answer D) is unlikely in this patient, as she had a diffuse goiter and elevated thyroid-stimulating immunoglobulin. A thyroid uptake and scan can distinguish between Graves disease (Answer C) and a hot nodule. In Graves disease, the uptake is increased throughout the gland, whereas in a hot nodule it is increased only in the nodule and is low in the rest of the gland. Given this patient's elevated thyroid-stimulating immunoglobulin, which was negative in the past, she most likely has Graves disease, although she did not have characteristic eye findings or a bruit. A number of cases of Graves disease have been reported following Hashimoto thyroiditis, either with or without a painful gland, with most occurrences in adults.

Hashitoxicosis (Answer A) is characterized by a brief period (a few weeks or less than 3 months) of hyperthyroidism that presents early in the course of Hashimoto thyroiditis. It does not present late in the course, and it occurs without elevated thyroid-stimulating immunoglobulin.

Silent subacute thyroiditis (Answer B) is a possibility in this patient, but her weight loss over 5 months and elevated thyroid-stimulating immunoglobulin make this an unlikely diagnosis. In subacute thyroiditis, there is decreased iodine uptake during the transient hyperthyroid phase.

Exogenous ingestion of levothyroxine (Answer E) is incorrect, as it is not expected to result in such a high total T_3 level and it is not associated with high thyroid-stimulating immunoglobulin.

Educational Objective
Diagnose Graves disease in a patient who has had Hashimoto thyroiditis for several years.

Reference(s)

Ohye H, Nishihara E, Sasaki I, et al. Four cases of Graves' disease which developed after painful Hashimoto's thyroiditis. *Intern Med*. 2006;45:385-389. PMID: 16617190

Takasu N, Yamada T, Sato A, et al. Graves' disease following hypothyroidism due to Hashimoto's disease: studies of eight cases. *Clin Endocrinol (Oxf)*. 1990;33(6):687-698. PMID: 1982861

30 ANSWER: C) GH-stimulation test

Endocrine consequences of radiation therapy for CNS malignancies depend on the anatomic site of cranial radiation, radiation dose, fractionation, and age at the time of treatment. Radiation directed to the hypothalamic-pituitary region, as was the case for the child in this vignette, is more likely to induce endocrine abnormalities involving the hypothalamic-pituitary axis. The hypothalamus is more sensitive than the pituitary gland to radiation. However, the somatotrophs (the GH-secreting cells of the pituitary gland) are more sensitive to radiation than the gonadotrophs, thyrotrophs, or corticotrophs. As a result, GH deficiency is more likely to occur after irradiation of the hypothalamic-pituitary region even with a lower dose (such as ≥10 Gy single fraction total body or ≥12 Gy fractionated total body), intermediate dose (≥18 Gy and ≤30 Gy cranial radiation), or higher dose (≥30 Gy cranial radiation), while deficiencies of LH, FSH, TSH, and ACTH are less likely to occur at lower or intermediate doses, but are more likely to occur after higher doses of cranial radiation (≥30 Gy). Interestingly, intermediate doses of cranial radiation (≥18 Gy and ≤30 Gy) may induce precocious puberty as opposed to LH/FSH deficiency, possibly due to disruption of hypothalamic physiologic inhibition of pubertal onset.

The child in this vignette has evidence of activation of the hypothalamic-pituitary-gonadal axis as manifested by testicular volume consistent with Tanner stage 2 to 3, which, at an age younger than 9 years in a boy is consistent with central precocious puberty. Therefore, it is unnecessary to perform a GnRH-stimulation test (Answer A).

Secondary sexual characteristics, such as pubic hair and penile enlargement, may be related to adrenarche or to endogenous testosterone of testicular origin. However, despite the degree of pubertal development, his growth velocity has remained normal (prepubertal). The lack of linear growth deceleration may be confusing, as it would not prompt the clinician to think about GH deficiency. However, in the presence of precocious puberty, growth deceleration may not be obvious. IGF-1 levels may not appear low in the face of precocious puberty and therefore are not a reliable indicator in this patient. Additionally, based on the history of 20 Gy of radiation delivered to the hypothalamic-pituitary region, the possibility of GH deficiency should be entertained. Evaluation for GH deficiency with a GH-stimulation test (Answer C) is the best next step.

Brain MRI (Answer D) is not indicated in this patient, as it would not change his management. His previous tumor is not associated with central precocious puberty, and the effects of the radiation would not be seen on MRI.

Testicular ultrasonography (Answer E) could be performed to look for a peripheral source for testosterone. However, with measurable gonadotropins, it is not the best option.

A low-dose cosyntropin-stimulation test (Answer B) is not the best next step, as there are no clinical manifestations described in the vignette to support central adrenal insufficiency and the patient had a normal 8-AM cortisol concentration. ACTH deficiency is unlikely to occur with low or intermediate doses of cranial radiation.

Educational objective
Describe the pitfalls in diagnosing GH deficiency when there is simultaneous precocious puberty in children receiving radiation therapy to the hypothalamic-pituitary region.

Reference(s)

Rutter MM, Rose SR. Long-term endocrine sequelae of childhood cancer. *Curr Opin Pediatr.* 2007;19(4):480-487. PMID: 17630615

Sklar CA, Antal Z, Chemaitilly W, et al. Hypothalamic-pituitary and growth disorders in survivors of childhood cancer: an Endocrine Society clinical practice guideline. *J Clin Endocrinol Metab.* 2018;103(8):2761-2784. PMID: 29982476

31 ANSWER: C) Perform a ^{99}Tc sestamibi scan

This patient has hyperparathyroidism as evidenced by elevated serum calcium, low phosphate, and inappropriately high-normal PTH. PTH is exquisitely sensitive to calcium such that any elevation in the serum calcium concentration should result in PTH suppression. High PTH levels, even in the mid- to upper-normal range, in the setting of hypercalcemia establish the diagnosis of primary hyperparathyroidism. The next step is to determine whether she has a parathyroid adenoma or hyperplasia. A sestamibi scan (Answer C) is helpful in making this distinction.

Autosomal dominant inactivating pathogenic variants in the gene encoding the calcium-sensing receptor (*CASR*) can present with hyperparathyroidism. Adolescents or adults with this condition are generally asymptomatic, but there have been associations with pancreatitis or chondrocalcinosis. The biochemical profile can be similar to primary hyperparathyroidism with elevated calcium and an inappropriately normal or slightly elevated PTH level; however, the urinary calcium-to-creatinine ratio is usually less than 0.01 and the phosphate is normal. This disorder is known as familial hypocalciuric hypercalcemia, and parathyroidectomy is not recommended in this setting. Conversely, total parathyroidectomy is recommended for patients with homozygous inactivating pathogenic variants in *CASR*, as this typically presents with profound hypercalcemia, very high PTH levels, and severe bone disease, including multiple fractures and hypotonia in the neonatal period. This patient is unlikely to have familial hypocalciuric hypercalcemia, and genetic testing (Answer A) is not the best next step.

While thiazide diuretics can cause hypercalcemia due to inability to excrete calcium in the urine, the physiologic response would be to suppress PTH. In this vignette, PTH was even higher on the thiazide diuretic. Thus, stopping the thiazide diuretic and repeating laboratory tests (Answer E) is inappropriate.

Hyperparathyroidism has a more profound effect on cortical bone mineral density than on trabecular bone, which may explain, in part, this patient's normal lumbar spine bone mineral density. The one-third distal radius is primarily cortical bone, and DXA (Answer D) may be useful in assessing the degree of skeletal involvement. However, it would not be useful in determining the etiology of hyperparathyroidism. In adult patients, this may guide surgical decision-making, whereas in younger patients (<50 years) parathyroidectomy is usually indicated, even in asymptomatic patients.

The most common cause of hyperparathyroidism is a benign adenoma (80%). The 2 most common techniques to localize parathyroid adenomas are parathyroid ultrasonography (Answer B) or a technetium ^{99}Tc sestamibi scan (Answer C). Single-photon emission CT (SPECT) has also been used to localize parathyroid adenomas, but this approach is generally better for ectopic parathyroid tissue and carries the risk of radiation exposure. Parathyroid ultrasonography is technician dependent and may be more challenging in pediatric patients in whom this is a more rare condition. Technetium ^{99}Tc sestamibi scans have a higher positive predictive value, although they may miss small adenomas and are not ideal for multiglandular disease (hyperplasia). This is because the technique relies on the preferential retention of the radiotracer in the mitochondrial-rich oxyphil cells of the hyperfunctioning gland. If all glands are functioning with a similar intensity, they will all experience similar washout and the overall result of the scan will be negative. It is important to therefore remember that a ^{99}Tc sestamibi scan is not used to diagnose hyperparathyroidism, but rather to determine whether it is caused by a parathyroid adenoma and to guide the surgical approach.

Educational Objective

Recommend ^{99}Tc sestamibi scanning to determine whether hyperparathyroidism is secondary to a solitary parathyroid adenoma and to guide surgical management in young patients.

Reference(s)

Davies JH. Approach to the child with hypercalcaemia. *Endocr Dev.* 2015;28:101-118. PMID: 26138838

Wermers RA, Kearns AE, Jenkins GD, Melton LJ 3rd. Incidence and clinical spectrum of thiazide-associated hypercalcemia. *Am J Med.* 2007;120(10):911.e9-e15. PMID: 17904464

Hughes DT, Sorensen MJ, Miller BS, Cohen MS, Gauger PG. The biochemical severity of primary hyperparathyroidism correlates with the localization accuracy of sestamibi and surgeon-performed ultrasound. *J Am Coll Surg.* 2014;219(5):1010-1009. PMID: 25086814

32 ANSWER: E) Undernutrition

This patient presents with marked weight loss, growth deceleration, elevated GH, and low IGF-1 levels. Her history is concerning for a restrictive eating disorder. IGF-1, which is primarily produced in the liver, is regulated by GH secretion. IGF-1 secretion is also altered by nutritional status. In states of undernutrition or starvation, GH levels are normal or elevated in the setting of low IGF-1 levels. This state of GH resistance may represent an adaptive response to decreased energy intake, a mechanism to preserve energy during periods of starvation. In animal models of starvation, low IGF-1 levels are seen along with decreased GH receptor mRNA and decreased GH binding, suggesting that down-regulation of GH receptors in the liver contributes to the GH resistance. Elevated GH levels may be necessary to mobilize fat stores and maintain euglycemia, and low IGF-1 levels may lead to decreased energy expenditure for growth. Therefore, undernutrition (Answer E) is the most likely cause of this patient's growth delay.

Craniopharyngiomas (Answer A) are rare intracranial tumors that account for 6% to 9% of all childhood brain tumors and have a peak incidence in children aged 5 to 14 years. Affected children may present with signs of increased intracranial pressure, endocrine deficits (52%-87%), and vision impairment (62%-84%). The growth deceleration is this setting is due to GH deficiency, which would be associated with low IGF-1 and GH levels.

GH insensitivity syndrome (Answer B), also known as Laron dwarfism, is associated with marked short stature with preservation of weight, a history of a relatively normal birth size, very low IGF-1 levels, and elevated GH levels. This child had normal growth until recently, and, unlike individuals with Laron dwarfism, she has had weight loss and is underweight.

Addison disease (Answer C), or primary adrenal insufficiency, can be acute or chronic in presentation. Chronic adrenal insufficiency is characterized by poor weight gain or weight loss, weakness, fatigue, nausea or vague gastrointestinal complaints, and salt craving. Skin hyperpigmentation is common and is due to elevated ACTH binding to the melanocortin 1 receptor. Height growth is generally normal in persons with Addison disease. Hypotension, tachycardia, hyponatremia, and hyperkalemia are frequently present. While Addison disease should be considered in this patient, her height growth has slowed, she has no hyperpigmentation on examination and no information is given about her cortisol or ACTH levels.

This patient has a strong family history of constitutional delay of maturity (Answer D). She has no breast development on examination and her bone age is delayed. However, children with constitutional delay would not be expected to have dramatic weight loss, growth deceleration, or elevated GH levels.

Educational Objective
Explain how deficiencies in nutrition can cause functional GH resistance.

Reference(s)

Fazeli PK, Klibanski A. Determinants of GH resistance in malnutrition. *J Endocrinol.* 2014;220(3):R57-R65. PMID: 24363451

Savage MO, Attie KM, David A, Metherell LA, Clark AJ, Camacho-Hübner C. Endocrine assessment, molecular characterization and treatment of growth hormone insensitivity disorders. *Nat Clin Pract Endocrinol Metab.* 2006;2(7):395-407. PMID: 16932322

33 ANSWER: D) Retained portion of histrelin implant, which is continuing to suppress puberty

Silver-Russell syndrome is characterized by prenatal and postnatal growth retardation, feeding difficulties, and recurrent hypoglycemia. Individuals with Silver-Russell syndrome are at increased risk for premature adrenarche and early and rapid central puberty, which can lead to early closure of epiphyses and limited growth.

The patient in this vignette presents with pubertal delay and a height velocity that has decreased over the past year despite GH treatment. Effective GH dosages for children with a history of being small for gestational age are higher than those for children with GH deficiency; thus, there may be a degree of GH resistance. However, his IGF-1 value is at the upper end of the reference range for his age, so it is unlikely that poor adherence to GH treatment (Answer A) is responsible for slowing his growth rate.

In Silver-Russell syndrome, puberty typically starts at the early end of the normal range and progresses rapidly. Delayed puberty has not been reported in Silver-Russell syndrome, and, anecdotally, it was not observed by a group that studied a large cohort of patients with Silver-Russell syndrome. In one cohort, puberty began, on average, 1 year earlier in children with Silver-Russell syndrome vs children who were small for gestational age but did not have Silver-Russell syndrome. While there is a history of constitutional growth delay in this patient's father, delayed puberty (Answer C) is highly unlikely in the setting of Silver-Russell syndrome. Gonadotropin deficiency (Answer B) is possible, but it has not been described as a feature of Silver-Russell syndrome and is an unlikely explanation for his lack of pubertal progression.

Children with Silver-Russell syndrome experience acceleration of bone age advancement, most likely due to premature adrenarche and early and rapid pubertal progression, as well as other factors not yet identified. Untreated, this leads to attenuation of the pubertal growth spurt and compromised adult height. As such, bone age cannot be used to make accurate adult height predictions in children with Silver-Russell syndrome. However, bone age can be expected to correlate with timing of peak growth velocity. A height velocity of 7 to 8 cm/y would be expected with a bone age of 14 years. Thus, early epiphyseal closure (Answer E) is unlikely to be a factor in this patient's growth pattern.

Recommendations in a consensus statement on the diagnosis and management of Silver-Russell syndrome include considering treatment with a GnRH agonist for at least 2 years in children with evidence of central puberty (starting no later than 12 years in girls and 13 years in boys) to preserve adult height potential. One study reported a high rate of procedural difficulties with implant removal, citing implant fracture during removal in 16 of 58 cases (28%). Implant fracture is more likely in implants that have remained in place longer. While there are no formal guidelines for management of this situation, removing retained portions of an implant may not be practical, and the recommendation is to allow the medication to wear off over time.

For the patient in this case, the continued suppression of puberty and length of time the implant remained in place suggest that the implant may have fractured on removal, with retained histrelin continuing to suppress puberty (Answer D). This may be underrecognized clinically and should be considered when puberty fails to resume with removal of a histrelin implant. Single histrelin implants have been shown to consistently suppress puberty for at least 2 years, thus the duration of action of retained fragments of implant may be significantly longer.

Educational Objective
Identify characteristic variations in timing of pubertal events in individuals with Silver-Russell syndrome.

Reference(s)
Wakeling EL, Brioude F, Lokulo-Sodipe O, et al. Diagnosis and management of Silver-Russell syndrome: first international consensus statement. *Nat Rev Endocrinol.* 2017;13(2):105-124. PMID: 27585961

Davis JS, Alkhoury F, Burnweit C. Surgical and anesthetic considerations in histrelin capsule implantation for the treatment of precocious puberty. *J Pediatr Surg.* 2014;49(5):807-810. PMID: 24851775

Lewis KA, Goldyn AK, West KW, Eugster EA. A single histrelin implant is effective for 2 years for treatment of central precocious puberty. *J Pediatr.* 2013;163(4):1214-1216. PMID: 23809043

34   ANSWER: B) MRI of the pancreas

This case illustrates a rare presentation of an insulinoma. Insulinomas are extremely rare in children, often diagnosed after a long duration of symptoms. In various case reports, affected children are often misdiagnosed as having refractory seizures, insomnia, and migraine headaches. Insulinoma recurrence is 4 times more common within 10 years in individuals who have a pathogenic variant in the *MEN1* gene (associated with multiple endocrine neoplasia type 1) than in those who do not.

Hypoglycemia in infancy can be a presentation of congenital hyperinsulinism, GH deficiency, or adrenal insufficiency. Insulinoma should be considered in children presenting with nonketotic hypoglycemia beyond the age of infancy, as hypopituitarism does not usually present with isolated hypoglycemia in older children. GH and cortisol may not increase if hypoglycemia is insidious or if there are frequent episodes of hypoglycemia as observed in this case. Inappropriately high insulin and C-peptide in the presence of nonketotic hypoglycemia indicate a β-islet–cell lesion. Other causes of nonketotic hypoglycemia are carnitine deficiency or β-oxidation defects such as MCAD (medium-chain acyl-coenzyme A dehydrogenase deficiency) presenting with low insulin levels, hepatomegaly, increased anion gap, hyperuricemia, elevated liver transaminases, and hyperammonemia.

Localization of an insulinoma is challenging due to the probability of multiple, diffuse, or extrapancreatic lesions. Up to 10% of insulinomas are malignant and 6% are associated with multiple endocrine neoplasia type 1. Different invasive and noninvasive imaging modalities are used to localize the lesion, although the sensitivities and specificities are not documented in children. Invasive modalities include (1) arterial stimulation and venous sampling, in which different arteries supplying pancreatic tissue are infused with calcium followed by hepatic venous sampling to detect a rise in insulin; (2) transhepatic portal venous sampling; and (3) endoscopic ultrasonography. Peranteau et al reported 8 cases of insulinoma in children; one had arterial stimulation and venous sampling and another had transhepatic portal venous sampling. Both modalities accurately localized the lesion, whereas endoscopic ultrasonography localized the lesion in 2 of 5 cases.

MRI is a noninvasive modality with high sensitivity and specificity for detecting insulinoma in adults. Peranteau et al reported a detection rate of 50% (3/6) while Padidela et al reported accurate localization in 88% (7/8) with MRI. Octreotide scans have poor detection rates for insulinoma, as these tumors usually do not express enough somatostatin receptors. ^{18}F-DOPA is taken up by neuroendocrine cells and is used to distinguish between focal and diffuse lesions in congenital hyperinsulinism. The ^{18}F-DOPA PET scan is inconsistent in localizing insulinoma in children (100% [3/3] in one series and 50% [2/4] in another). GLP-1 receptor imaging is a new noninvasive modality that has shown 100% successful localization in a small study of 6 cases. Radiolabeled peptides have shown promising results in localizing the lesions in oncology and endocrinology cases. GLP-1 binds to specific receptors on β-islet cells to induce insulin release. GLP-1 receptors are expressed on insulinomas in large quantity. In this patient, MRI of the pancreas (Answer B) detected the lesion correctly at first presentation, as well as at recurrence. An octreotide scan performed at first presentation and PET scan performed at the time of recurrence both detected the lesion correctly.

Sulfonylureas are used extensively for treating type 2 diabetes. Sulfonylurea poisoning can produce sustained and profound hypoglycemia refractory to intravenous dextrose, particularly in children and elderly patients. A sulfonylurea screen (Answer A) could be considered, but there is no suggestion in the vignette that this child has access to a sulfonylurea. The history of rapid weight gain also favors chronicity of insulin secretion vs an acute elevation due to ingestion.

One should also consider factitious hypoglycemia due to exogenous insulin administration. Endogenous insulin is synthesized as a precursor, proinsulin, which undergoes enzymatic cleavage to produce insulin and C-peptide in equimolar amounts. Therefore, factitious hypoglycemia produced by exogenous insulin administration leads to suppressed C-peptide levels. In addition, proinsulin levels are poorly suppressible in patients with insulinoma in contrast to those without insulinoma. In patients with surreptitious use of insulin or an oral hypoglycemic agent, the proinsulin level is either normal or decreased.

Diazoxide is a benzothiazine derivative that acts as a potent β-cell K_{ATP} channel opener. The stabilization of open K_{ATP} channels leads to the inhibition of insulin secretion. Diazoxide challenge (Answer C) would not provide any diagnostic value in this case, but it could help manage hypoglycemia until surgical intervention.

After a second critical sample, obtaining a third critical sample (Answer D) is not necessary.

Genetic testing (Answer E) is relevant to establish the diagnosis of multiple endocrine neoplasia type 1 (*MEN1* pathogenic variant). However, it is not the best next step in establishing the diagnosis of insulinoma in this case.

Educational Objective
Guide the evaluation to localize an insulinoma in a child.

Reference(s)

Padidela R, Fiest M, Arya V, et al. Insulinoma in childhood: clinical, radiological, molecular and histological aspects of nine patients. *Eur J Endocrinol.* 2014;170(5):741-747. PMID: 24599222

Peranteau WH, Palladino AA, Bhatti TR, et al. The surgical management of insulinomas in children. *J Pediatr Surg.* 2013;48(12):2517-2524. PMID: 24314196

Kao KT, Simm PJ, Brown J. Childhood insulinoma masquerading as seizure disorder. *J Paediatr Child Health.* 2014;50(4):319-322. PMID: 24698060

Gozzi Graf T, Brändle M, Clerici T, l'Allemand D. Insulinoma: only in adults?-case reports and literature review. *Eur J Pediatr.* 2014;173(5):567-574. PMID: 23604412

Service FJ, McMahon MM, O'Brien PC, Ballard DJ. Functioning insulinoma—incidence, recurrence, and long-term survival of patients: a 60-year study. *Mayo Clin Proc.* 1991;66(7):711-719. PMID: 1677058

Miralliè E, Pattou F, Malvaux P, et al. Value of endoscopic ultrasonography and somatostatin receptor scintigraphy in the preoperative localization of insulinomas and gastrinomas. Experience of 54 cases. *Gastroenterol Clin Biol.* 2002;26(4):360-366. PMID: 12070411

Christ E, Wild D, Forrer F, et al. Glucagon-like peptide-1 receptor imaging for localization of insulinomas. *J Clin Endocrinol Metab.* 2009;94(11):4398-4405. PMID: 19820010

Sweet CB, Grayson S, Polak M. Management strategies for neonatal hypoglycemia. *J Pediatr Pharmacol Ther.* 2013;18(3):199-208. PMID: 24052783

35 ANSWER: B) Calcium supplementation and calcitriol

This patient has a classic presentation of rickets, including a prominent forehead, rachitic rosary of the ribs, limb deformities, widening of the wrists, and poor growth/short stature. In addition to history and physical examination findings, biochemical and radiologic findings (*see images*) are helpful in the diagnosis. Management of a patient with rickets depends on the underlying cause (*see table*). This patient had a low calcium level, low phosphate level, normal 25-hydroxyvitamin D level, and inappropriately low normal 1,25-dihydroxyvitamin D level, especially in the setting of elevated PTH. This pattern is consistent with the diagnosis of 1α-hydroxylase deficiency leading to vitamin D–dependent rickets type 1A. The appropriate treatment is calcitriol with or without calcium supplementation (Answer B).

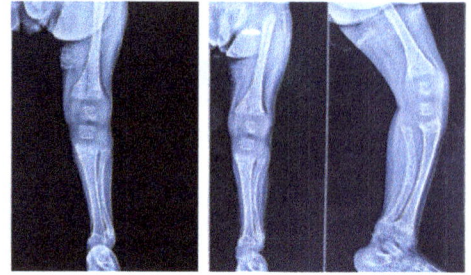

Table. Causes of Calcipenic or Hypophosphatemic Rickets (not all inclusive)

Serum calcium	Serum phosphate	25-Hydroxy-vitamin D	1,25-Dihydroxy-vitamin D	Diagnosis	Treatment
⇓⇔	⇓⇔	⇔	⇑	Nutritional calcium deficiency	Calcium
⇓⇔	⇓⇔	⇓	⇓⇔	Nutritional vitamin D deficiency	Calciferol ± calcium
⇓⇔	⇓⇔	⇓⇓ Despite adequate calciferol intake	⇓	25-Hydroxylase deficiency (vitamin D–dependent rickets type 1B)	Calcitriol ± calcium
⇓⇔	⇓⇔	⇔	⇓ or low-normal	1α-Hydroxylase deficiency (vitamin D–dependent rickets type 1A)	Calcitriol ± calcium
⇓⇔	⇓⇔	⇓	⇑	Hereditary 1,25-dihydroxyvitamin D–resistant rickets due to pathogenic variants in the VDR gene (vitamin D–dependent rickets type 2) or to overexpression of a vitamin D response element VDRE (vitamin D–dependent rickets type 2B)	High dosages of calcitriol ± calcium
⇑⇔	⇓ • Low urine phosphate • Low or normal serum FGF-23	⇔	⇑⇔	Nutritional phosphate deficiency	Phosphorus supplementation
⇔	⇓ • High urine phosphate • High serum FGF-23	⇔	⇓	FGF-23–dependent hypophosphatemic rickets • XLH (*PHEX* pathogenic variant) • ADHR (*FGF23* pathogenic variant) • ARHR (*DMP1* or *ENPP1* pathogenic variant)	Calcitriol and phosphorus supplementation or burosumab therapy
⇔	⇓ • High urine phosphate • Low or normal serum FGF-23	⇔	⇑⇔	FGF-23–independent hypophosphatemic rickets • Low or normal FGF-23 level • Pathogenic variants in SLC34A1 (encoding sodium-dependent phosphate transport protein 2A [NPT2A]) • Pathogenic variants in SLC34A3 (encoding NTP2C), causing hereditary hypophosphatemic rickets with hypercalciuria	Phosphorus supplementation

Note: Images in this vignette provided courtesy of Dr. Sirisha Kusuma, Rainbow Children's Hospital, Hyderabad and Vijayawada, India.

Treating with calcium alone (Answer D) or with calcium and ergocalciferol (Answer A) is not enough in this patient, as he has a normal vitamin D concentration and cannot convert that to 1,25-dihydroxyvitamin D given his diagnosis of 1α-hydroxylase deficiency. Improving the 1,25-dihydroxyvitamin D level by administering calcitriol is necessary, so he can absorb enteral calcium intake through diet and supplementation. Calcitriol and phosphorus supplementation (Answer C) or treatment with the human monoclonal antibody burosumab (Answer E) would be options for patients with X-linked hypophosphatemic rickets who have a normal serum calcium level.

Educational Objective
Diagnose and treat vitamin D–dependent rickets type 1A.

Reference(s)

Carpenter TO, Shaw NJ, Portale AA, Ward LM, Abrams SA, Pettifor JM. Rickets. *Nat Rev Dis Primers*. 2017;3:17101. PMID: 29265106

Thacher TD, Levine MA. CYP2R1 mutations causing vitamin D-deficiency rickets. *J Steroid Biochem Mol Biol*. 2017;173:333-336. PMID: 27473561

Goldsweig BK, Carpenter TO. Hypophosphatemic rickets: lessons from disrupted FGF23 control of phosphorus homeostasis. *Curr Osteoporos Rep*. 2015;13(2):88-97. PMID: 25620749

Razali NN, Hwu TT, Thilakavathy K. Phosphate homeostasis and genetic mutations of familial hypophosphatemic rickets. *J Pediatr Endocrinol Metab*. 2015;28(9-10):1009-1017. PMID: 25894638

Munns CF, Shaw N, Kiely M, et al. Global consensus recommendations on prevention and management of nutritional rickets. *J Clin Endocrinol Metab*. 2016;101(2):394-415. PMID: 26745253

36   ANSWER: A) Discontinue methimazole and discuss thyroidectomy

Thyrotoxicosis is a clinical condition caused by increased thyroid hormone action. Hyperthyroidism is thyrotoxicosis secondary to increased synthesis of thyroid hormones by the thyroid gland. The most common cause of hyperthyroidism in children is Graves disease. Graves disease is an autoimmune thyroid disease. The pathophysiology of autoimmune thyroid disease involves diffuse infiltration of T-cell lymphocytes into the thyroid gland, while B-cell lymphocytes produce different autoantibodies (most commonly against the TSH receptor (TSHR), thyroglobulin, and TPO. In Graves disease, the predominant antibodies are directed against the TSHR (TRAb), with predominant activating-type antibodies.

In children and adolescents, Graves disease can be treated with methimazole, radioactive iodine therapy, or thyroidectomy. However, the use of radioactive iodine is not recommended for children younger than 5 years because of the higher risk of thyroid cancer in this population after external radiation. Medical treatment is considered first-line therapy in children and adolescents because some children go into remission.

Antithyroid drugs used in the United States include methimazole and propylthiouracil. In Europe, carbimazole, a methimazole pro-drug, is also available. Antithyroid drugs peak in serum within 1 to 2 hours after ingestion and antithyroid effects last 12 to 24 hours. Their primary effect is to inhibit thyroid hormone synthesis by blocking TPO. Propylthiouracil also blocks the peripheral conversion of T_4 into T_3, and these drugs have also been shown to have immunomodulatory effects.

Methimazole is the recommended drug in children and adolescents, while propylthiouracil is contraindicated in this population because of the high risk of hepatotoxicity (liver failure in 1 in 2000 to 1 in 4000 children). Methimazole can be given once daily, as it has a longer duration than propylthiouracil, and the dosage used ranges between 0.1 and 1.0 mg/kg per day, usually 0.2 to 0.5 mg/kg per day. To maintain euthyroidism, the dosage is usually decreased as levels normalize. The approach of blocking with methimazole and replacing with levothyroxine is not currently recommended in the guidelines because this practice has been associated with higher dosages of methimazole and complications.

Antithyroid medications have mild and severe adverse effects. Mild adverse effects include rash, arthralgias, nausea, abnormal sense of taste or smell, and, very rarely, sialadenitis. Rash can be managed by concurrent administration of antihistamine. Major complications include agranulocytosis, hepatitis, cholestasis, liver failure, ANCA-positive vasculitis, and polyarthritis. Very rarely thrombocytopenia and aplastic anemia and pancreatitis may also develop.

Most adverse effects of methimazole are dosage dependent; therefore, lower dosages are recommended except in cases of severe hyperthyroidism. However, reactions can occur even at lower dosages and all patients must be warned about adverse effects.

Adverse effects in children have been reported in 6% to 35%, usually in the first 3 months of treatment, although they can occur at any time.

Mild granulocytopenia and mild elevation of liver enzymes can be seen in patients with Graves disease. Therefore, obtaining baseline levels before starting treatment is a good practice, as illustrated in this patient.

Complete blood cell count with differential should be ordered immediately if the patient develops fever, sore throat, arthralgias, mouth sores, or malaise. Liver enzymes must be measured immediately if the patient develops abdominal pain, nausea, vomiting, jaundice, dark urine, light-colored stools, pruritus, anorexia, or malaise.

Patients and their caregivers should be educated on the adverse effects of antithyroid drugs, preferably in writing, and they should be advised to stop the medication immediately and to contact their physician if they develop any of the symptoms associated with major complications of antithyroid medications. Antithyroid medications should be discontinued if transaminase levels (in asymptomatic or symptomatic patients) are 2 to 3 times the upper normal limit. After discontinuing the drug, levels must be monitored weekly until they resolve. If there is no evidence of improvement, referral to gastroenterology is indicated. This patient's levels are already 2 to 3 times above the upper normal limit, and they are rising. Decreasing the methimazole dosage (Answers C and E) is not recommended. Although the patient may benefit from seeing a gastroenterologist/hepatologist (Answers D and E) if liver enzymes do not improve following discontinuation of methimazole, referring her to gastroenterology before discontinuing the drug is incorrect.

This patient has developed a severe reaction to methimazole and the drug must be discontinued. She needs definitive treatment for Graves disease. In view of her age, total thyroidectomy in the hands of a high-volume surgeon (Answer A) is the best course of action. Radioactive iodine (Answer B) is not recommended in children younger than 5 years. She will need supersaturated potassium iodine drops (SSKI, 50 mg iodine/drop), 1 to 2 drops 3 times daily for 10 days before surgery.

Educational Objective
Summarize the medical management of Graves disease with antithyroid drugs, including pharmacologic actions, dosage, monitoring, adverse effects, and indications for seeking alternative treatments.

Reference(s)

Ross DS, Burch HB, Cooper DS, et al. 2016 American Thyroid Association guidelines for diagnosis and management of hyperthyroidism and other causes of thyrotoxicosis. *Thyroid.* 2016;26(10):1343-1421. PMID: 27521067

Rivkees SA. Controversies in the management of Graves' disease in children. *J Endocrinol Invest.* 2016;39(11):1247-1257. PMID: 27153850

Bauer AJ. Approach to the pediatric patient with Graves' disease: when is definitive therapy warranted? *J Clin Endocrinol Metab.* 2011;96(3):580-588. PMID: 21378220

Cooper DS. Antithyroid drugs. *N Engl J Med.* 2005;352(9):905-917. PMID: 15745981

37 ANSWER: C) Brain and pituitary MRI

Brain and pituitary MRI (Answer C) would be the most useful next test to determine the position and morphology of the pituitary gland (both anterior and posterior) and pituitary stalk, as well as presence or absence of the septum pellucidum, optic nerve appearance, midline defects, or masses. MRI of the brain and pituitary is the most sensitive method to image the hypothalamic-pituitary axis. In this newborn, brain MRI was normal, thus excluding any structural or space-occupying lesions that may affect the hypothalamic-pituitary axis.

The diagnosis of secondary adrenal insufficiency is clear in view of the undetectable serum cortisol and inappropriately normal plasma ACTH concentrations during a documented hypoglycemic episode. Therefore, performing either a standard dose (Answer A) or low-dose (Answer B) cosyntropin-stimulation test is not necessary. Identification of additional pituitary hormone deficiencies (TSH, GH, gonadotropin, diabetes insipidus) is important, although this can be challenging during the neonatal period. In this vignette, the normal free T$_4$, TSH, and GH levels during a hypoglycemic episode make deficiencies in TSH and GH unlikely now. Gonadotropin measurement would be helpful to detect mini puberty and to exclude congenital hypogonadotropic hypogonadism. The recommendation is to perform gonadotropin hormone profiling at 4 to 8 weeks of life. Prolactin levels should also be assessed, as some genetic forms of congenital hypopituitarism are associated with prolactin deficiency. Central diabetes insipidus should always be considered, especially in neonates and children with midline defects. In this child, the lack of polyuria and hypernatremia is reassuring. It is important to remember that diabetes insipidus can be masked in patients with ACTH deficiency, as cortisol is essential for water excretion, and diabetes insipidus may only present clinically following treatment with hydrocortisone.

Measuring 17-hydroxyprogesterone (Answer D) and performing ultrasonography of the adrenal glands (Answer E) are unhelpful in the situation of secondary adrenal insufficiency.

Secondary adrenal insufficiency can be congenital or acquired and either isolated or combined with other pituitary hormone deficiencies. Genetic workup should be performed in all patients with congenital secondary adrenal insufficiency. Recessive pathogenic variants in the *TBX19* gene (formerly *TPIT*) are the main cause of congenital isolated ACTH deficiency. In this particular case, a homozygous frameshift mutation in exon 6 (782delA) was identified. ACTH deficiency has also been described in other congenital forms of hypopituitarism associated with pathogenic variants in the following genes: *PROP1, LHX3, FGF8, LHX4, ARNT2, GLI2, PCSK1*, and *POMC*. Both *PCSK1* and *POMC* are associated with weight gain and hypopigmentation. With several of these conditions, such as *PROP1* pathogenic variants, ACTH deficiency can evolve with time, so continuous monitoring and assessment are required. An important acquired cause of secondary adrenal insufficiency is the use and subsequent withdrawal of glucocorticoid-containing drugs. Other causes of secondary adrenal insufficiency include trauma (prenatal or postnatal), infection or inflammation (eg meningitis, sarcoidosis, tuberculosis, autoimmune), infiltrative causes (eg, Langerhans cell histiocytosis, hemochromatosis), tumors (eg, craniopharyngiomas), or pituitary surgery or radiotherapy.

Diagnosis of secondary adrenal insufficiency can be challenging, especially in the first 9 months of life before the establishment of a circadian rhythm (eg, asymptomatic neonates with midline defects at risk of adrenal insufficiency). In such circumstances, multiple paired cortisol and ACTH measurements may point towards a diagnosis. A standard cosyntropin-stimulation test is safe and easy to perform. Once a circadian rhythm has been established, the combination of an 8-AM serum cortisol measurement greater than 6.3 µg/dL (>175 nmol/L) and a 30-minute serum cortisol value greater than 18.1 µg/dL (>500 nmol/L) on standard cosyntropin-stimulation testing have a sensitivity of 69% and a specificity of 100% in excluding ACTH deficiency. The low-dose cosyntropin-stimulation test has been proposed as a more sensitive test for diagnosing secondary adrenal insufficiency although there is no consensus and it is not performed universally. The corticotropin-releasing hormone test (corticotropin-releasing hormone 1 mcg/kg, maximum dose 100 mcg) has been suggested to distinguish hypothalamic from pituitary disease in secondary adrenal insufficiency. However, because of variable responses and undefined normal ranges, the usefulness of this test is unclear.

Treatment of secondary adrenal insufficiency consists of glucocorticoid replacement. Endocrine Society guidelines suggest a starting dosage of 8 mg/m² per day in 3 to 4 divided doses to be titrated according to individual need. The American Academy of Pediatrics suggests a dosage of 9 to 12 mg/m² per day to compensate for incomplete intestinal absorption and hepatic metabolism. Hydrocortisone is preferred in children over other types of glucocorticoid (prednisolone and dexamethasone) to avoid adverse effects and to be able to titrate treatment more accurately. Depending on the cause and associated pituitary deficiency, additional hormone replacement may be required at varying time points in childhood. Before thyroid hormone replacement is initiated, it is important to ensure that glucocorticoid deficiency is adequately treated. Furthermore, patients with combined pituitary hormone deficiencies who start glucocorticoid replacement should be carefully monitored for development of diabetes insipidus. Like all forms of adrenal insufficiency, primary or secondary emergency management during illnesses and trauma, along with patient and family education is critical. Apart from individuals with isolated ACTH deficiency due to pathogenic variants in the *TBX19* gene, other causes of secondary adrenal insufficiency are likely to require long-term surveillance and assessment of progressive involvement of other pituitary hormones.

Educational Objective
Develop an approach to the diagnosis and evaluation of secondary adrenal insufficiency.

Reference(s)
Patti G, Guzzeti C, Di lorgi N, et al. Central adrenal insufficiency in children and adolescents. *Best Pract Res Clin Endocrinol Metab.* 2018;32(4):425-444. PMID: 30086867

Alatzoglou KS, Dattani MT. Genetic forms of hypopituitarism and their manifestation in the neonatal period. *Early Hum Dev.* 2009;85(11):705-712. PMID: 19762173

Couture C, Saveanu A, Barlier A, et al. Phenotypic homogeneity and genotypic variability in a large series of congenital isolated ACTH-deficiency patients with TPIT gene mutations. *J Clin Endocrinol Metab.* 2012;97(3):E486-E495. PMID: 22170728

Higham CE, Johannsson G, Shalet SM. Hypopituitarism. *Lancet.* 2016;388(10058):2403-2415. PMID: 27041067

Shulman DI, Palmert MR, Kemp SF; Lawson Wilkins Drug and Therapeutics Committee. Adrenal insufficiency: still a cause of morbidity and death in childhood. *Pediatrics.* 2007;119(2):e484-e494. PMID: 17242136

Bornstein SR, Allolio B, Arlt W, et al. Diagnosis and treatment of primary adrenal insufficiency: an Endocrine Society clinical practice guideline. *J Clin Endocrinol Metab.* 2016;101(2):364-389. PMID: 26760044

38 ANSWER: E) Heterozygous inactivating pathogenic variant in *NPR2* in the patient and homozygous inactivating pathogenic variants in *NPR2* in her brother

The 4-year-old girl in this vignette has mild short stature, normal bone age, and normal laboratory results. These findings would be consistent with possible diagnoses of familial short stature (as her parents are short) or idiopathic short stature. However, her family history is revealing in that there is parental consanguinity, which may increase the possibility of autosomal recessive disorders. In fact, her brother has severe disproportionate short stature with dysmorphic features consistent with acromesomelic dysplasia Maroteaux type (short stature with shortening of the distal and midsegments of the extremities, prominent forehead, wide and depressed nasal bridge, prominent lips) and normal intellect. This condition is due to homozygous inactivating pathogenic variants in the *NPR2* gene, which encodes natriuretic peptide receptor B, one of the receptors for C-natriuretic peptide. C-natriuretic peptide, through its interaction with natriuretic peptide receptor B, stimulates growth plate chondrogenesis and, therefore, promotes linear growth. Homozygous inactivating pathogenic variants in *NPR2* are responsible for acromesomelic dysplasia Maroteaux type, while heterozygous inactivating pathogenic variants have been described in individuals with idiopathic short stature without significant dysmorphism except for slightly short extremities, as manifested by an arm span that is slightly shorter than the height of this 4-year-old girl. Thus, Answer E is correct. Both parents have mild-to-moderate short stature and are obligate carriers of *NPR2* inactivating pathogenic variants. As such, with each pregnancy, they have a 25% chance of having a child with acromesomelic dysplasia Maroteaux type (homozygous *NPR2* pathogenic variants), a 50% chance of having a child with isolated short stature of mild-to-moderate degree (heterozygous *NPR2* pathogenic variant), and a 25% chance of having an unaffected child (normal biallelic *NPR2* gene). Activating pathogenic variants in the *NPR2* gene (Answer B) would be expected to lead to an overgrowth condition. This has been indirectly demonstrated in animals overexpressing the C-natriuretic peptide gene.

Inactivating *FGFR3* pathogenic variants (Answer C) result in overgrowth conditions. Achondroplasia (Answer A) results from heterozygous activating pathogenic variants in the *FGFR3* gene. Achondroplasia is inherited in an autosomal dominant manner or arises by de novo mutation. The condition is characterized by rhizomelic (proximal [ie, humeral and femoral]) limb shortening, macrocephaly, midface hypoplasia, and trident hand configuration, which are easily recognized at birth. Achondroplasia differs from acromesomelic dysplasia Maroteaux type in which the limb segments that appear short are the mid and distal segments and the shortening is not manifested at birth but becomes evident postnatally. Pseudoachondroplasia is an unrelated disorder due to heterozygous (autosomal dominant) pathogenic variants in the *COMP* gene (cartilage oligomeric matrix protein), which lead to accumulation of an abnormal version of this protein in the endoplasmic reticulum that induces endoplasmic reticulum stress and death of the chondrocytes. Clinical manifestations include disproportionate short stature, deformities of the lower extremities, short fingers, laxity of ligaments, and progressive osteoarthritis.

Although Turner syndrome could be a consideration in this 4-year-old girl, even in the absence of stigmata suggestive of this condition, it is unlikely that the severe short stature and multiple dysmorphic features of the 8-year-old brother are due to *SHOX* haploinsufficiency (Answer D), where mesomelic (midsegment) limb shortening along with Madelung deformity are more characteristic.

Educational Objective
Identify heterozygous inactivating pathogenic variants in the *NPR2* gene as a cause of idiopathic short stature and homozygous pathogenic *NPR2* variants as the cause of acromesomelic dysplasia Maroteaux type.

Reference(s)
Olney R, Bükülmez H, Bartels C, et al. Heterozygous mutations in natriuretic peptide receptor-B (NPR2) are associated with short stature. *J Clin Endocrinol Metab.* 2006;91(4):1229-1232. PMID: 16384845

Wang SR, Jacobsen CM, Carmichael, et al. Heterozygous mutations in natriuretic peptide receptor-B (NPR2) gene as a cause of short stature. *Hum Mutat.* 2015;36(4):474-481. PMID: 25703509

Pauli RM. Achondroplasia: a comprehensive clinical review. *Orphanet J Rare Dis.* 2019;14(1):1-49. PMID: 30606190

39

ANSWER: D) BMI percentile

Bariatric procedures are increasingly used as a means of effectively inducing weight loss and avoiding complications of extreme obesity in adolescents. The American Academy of Pediatrics developed guidelines to help determine which patients are appropriate candidates for bariatric surgery. The December 2019 policy statement recommends that pediatric patients with the following findings be considered for bariatric surgery:

- Class 2 obesity, BMI ≥35 kg/m² or 120% of the 95th percentile for age and sex (whichever is lower), with clinically significant comorbidities (including obstructive sleep apnea [apnea-hypopnea index >5], type 2 diabetes, idiopathic intracranial hypertension, nonalcoholic steatohepatitis, Blount disease, slipped capital femoral epiphysis, gastroesophageal reflux disease, and hypertension)

OR

- Class 3 obesity, BMI ≥40 kg/m² or 140% of the 95th percentile for age and sex (whichever is lower), with or without comorbidities

BMI and BMI percentile (Answer D) are considered one of the criteria to determine whether a pediatric patient should be considered for bariatric surgery. This patient's BMI of 38 kg/m², however, does not meet criteria for recommending bariatric surgery, as he has no qualifying comorbidities.

Dyslipidemia (Answer A) is not considered to be a clinically significant comorbidity according to the guidelines. Neither family history of bariatric surgery (Answer C) nor history of participating in a formal weight-loss program (Answer E) is a consideration for bariatric surgery eligibility according to the American Academy of Pediatrics.

Completion of pubertal growth (Answer B) is not necessary in order to proceed with a bariatric procedure. Therefore, this patient's age does not disqualify him from being considered for bariatric surgery. Previously, clinicians were concerned that the procedure might accelerate and limit further linear growth in adolescent patients. In fact, studies, including a prospective study by Olbers et al, have shown that patients who have the procedure continue to grow afterwards.

Educational Objective
Identify criteria to recommend bariatric procedures in adolescents.

Reference(s)
Armstrong AC, Bolling CF, Michalsky MP, Reichard KW; Section on Obesity, Section on Surgery. Pediatric metabolic and bariatric surgery: evidence, barriers, and best practices. *Pediatrics.* 2019;144(6):e20193223, PMID: 31656225

Alqahtani A, Elahmedi M, Qahtani AR. Laparoscopic sleeve gastrectomy in children younger than 14 years: refuting the concerns. *Ann Surg.* 2016;263(2):312-319. PMID: 26496081

Pratt JSA, Browne A, Browne NT, et al. ASMBS pediatric metabolic and bariatric surgery guidelines, 2018. *Surg Obes Relat Dis.* 2018;14(7):882-901. PMID: 30077361

Olbers T, Beamish AJ, Gronowitz E, et al. Laparoscopic Roux-en-Y gastric bypass in adolescents with severe obesity (AMOS): a prospective, 5-year, Swedish nationwide study [published correction appears in *Lancet Diabetes Endocrinol.* 2017;5(5):e3]. *Lancet Diabetes Endocrinol.* 2017;5(3):174-183. PMID: 28065734

40

ANSWER: D) Ovarian failure due to follicle depletion

This patient has hypergonadotropic hypogonadism, as indicated by elevated FSH and LH and low serum estradiol. This most often falls under the category of primary ovarian insufficiency (POI). POI is defined as ovarian failure before age 40 years and has an incidence of approximately 1%. In this vignette, lack of pubertal development suggests absent ovarian function before onset of central puberty.

In POI, ovarian failure is due to either ovarian follicle dysfunction or accelerated ovarian depletion, without clear etiology approximately 90% of the time. As such, ovarian follicle depletion (Answer D) is the most likely etiology of the options listed. Other causes of POI include autoimmunity, galactosemia, and fragile X premutation.

An increased number of CGG triplet repeats in the *FMR1* gene (Answer A) is associated with both fragile X syndrome and fragile X premutation. Normally, this DNA segment is repeated 5 to 40 times. In fragile X syndrome, the segment is repeated more than 200 times, which causes loss of the FMR1 protein. Small CGG repeat expansions in the range of 55 to 200 repeats, classified as a fragile X premutation, causes production of a dysfunctional protein. Fragile X premutations are identified in approximately 5% of patients of POI. Individuals with fragile X syndrome, however, have the same risk of POI as the general population.

Excess ovarian androgen production (Answer B) can cause anovulation, but lack of pubertal development would not be expected. Individuals with polycystic ovary syndrome have an elevated LH-to-FSH ratio, but within normal range and not suggestive of POI, as in this case. This patient lacks other features associated with polycystic ovary syndrome such as hirsutism, and hyperandrogenemia would be an unlikely explanation for her examination and laboratory findings.

Elevated prolactin has a number of causes, including pituitary adenoma, other hypothalamic and pituitary disorders, hypothyroidism, renal or liver failure, or autoimmune disorders. Hyperprolactinemia is a fairly common cause of amenorrhea; however, the mechanism is due to inhibition of LH pulses, so the expected hormone profile would show low levels of FSH and LH. As such, elevated prolactin levels (Answer E) would not be consistent with this case presentation.

Several chromosomal abnormalities (Answer C) are associated with POI, including Turner syndrome and tetrasomy X. Short stature is a nearly universal finding in Turner syndrome. This patient is growing well along higher percentiles and has no other features consistent with Turner syndrome. While half of females with tetrasomy X develop POI, most have other identifiable features, including dysmorphic facial features, cleft palate, dental abnormalities, hypotonia, scoliosis, developmental delays, hearing and vision problems, cardiac defects, and seizures. While a karyotype would be indicated in any female patient with POI, the patient in this vignette is unlikely to have a chromosomal abnormality as an explanation for her hypogonadism.

Educational Objective
Identify the underlying etiology of primary ovarian insufficiency in an adolescent girl.

Reference(s)
Nelson LM. Clinical practice. Primary ovarian insufficiency. *N Engl J Med.* 2009;360(6):606-614. PMID: 19196677

Torrealday S, Kodaman P, Pal L. Premature ovarian insufficiency - an update on recent advances in understanding and management. *F1000Res.* 2017;6:2069. PMID: 29225794

41 ANSWER: B) Thyroglobulin measurement and assessment of thyroglobulin antibodies
In most cases of hyperthyroidism, total T_3, total T_4, and free T_4 are elevated. Some patients with Graves disease, for example, present with T_3 thyrotoxicosis, but free T_4 would not be in the low-normal range as it is in this patient, and the discrepancy between T_4 and T_3 would not be as great as it is in this vignette. The clinician must determine whether this patient has subacute thyroiditis or exogenous intoxication, most likely from the diet pills.

A complete blood cell count with differential (Answer A) would not help distinguish between the 2 diagnoses. Measuring calcitonin (Answer C) is not indicated. Procalcitonin measurement (Answer D) could help assess whether there is a bacterial infection (which could also explain an elevated erythrocyte sedimentation rate), but it would not be helpful in this case, as subacute thyroiditis is often associated with preceding viral illnesses. Thyroid ultrasonography (Answer E) may be helpful in imaging a hot nodule, but a focus of intense uptake would have been visible on the thyroid scan if that were the case.

The best next step is to measure thyroglobulin (Answer B), which would be low in the setting of exogenous intoxication and normal in subacute thyroiditis. Measuring thyroglobulin antibodies would help ensure that the thyroglobulin level reported is not artificially low due to an elevated antibody titer. Specialized thyroglobulin assays (liquid chromatography/tandem mass spectrometry) used to monitor patients with thyroid cancer can also be used in the setting of elevated thyroglobulin antibodies.

This patient was indeed receiving exogenous T_3 from her diet pills, which explains the very high T_3 and normal free T_4. She obtained the pills while on vacation in Mexico. Such pills are banned by the US FDA, but they can still be purchased outside the United States. The diet pills she took each contained 75 mcg of liothyronine, as well as norpseudoephedrine, atropine, aloin, and diazepam, which can mask or alter some of the symptoms of thyrotoxicosis.

Educational Objective
Distinguish between subacute thyroiditis and exogenous intoxication in a patient with hyperthyroidism.

Reference(s)

Graves CL, Newfield RS. Dangerous dieting – Mexican diet pills and T3 thyrotoxicosis. *J Case Rep Images Pediatr.* 2018;1:100002Z19CG2018.

Pacifico L, Osborn JF, Natale F, Ferraro F, De Curtis M, Chiesa C. Procalcitonin in pediatrics. *Adv Clin Chem.* 2013;59:203-263. PMID: 23461137

42   ANSWER: E) Vitamin D supplementation, 2000 IU daily; enteral calcium, 50 mg/kg per day; and intravenous calcium gluconate as needed

In general, infants double their birth weight by 4 months of age. This infant has failed to do so by 6 months of age, most likely because of insufficient caloric intake from a primarily plant-based diet. Individuals who follow a vegan diet are at risk for protein, vitamin D, and calcium deficiencies in addition to insufficient intake of other micronutrients and macronutrients. This patient has evidence of significant malnourishment, as well as calcium and phosphorus deficiencies secondary to severe vitamin D deficiency. Although his 1,25-dihydroxyvitamin D level is also low, this is most likely secondary to profound hypovitaminosis D as opposed to an inhibition of 1α-hydroxylase. Calcitriol supplementation is not recommended as part of the initial management of hypocalcemia because endogenous levels of 1,25-dihydroxyvitamin D will rise substantially within 72 hours. Providing a maintenance dosage of calcitriol (Answers B and C) can prevent this rise and actually impede the treatment of hypocalcemia. In addition, normal infant formula generally has sufficient phosphorus, so additional supplementation is not necessary. It is also important to recognize that intravenous calcium gluconate will temporarily increase serum calcium levels, but the concentration will drop again within 2 to 3 hours if enteral calcium is not provided. Intravenous calcium (Answer C) can be used as an adjunct to enteral calcium when symptoms are severe or patients are not able to tolerate enteral calcium, but it should not be the sole source of calcium supplementation.

In Answer A, the vitamin D supplementation only provides the recommended daily allotment (RDA) for infants. This is not sufficient to adequately replete the vitamin D stores in this patient. While breastfeeding should be supported when possible, and studies have shown that maternal high-dosage vitamin D supplementation of 5000 to 10,000 IU daily (Answer D) results in normal infant serum 25-hydroxyvitamin D levels without direct infant supplementation, this also would be appropriate for maintaining vitamin D levels, not increasing them to normal from a deficient state. In addition, the concentration of both calcium and phosphorus in maternal breast milk at 6 months postpartum is low.

Severe vitamin D deficiency and hypocalcemia can cause significant cardiac effects, including prolonged QTc interval (present in this patient), as well as dilated cardiomyopathy secondary to ventricular dilatation. In a case series of 16 infants with vitamin D–associated dilated cardiomyopathy, 6 presented with cardiac arrest and 10 presented in heart failure. Fifty percent of patients required mechanical ventilation. Nearly 20% (3/16) of the children died. The child in this vignette has profound hypocalcemia with electrocardiographic changes, increasing his risk for dilated cardiomyopathy. These findings warrant urgent intervention with intravenous calcium and ongoing monitoring of telemetry. Enteral calcium must be introduced simultaneously with intravenous calcium to allow for sustained repletion of calcium stores. High-dosage vitamin D supplementation is necessary to allow absorption of enteral calcium. Monitoring the patient's other electrolytes during refeeding is also reasonable. Thus, Answer E provides the best approach for treating the manifestations of severe vitamin D deficiency in this infant.

Educational Objective

Recognize that severe vitamin D deficiency in infancy can present with cardiac changes, including prolonged QTc interval, dilated cardiomyopathy, laryngospasm, and seizures.

Reference(s)

Maiya S, Sullivan I, Allgrove J, et al. Hypocalcaemia and vitamin D deficiency: an important, but preventable, cause of life-threatening infant heart failure. *Heart.* 2008;94(5):581-584. PMID: 17690157

Hollis BW, Wagner CL, Howard CR, et al. Maternal versus infant vitamin D supplementation during lactation: a randomized controlled trial. *Pediatrics.* 2015;136(4):625-634. PMID: 26416936

43

ANSWER: C) Thyroid C-cell tumors: contraindicated in patients with a personal or family history of medullary thyroid cancer or in patients with multiple endocrine neoplasia type 2

A "black box" warning is the strictest warning put in the labeling of a prescription drug by the US FDA when there is reasonable evidence of an association of a serious hazard with the drug. First implemented in 1979, black box warnings highlight serious and sometimes life-threatening adverse drug reactions within the labeling of prescription drug products.

Liraglutide is a GLP-1 receptor agonist. GLP-1 is a peptide hormone that increases insulin secretion and decreases glucagon secretion from the pancreas in a glucose-dependent manner. GLP-1 receptor agonists provide pharmacologic levels of GLP-1, which reduce glucose and weight by increasing glucose-dependent insulin secretion, decreasing glucagon secretion, delaying gastric emptying, and increasing satiety. All of the GLP-1 receptor agonist agents are administered as subcutaneous injections.

Liraglutide is indicated as an adjunct to diet and exercise to improve glycemic control in patients aged 10 years and older with type 2 diabetes. It reduces the risk of major adverse cardiovascular events in adults with type 2 diabetes and established cardiovascular disease.

Liraglutide causes thyroid C-cell tumors at clinically relevant exposures in both sexes of rats and mice. It is unknown whether liraglutide causes thyroid C-cell tumors, including medullary thyroid carcinoma, in humans. The human relevance of liraglutide-induced rodent thyroid C-cell tumors has not been determined. However, liraglutide has a black box warning and is contraindicated in patients with a personal or family history of medullary thyroid carcinoma or in patients with multiple endocrine neoplasia type 2. Physicians who prescribe liraglutide should counsel patients regarding the potential risk of medullary thyroid carcinoma and the symptoms of thyroid tumors (Answer C).

Other warnings and precautions include:
- Pancreatitis (Answer A): Postmarketing reports, including fatal and nonfatal hemorrhagic or necrotizing pancreatitis. Discontinue promptly if pancreatitis is suspected. Do not restart if pancreatitis is confirmed.
- Serious hypoglycemia (Answer D): When liraglutide is used with an insulin secretagogue (eg, a sulfonylurea) or insulin, consider lowering the dosage of the insulin secretagogue or insulin to reduce the risk of hypoglycemia. The risk of hypoglycemia is higher in pediatric patients 10 years and older regardless of concomitant antidiabetes therapies.
- Renal impairment (Answer B): Postmarketing reports, usually in association with nausea, vomiting, diarrhea, or dehydration that may sometimes require hemodialysis. Use caution when initiating or escalating doses of liraglutide in patients with renal impairment.
- Hypersensitivity (Answer E): Postmarketing reports of serious hypersensitivity reactions (eg, anaphylactic reactions and angioedema). Liraglutide should be discontinued and the patient should promptly seek medical advice.
- Acute gallbladder disease: If cholelithiasis or cholecystitis is suspected, gallbladder studies are indicated.

Liraglutide was evaluated in a 26-week, double-blind, randomized, parallel group, placebo-controlled, multicenter trial in 134 pediatric patients with type 2 diabetes aged 10 years and older. Patients were randomly assigned to liraglutide once daily or placebo once daily in combination with metformin with or without basal insulin treatment. All patients were on a metformin dosage of 1000 to 2000 mg daily before randomization. The basal insulin dose was decreased by 20% at randomization and liraglutide was titrated weekly by 0.6 mg for 2 to 3 weeks based on tolerability and an average fasting plasma glucose goal of 110 mg/dL or less (≤6.1 mmol/L). At week 26, treatment with liraglutide was superior to placebo in reducing hemoglobin A_{1c} from baseline. The estimated treatment difference in hemoglobin A_{1c} reduction from baseline between liraglutide and placebo was –1.06% with a 95% confidence interval of –1.65% to –0.46%.

Educational Objective
Explain the risks associated with use of liraglutide to treat children with type 2 diabetes mellitus.

Reference(s)
Tamborlane WV, Barrientos-Pérez M, Fainberg U, et al; Ellipse Trial Investigators. Liraglutide in children and adolescents with type 2 diabetes. *N Engl J Med.* 2019;381(7):637-546. PMID: 31034184

44

ANSWER: D) LH, high; FSH, high; testosterone, normal or low; inhibin B, undetectable

This boy has Klinefelter syndrome (47,XXY), which occurs in approximately 1 in 600 newborn boys. It was first described in 1942 by Harry F. Klinefelter and is characterized by gynecomastia, small testes, Sertoli-cell dysfunction with absent or reduced spermatogenesis, normal to moderately reduced Leydig-cell function, and increased FSH secretion. Klinefelter syndrome is a frequent genetic cause of infertility in men. Additional findings can include delayed or incomplete puberty, decreased muscle mass, reduced body and facial hair, language delay, learning disabilities, and behavioral issues. However, the clinical features of Klinefelter syndrome vary widely. Like the patient in this vignette, individuals with Klinefelter syndrome may have evidence of normal virilization on examination because of relatively normal Leydig-cell function. However, testicular size is small due to a decline in germ cells, hyalinization of the tubules, and degeneration of Sertoli cells.

Inhibin is a glycoprotein hormone made primarily by the gonads. It is a disulfide-linked dimer with a common α subunit and either a βA subunit forming inhibin A or a βB subunit forming inhibin B. Dimers of these β subunits form the activins (activin A βA- βA, activin B βB- βB, activin AB βA-βB). Inhibins and activins are members of the transforming growth factor-β (TGF-β) family. Inhibin A and inhibin B suppress FSH secretion at the pituitary in a classic feedback loop and may also have paracrine effects in the gonads. Although activins share a common β subunit with inhibin, they have the opposite effect, stimulating FSH release. Inhibin B is the circulating form of inhibin in males. It is primarily produced by the Sertoli cells of the testis. In normal men, inhibin B levels are positively correlated with Sertoli-cell function and sperm number and negatively correlated with FSH levels.

Inhibin A is mainly secreted by the corpus luteum and may serve as a prognostic factor for predicting the return of ovarian function in women. During pregnancy, the placenta becomes the major source for inhibin A secretion, also produced by the corpus luteum. Measurement of inhibin A has clinical value in women in early pregnancy with impending abortion or hydatiform mole. Inhibin B is secreted by antral follicles in response to FSH, and it is the major marker of follicular growth. Therefore, inhibin B levels in women may serve as a marker of ovarian function.

Prepubertal boys with Klinefelter syndrome generally have normal serum levels of FSH, LH, testosterone, and inhibin B until onset of puberty. During puberty, testosterone levels increase initially but then plateau and remain in the low-normal range, while LH and FSH levels rise to hypergonadotropic levels by adulthood. Inhibin B levels simultaneously decrease. In most adults with Klinefelter syndrome, serum inhibin B levels are undetectable. Therefore, the most likely laboratory findings in this patient are represented in Answer D.

Educational Objective
Explain the effects of the inhibins and activins on gonadotropin synthesis and secretion.

Reference(s)
Luisi S, Florio P, Reis FM, Petraglia F. Inhibins in female and male reproductive physiology: role in gametogenesis, conception, implantation and early pregnancy. *Hum Reprod Update.* 2005;11(2):123-135. PMID: 15618291

O'Connor AE, De Kretser DM. Inhibins in normal male physiology. *Semin Reprod Med.* 2004;22(3):177-185. PMID: 15319820

45

ANSWER: E) Treat with [131]I 120 mCi (4440 MBq) and perform posttreatment scan 4 to 7 days later

This patient has a high recurrence risk, as evidenced by regional extensive disease (N1b), tumor size, and extrathyroidal extension. She also has an aggressive type of papillary thyroid carcinoma. Although having the stimulated thyroglobulin level would further assist in medical decision-making, she would most likely benefit from radioactive iodine treatment since she has multifocal T3 tumor with extensive nodal disease and a high-risk variant of thyroid cancer.

While her diagnostic ^{123}I scan did not identify remnant nodal disease, some studies show that lymph node metastasis is sometimes only found on the posttreatment scan. For these reasons, reassuring the family based on ^{123}I uptake alone (Answers A, B, and C) is not appropriate.

A recent study provides guidelines for adults regarding use of whole-body scanning and thyroglobulin measurement to guide the dose of ^{131}I to decrease recurrence risk in patients with radioactive-avid differentiated thyroid cancer. Doses of radioactive iodine less than 50 mCi (1850 MBq) (Answer D) are generally used in adults for thyroid remnant ablation, when there is a low risk for regional or distant metastatic disease. Therapeutic doses used in adults at high recurrence risk are usually 100 to 150 mCi (3700-5180 MBq) or higher.

In children, radioactive iodine administration is usually determined based on empiric doses or may be based on whole-body dosimetry. As nicely reviewed in the management guidelines for children with thyroid nodules and differentiated thyroid cancer, for empiric dosing, there are several approaches:

1. ^{131}I may be adjusted according to weight or body surface area, giving a fraction of the adult dose (eg, correcting for a 70-kg adult with similar extent of disease)
2. The dose may be adjusted based on body weight alone using a dose between 1.0 and 1.5 mCi/kg (37-56 MBq/kg)
3. A general rule based on age may be used, assuming that a 15-year-old child needs five-sixths of the adult activity, a 10-year-old child needs one-half of the adult activity, and a 5-year-old child may need only one-third of the adult dose for equivalent disease.

However, current guidelines recommend that all activities of ^{131}I should be calculated by experts with experience in dosing children. For children with extensive metastatic disease or diffuse lung uptake or in whom multiple doses are anticipated or who may have bone marrow disease, dosimetry is recommended.

This patient would benefit from radioactive iodine treatment at a therapeutic dose to minimize the need of future exposure to radioactive iodine. An adult with similar extent of disease would receive about 150 mCi (5180 MBq). Of the options provided, 120 mCi (4440 MBq) (Answer E) is the best answer for this 15-year-old patient, which corresponds to five-sixths of the adult dose.

Her stimulated thyroglobulin level was 43 ng/mL (43 µg/L) with negative antibodies. She received 120 mCi (4440 MBq) of ^{131}I. A posttreatment scan showed mild residual activity in the thyroid bed and uptake in bilateral cervical lymph nodes with no evidence of distant metastasis. Nonstimulated thyroglobulin levels have decreased over 6 months to 0.2 ng/mL (athyreotic level <0.1 ng/mL) and antibodies have remained negative. Findings on neck ultrasonography have been negative.

Educational Objective
Make recommendations based on the guidelines for medical management following surgery for thyroid cancer.

Reference(s)
Antonelli A, Miccoli P, Fallahi P, et al. Role of neck ultrasonography in the follow-up of children operated on for thyroid papillary cancer. *Thyroid.* 2003;13(5):479-484. PMID: 12855015

Francis GL, Waguespack SG, Bauer AJ, et al. Management guidelines for children with thyroid nodules and differentiated thyroid cancer. *Thyroid.* 2015;25(7):716-759. PMID: 25900731

Jarzab B, Handkiewicz-Junak D, Wloch J. Juvenile differentiated thyroid carcinoma and the role of radioiodine in its treatment: a qualitative review. *Endocr Relat Cancer.* 2005;12(4):773-803. PMID: 16322322

Jin Y, Ruan M, Cheng L, et al. Radioiodine uptake and thyroglobulin-guided radioiodine remnant ablation in patients with differentiated thyroid cancer: a prospective, randomized, open-label, controlled trial. *Thyroid.* 2019;29(1):101-110. PMID: 30560716

46 ANSWER: A) Redraw a fasting lipid panel in 3 months

This patient is considered to be at risk for cardiovascular disease due to her very elevated LDL-cholesterol level. However, guidelines recommend repeating a fasting lipid panel (Answer A) before diagnosing dyslipidemia.

Cardiovascular disease remains the most common cause of death in the United States. Beyond discontinuation of cigarette smoking, statin medications to lower LDL cholesterol have had an important role in recent improvements in cardiovascular mortality. LDL cholesterol–related atherosclerosis often has its roots in early childhood, with autopsy studies revealing strong correlations between atherosclerotic plaques and LDL-cholesterol levels, even during early childhood. Genetic conditions such as familial hypercholesterolemia are relatively common causes of high cholesterol levels, with a carrier rate of 1 in 500. Heterozygotes may have LDL-cholesterol levels up to 300 to 400 mg/dL (7.77-10.36 mmol/L), although they often have lower levels. This is the main basis for current recommendations regarding universal LDL-cholesterol screening.

In most lipid panel assessments, direct measurements are made of total cholesterol and HDL cholesterol, while triglycerides are estimated from direct measurement of serum glycerol levels. LDL cholesterol is calculated using the Friedewald equation (as long as triglycerides are <400 mg/dL [<4.52 mmol/L]):

$$LDL = total\ cholesterol - HDL - 1/5\ triglycerides$$

Total cholesterol and HDL cholesterol are stable in the serum regardless of fasting status, while triglycerides can be greatly elevated after meal ingestion.

Current guidelines that have been in place for more than 25 years are to treat children 10 years and older with medical therapy if they have an LDL-cholesterol level greater than 160 mg/dL (>4.14 mmol/L) plus a family history of early heart disease and to treat children 10 years and older if they have an LDL-cholesterol level greater than 190 mg/dL (>4.92 mmol/L) but no relevant family history or unknown family history and if 6 months of dietary and exercise treatment have not been successful. This patient is 7 years old and while her lipid levels are suspicious for familial hypercholesterolemia, she does not meet the high-risk criteria for initiating a statin (Answer D) with a low-risk family history.

It should be noted that these guidelines are not based on long-term trials demonstrating efficacy in avoiding future cardiovascular disease, but instead are based on expert opinion given the strong relationships between LDL-cholesterol levels and clinically significant cardiovascular disease in adult cohorts.

In this vignette, initiating the CHILD-2 diet (Answer B) without first attempting the CHILD-1 diet would be incorrect. The Cardiovascular Health Integrated Lifestyle Diet (CHILD-1 diet) is the initial step recommended by nutritionists to achieve a healthy lifestyle. The recommendations are age-based and vary for very young to older adolescents. The initial dietary recommendation is restricting saturated fat to less than 10% of daily caloric intake and reducing cholesterol consumption to less than 300 mg daily. It is also recommended to reduce consumption of sugary beverages. If a patient is unable to achieve the laboratory or BMI goals after a 3-month trial, the CHILD-2 diet is recommended. It further restricts saturated fat (<7% of total caloric intake) and cholesterol (<200 mg daily), and may introduce plant sterol and stanol esters, water-soluble psyllium fiber, or omega-3 fatty acids to reduce lipid levels.

While fibrates (Answer C) have been used as cholesterol-lowering agents, their use is not indicated at this time without a repeated lipid panel and an attempt at nutritional intervention.

Fish oil (Answer E) has been recommended to treat hypertriglyceridemia; however, experts recommend its use only after strict lifestyle intervention and for a triglyceride concentration greater than 500 mg/dL (>5.65 mmol/L).

Educational Objective
Interpret nonfasting lipid measurements and recommend management for children with elevated LDL-cholesterol levels.

Reference(s)

de Ferranti SD, Steinberger J, Ameduri R, et al. Cardiovascular risk reduction in high-risk pediatric patients: a scientific statement from the American Heart Association. *Circulation.* 2019;139(13):e603-e634. PMID: 30798614

Expert Panel on Integrated Guidelines for Cardiovascular Health and Risk Reduction in Children and Adolescents; National Heart, Lung, and Blood Institute. Expert panel on integrated guidelines for cardiovascular health and risk reduction in children and adolescents: summary report. *Pediatrics.* 2011;128(Suppl 5):S213-S256. PMID: 22084329

de Ferranti SD. Familial hypercholesterolemia in children and adolescents: a clinical perspective. *J Clin Lipidol.* 2015;9(5 Suppl):S11-S19. PMID: 26343208

47 **ANSWER: B) C-type natriuretic peptide analogue**
Achondroplasia results from heterozygous activating pathogenic variants in the fibroblast growth factor receptor 3 gene (*FGFR3*) on chromosome 4p16.3. It can be inherited in an autosomal dominant manner or result from de novo mutation. The condition is characterized by rhizomelic (proximal [ie, humeral and femoral]) limb shortening, macrocephaly, midface hypoplasia, and trident hand configuration, which are usually easily recognized at birth.

Four fibroblast growth factor receptors are known in humans. They localize on the cell surface and are involved in cellular proliferation. Natural ligands for FGFR-3 include several fibroblast growth factors (FGFs). The net effect of the interaction of these FGFs with FGFR-3, which involves activation of a tyrosine kinase in the post receptor cascade, is a decrease in chondrogenesis by limiting the duration of the proliferative phase and accelerating the terminal differentiation. A constitutively active gain-of-function pathogenic variant in *FGFR3*, therefore, leads to decreased growth plate chondrogenesis, as seen in achondroplasia.

Acromesomelic dysplasia Maroteaux type is due to homozygous inactivating pathogenic variants in the *NPR2* gene, which encodes natriuretic peptide receptor B, one of the receptors for C-natriuretic peptide (CNP). CNP, through its interaction with natriuretic peptide receptor B, stimulates growth plate chondrogenesis and, therefore, promotes linear growth. CNP has been postulated to enhance growth plate chondrogenesis in achondroplasia through a pathway that does not involve the FGFR-3 protein, which is dysfunctional in these individuals. CNP analogues (Answer B), through activation of the natriuretic peptide receptor B pathway, have been shown to counteract the constitutively activated FGFR-3 signaling. Phase 3 studies are now underway for the management of short stature associated with achondroplasia.

Although recombinant human GH (Answer D) has been used for the management of short stature in achondroplasia and is approved in Japan for this indication, it induces a transient increase in growth velocity, which rapidly attenuates with prolongation of therapy. It is estimated that the net effect of GH therapy in individuals with achondroplasia is a height gain of 1.0 to 1.5 in (2.5-3.8 cm) after several years of treatment.

GH action is mediated by IGF-1 in the growth plate. While in vitro studies have shown that IGF-1 prevents apoptosis through phosphatidylinositol 3 kinase and MAPK and was expected to improve altered growth plate chondrogenesis in achondroplasia, the use of recombinant human IGF-1 (Answer A) in the clinical setting is not supported by the attenuated growth response seen during prolonged recombinant human GH therapy.

GnRH analogues and aromatase inhibitors (Answers C and E), although not standard of care for the management of growth disorders, have been used to slow down growth plate maturation and delay epiphyseal fusion in peripubertal individuals, while enhancing growth plate chondrogenesis with recombinant human GH in peripubertal or pubertal individuals with short stature. These interventions would not be appropriate for the patient described in this vignette.

Educational Objective
Describe new developments in the management of severe short stature associated with achondroplasia to appropriately guide parents who inquire about potential interventions.

Reference(s)
Pauli RM. Achondroplasia: a comprehensive clinical review. *Orphanet J Rare Dis.* 2019;14(1):1. PMID: 30606190

Harada D, Namba N, Hamioka Y, et al. Final adult height in long-term growth hormone-treated achondroplasia patients. *Eur J Pediatr.* 2017;176(7):873-879. PMID: 28501952

Koike M, Yamanaka Y, Inoue M, Tanaka H, Nishimura R, Seino Y. Insulin-like growth factor-1 rescues the mutated FGF receptor 3 (G380R) expressing ATDC5 cells from apoptosis through phosphatidylinositol 3-kinase and MAPK. *J Bone Miner Res.* 2003;18(11):2043-2051. PMID: 14606518

48 ANSWER: A) Perform a pubertal examination

A pubertal examination (Answer A) is the most immediate course of action in view of the high documented height velocity at 4 years of age. Determining bone age (Answer B), measuring 17-hydroxyprogesterone (Answer C), and increasing the hydrocortisone dosage (Answer D) all have merit, but pubertal examination is an essential first step. Reducing the fludrocortisone dosage (Answer E) would not have any effect on her growth, so it is irrelevant in this case. Children with congenital adrenal hyperplasia (CAH) are predisposed to development of central precocious puberty. This is more common in those who have poor control or are diagnosed late with virilizing forms of CAH. In this case, the child was appropriately prepubertal, having been diagnosed with CAH at birth and treated since that time.

Laboratory test results (sample drawn 2 hours after the morning dose of hydrocortisone):
   Androstenedione = 137.5 ng/dL (0-20.0 ng/dL) (SI: 4.8 nmol/L [0-0.7 nmol/L])
   DHEA-S = 14.8 μg/dL (0-18.5 μg/dL) (SI: <0.4 μmol/L [0-0.5 μmol/L])
   Testosterone = 17.3 ng/dL (<14.4 ng/dL) (SI: 0.6 nmol/L [<0.5 nmol/L])
   17-Hydroxyprogesterone = 10,656 ng/dL (SI: 322.9 nmol/L)
   Plasma renin activity = 4.5 ng/mL per h (<2.5 ng/mL per h for age 1-6 year old)
   Sodium = 138 mEq/L (133-146 mEq/L) (SI: 138 mmol/L [133-146 mmol/L])
   Potassium = 4.0 mEq/L (3.5-5.3 mEq/L) (SI: 4.0 mmol/L [3.5-5.3 mmol/L]).

The high serum 17-hydroxyprogesterone and androstenedione suggest poor control, either because of nonadherence or the need to intensify her current treatment. To assess her hydrocortisone dosage and interval, a 24-hour profile with 2 hourly serum measurements of cortisol, pre-dose 17-hydroxyprogesterone measurement, and androstenedione measurement was arranged.

The aim of monitoring in children with CAH is first to ensure adequate treatment, but not overtreatment, with hydrocortisone to minimize long-term overexposure to glucocorticoids and to allow suppression of adrenal androgens. The recommended hydrocortisone dosage in children with CAH is 10 to 15 mg/m² per day. Monitoring CAH treatment varies among different centers and is often dependent on availability of local services. However, published guidelines recommend that children with CAH be closely monitored in the first 3 months of life then every 3 months until 18 months old. After age 18 months, the recommendation is to monitor every 4 months. Monitoring incorporates regular clinical assessments and inquiring about history of adrenal crisis or salt-craving and symptoms of undertreatment or overtreatment. Clinical assessment includes measurement of growth velocity, weight, and blood pressure; assessment of pubertal status; assessment for evidence of virilization; and biochemical measurements to determine the adequacy of glucocorticoid and mineralocorticoid dosages.

Traditionally, 17-hydroxyprogesterone and androstenedione have been used as indicators of the adequacy of glucocorticoid treatment, although alternatives have been suggested such as 21-deoxycortisol and 11-oxysteroids. When using serum 17-hydroxyprogesterone as a guide to treatment, it is important to remember that complete suppression to the normal range is an indication of overtreatment.

Educational Objective
Develop an approach to the monitoring of treatment in children with congenital adrenal hyperplasia.

Reference(s)
Speiser PW, Azziz R, Baskin LS, et al; Endocrine Society. Congenital adrenal hyperplasia due to steroid 21-hydroxylase deficiency: an Endocrine Society clinical practice guideline [published correction appears in *J Clin Endocrinol Metab*. 2010;95(11):5137]. *J Clin Endocrinol Metab*. 2018;103(11):4043-4088. PMID: 20823466

Turcu AF, Mallappa A, Elman MS, et al. 11-Oxygenated androgens are biomarkers of adrenal volume and testicular adrenal rest tumors in 21-hydroxylase deficiency. *J Clin Endocrinol Metab*. 2017;102(8):2701-2710. PMID: 28472487

49 **ANSWER: A) Wait for the result of the T_3 measurement before adjusting the methimazole dosage**
This patient's thyroid laboratory results are quite typical of what is observed after methimazole therapy is initiated. Repeating the measurement of thyroid-stimulating immunoglobulin (Answer D) so soon after diagnosis is unlikely to demonstrate a drop and will not help guide methimazole dosing. Assessing T_3 uptake (Answer B) would help evaluate free T_4, but it is not indicated because her total T_4 concentration decreased almost 50% since starting methimazole. While her T_4 level is already normal, one must verify that the T_3 has normalized before reducing the methimazole dosage (thus, Answer A is correct and Answer C is incorrect). The methimazole dosage would most likely be reduced to 10 mg once daily. If the patient is already hypothyroid, the methimazole dosage could be reduced by 50%. As noted in the American Thyroid Association 2016 guidelines: "*Serum T_3 should be monitored because the serum free T_4 levels may normalize despite persistent elevation of serum total T_3. Serum TSH may remain suppressed for several months after starting therapy, and it is therefore not a good parameter for monitoring therapy early in the course.*" Because TSH stays suppressed early in the course, increasing the methimazole dosage now (Answer E) is incorrect. Methimazole is a thionamide that acts as an inhibitor of the TPO enzyme, and this decreases thyroid hormone synthesis. Higher doses may increase adverse effects and also cause her to become hypothyroid.

Educational Objective
Monitor effectiveness of therapy in a child with newly diagnosed Graves disease.

Reference(s)
Ross DS, Burch HB, Cooper DS, et al. 2016 American Thyroid Association guidelines for diagnosis and management of hyperthyroidism and other causes of thyrotoxicosis. *Thyroid*. 2016;26(10):1343-1421. PMID: 27521067

Chen JJ, Ladenson PW. Discordant hypothyroxinemia and hypertriiodothyroninemia in treated patients with hyperthyroid Graves' disease. *J Clin Endocrinol Metab*. 1986;63(1):102-106. PMID: 2423547

50

ANSWER: A) Refer to sports medicine for evaluation of running mechanics

In this case, recognizing and addressing the misinformation provided to the family is very important. In pediatric patients, the definition of osteoporosis is based on the presence of low-trauma vertebral compression fractures (regardless of bone mineral density) or a bone mineral density Z-score less than −2.0 and 2 pathologic long bone fractures before the age of 10 years or 3 pathologic long bone fractures before the age of 19 years. There are no criteria for osteopenia. This patient's bone density is within normal limits. Stress fractures are also not considered to reflect pathologic bone disease. Rather, they are secondary to excessive mechanical load on normal bone. While total body and hip DXA scans (Answer B) would give additional information and are reliable sites for children in this age group, this information would not aid in the diagnosis or treatment of this patient. In addition, DXA scans are not recommended for stress fractures alone. This patient's vitamin D level is mildly low, but his alkaline phosphatase concentration is actually normal for a young man in the midst of a pubertal growth spurt. Therefore, he is unlikely to have osteomalacia. Large meta-analyses have failed to show that raising vitamin D levels from the insufficient to sufficient range (Answer C) has a significant impact on bone density or fracture risk.

In adults, significant risk factors for fracture (previous fracture, cigarette smoking history, alcohol use, family history, secondary osteoporosis) in combination with bone mineral density can be used to calculate the 10-year probability of fracture (Fracture Risk Assessment Tool or FRAX) to guide the clinician in the initiation of prophylactic bisphosphonate therapy. This tool has not been validated in pediatric patients, and there are no studies showing efficacy of oral bisphosphonates in preventing fractures in otherwise healthy children with low bone density. Thus, starting prophylactic oral bisphosphonate therapy (Answer D) would be incorrect in this patient who has a normal bone density.

Although high-contact sports such as football, soccer, and lacrosse may increase risk for traumatic fractures, stress fractures occur from repetitive overuse. In patients with normal bone density, there is no reason to restrict physical activity (Answer E). Weight-bearing activity is important for bone mass accrual during childhood and maintaining bone density throughout adulthood. Running provides this mechanical stimulation; however, an evaluation by sports medicine (Answer A) may be helpful to identify gait abnormalities or areas of muscle weakness that are causing excessive mechanical strain on the bones leading to stress fracture. In addition, sports medicine physicians work closely with physical therapists and athletic trainers to help a young athlete safely return to sport. Of all the options, this is most likely to be beneficial in preventing further injuries both now and potentially during young adulthood as a military recruit.

On the basis of his age and examination findings, this young man most likely started puberty at the late end of normal or possibly after age 14 years. That being said, his current Tanner staging indicates that he is progressing through puberty. There is a known increase in fracture risk around the time of the pubertal growth spurt, possibly due to the lag in mineralization and the need for recorticalization that occurs as long bones are undergoing rapid elongation at the growth plate. While there are not recommendations to adjust bone mineral density Z-scores for pubertal status, it is important to recognize that most 16-year-old boys have completed their linear growth and thus are further into the process of peak bone mass accrual that occurs in the 6 to 12 months after peak linear growth velocity. Therefore, the family could be further reassured that bone density is most likely to continue to increase and fracture risk will continue to decrease over the next year as his linear growth velocity declines.

Educational Objective
Summarize the physiologic changes that occur during puberty and explain how the adolescent growth spurt correlates with peak fracture incidence in childhood and timing of peak bone mass accrual.

Reference(s)
Bishop N, Arundel P, Clark E, et al; International Society of Clinical Densitometry. Fracture prediction and the definition of osteoporosis in children and adolescents: the ISCD 2013 Pediatric Official Positions. *J Clin Densitom.* 2014;17(2):275-280. PMID: 24631254

Rauch F. Bone growth in length and width: the Yin and Yang of bone stability. *J Musculoskelet Neuronal Interact.* 2005;5(3):194-201. PMID: 16172510

Baxter-Jones AD, Faulkner RA, Forwood MR, Mirwald RL, Bailey DA. Bone mineral accrual from 8 to 30 years of age: an estimation of peak bone mass. *J Bone Miner Res.* 2011;26(8):1729-1739. PMID: 21520276

51
ANSWER: E) Offer reassurance and follow-up in 6 months

Pubertal gynecomastia is common (present in approximately 50% of boys) and is most often physiologic. Gynecomastia is generally caused by an imbalance between estrogen and androgen effects on glandular breast tissue. Estrogen levels rise more rapidly than testosterone levels during early puberty, which leads to a transiently elevated estrogen-to-androgen ratio. The patient in this scenario has evidence of puberty onset on examination without other findings suggestive of a pathologic cause for gynecomastia. Thus, reassurance and observation (Answer E) would be most appropriate at this point.

Karyotype analysis (Answer A) should be ordered if there is suspicion for Klinefelter syndrome in a pubertal or postpubertal boy (eg, tall stature, small testes, and/or other features). Gynecomastia is among the more common findings in individuals with Klinefelter syndrome and is caused by elevated LH, which stimulates estradiol secretion from Leydig cells out of proportion to testosterone production. While the patient in this vignette does have excessively tall stature for family background, the normal LH concentration and stage 2 testicular development are not consistent with Klinefelter syndrome and karyotype analysis would most likely not be helpful.

Assessing serum tumor markers (Answer B) would be appropriate if testicular tumors were suspected. Sertoli-cell tumors are rare but often present in boys younger than 13 years. In Sertoli-cell tumors, overexpression of p450 aromatase (CYP19A1) causes an increase in conversion of androstenedione to estrone, which is sufficient to advance skeletal maturation, accelerate linear growth, and cause gynecomastia. Ectopic β-hCG production from certain tumors (large cell lung carcinoma, gastric carcinoma, renal cell carcinoma, hepatoma) acts via the Leydig-cell LH receptor to stimulate testicular production of estrogen out of proportion to testosterone, which causes gynecomastia. The patient in this vignette does not have a testicular mass or other concerning findings that would warrant screening for an hCG-secreting tumor.

Boys can experience significant distress due to gynecomastia and are often referred to endocrinology for consideration of treatment. When identified, treatment of an underlying disorder or elimination of a medication or environmental exposure suspected of causing gynecomastia can lead to resolution. In the rare case of aromatase excess, which includes aromatase excess syndrome, Carney complex, and Peutz-Jeghers syndrome, aromatase inhibitors (Answer C) have been shown to be beneficial. However, the only randomized, double-blind, placebo-controlled trial of an aromatase inhibitor for pubertal gynecomastia showed no benefit of anastrozole over placebo.

It has recently been reported that pubertal boys with gynecomastia have a significantly higher estradiol-to-testosterone ratio compared with that of healthy boys with either pseudogynecomastia or no breast enlargement. While it is not currently possible to prospectively determine which individuals have a transient, reversible elevation in the estradiol-to-testosterone ratio, it is known that pubertal gynecomastia that persists beyond 3 years is unlikely to regress. In this situation, surgery may be a reasonable option, particularly if there is pain or a significant degree of distress or embarrassment associated with the gynecomastia. Given that up to 90% of adolescents with gynecomastia experience spontaneous regression of breast tissue over a 1- to 3-year period, it would be premature to recommend surgery (Answer D) in a younger patient.

Educational Objective
Distinguish between pathologic and physiologic causes of pubertal gynecomastia and recommend appropriate management.

Reference(s)

Ma NS, Geffner ME. Gynecomastia in prepubertal and pubertal boys. *Curr Opin Pediatr.* 2008;20(4):465-470. PMID: 18622206

Reinehr T, Kulle A, Barth A, Ackermann J, Lass N, Holterhus P-M. Sex hormone profile in pubertal boys with gynecomastia and pseudogynecomastia. *J Clin Endocrinol Metab.* 2020;105(4):1-8. PMID: 31996898

52
ANSWER: D) Pathogenic variant in the *MC4R* gene

Genetic testing should be considered in pediatric patients who exhibit early-onset, severe, rapid weight gain, particularly if other features such as hyperphagia or clinical findings that could indicate a genetic syndrome are evident. Monogenic obesity results from pathogenic variants in a single gene. Leptin deficiency, leptin receptor pathogenic variants, proopiomelanocortin (POMC) deficiency, and melanocortin 4 receptor (*MC4R* gene) pathogenic variants are all examples of monogenic obesity conditions. Most monogenic causes are located along the leptin-melanocortin pathway, which is critical for appetite and weight regulation. Significant hyperphagia is a hallmark of monogenic conditions. Of these, an *MC4R* pathogenic variant (Answer D) represents the most common cause of genetic early-onset obesity and is the most likely diagnosis for the patient in this vignette. The prevalence of *MC4R* pathogenic variants varies between 0.5% and 6%, depending on the population studied. In most cases, it is an autosomal dominant mode of transmission. Children with an *MC4R* pathogenic variant have hyperphagia that is evident early in life. Additionally, they have linear growth acceleration and are tall for age, but they do not demonstrate dysmorphic features and do not have intellectual impairment.

The other monogenic obesity syndromes listed below all have distinct phenotypic features that the patient in this vignette does not demonstrate.

Bardet-Biedl syndrome is a rare syndromic form of obesity characterized by retinal degeneration, early-onset obesity, polydactyly, learning problems, kidney abnormalities, and hypogonadism. There are at least 19 different genes associated with Bardet-Biedl syndrome, but pathogenic variants in *BBS1* (Answer A) account for about 25% of all cases. These variants lead to defective structure and function of cilia.

Leptin deficiency is an extremely rare cause of monogenic obesity with fewer than 100 cases reported worldwide. It is due to pathogenic variants in the *LEP* gene (Answer B) and is inherited in an autosomal recessive fashion. Children with congenital leptin deficiency have early-onset obesity and hyperphagia and may be predisposed to increased risk of serious bacterial infections and hypogonadotropic hypogonadism.

The most common cause of syndromic obesity is Prader-Willi syndrome, with a prevalence of 1 in 15,000 to 1 in 25,000 births. Prader-Willi syndrome is an imprinting disorder. Up to 70% of cases are due to deletions in the paternal copy of the Prader-Willi critical region, which is located on chromosome 15q11.2-q13 (Answer C). Features of Prader-Willi syndrome may include severe hypotonia in infancy, dysmorphic features, intellectual impairment, behavioral challenges, endocrine dysfunction, and nutritional phases that range from poor feeding in infancy to hyperphagia and food-seeking in childhood.

Alstrom syndrome is a rare cause of syndromic obesity that, in addition to early-onset obesity, is characterized by progressive loss of vision and hearing, short stature, cardiomyopathy, early-onset type 2 diabetes, and endocrine dysfunction. It is caused by pathogenic variants in the *ALMS1* gene (Answer E).

Proopiomelanocortin (POMC) deficiency is another very rare cause of severe, early-onset obesity in childhood. It is inherited in an autosomal recessive manner and is caused by loss-of-function pathogenic variants in the *POMC* gene. In addition to obesity and hyperphagia, affected patients tend to have fair skin and red hair. Patients with POMC deficiency are also at risk for secondary adrenal insufficiency, which requires glucocorticoid treatment to avoid potential adrenal crisis.

Educational Objective
Differentiate among genetic syndromes that cause early-onset obesity and diagnose *MC4R* deficiency on the basis of clinical presentation.

Reference(s)
Thaker VV. Genetic and epigenetic causes of obesity. *Adolesc Med State Art Rev.* 2017;28(2):379-405. PMID: 30416642

Mason K, Page L, Balikcioglu PG. Screening for hormonal, monogenic, and syndromic disorders in obese infants and children. *Pediatr Ann.* 2014;43(9):e218-e224. PMID: 25198446

Huvenne H, Dubern B, Clément K, Poitou C. Rare genetic forms of obesity: clinical approach and current treatments in 2016. *Obes Facts.* 2016;9(3):158-173. PMID: 27241181

53 ANSWER: B) Elevated serum sodium
This newborn has lobar holoprosencephaly and cleft lip and palate. Had this mother received prenatal care, these findings would most likely have been noted on fetal ultrasonography. Holoprosencephaly is a congenital brain malformation that results from failure of the forebrain to bifurcate into 2 hemispheres, with alobar holoprosencephaly being the most severe form. Due to the midline malformation, children with holoprosencephaly commonly have endocrinopathies from variable abnormalities of the hypothalamus and pituitary gland. The most common endocrinopathy is diabetes insipidus. In a study of 117 children with classic holoprosencephaly, 70% had diabetes insipidus. The severity of diabetes insipidus has been correlated with the severity of the holoprosencephaly, and it is believed to be due to abnormal development of the hypothalamus. Diabetes insipidus in this setting can present with severe hypernatremia and dehydration, but it may also evolve slowly and can be relatively asymptomatic, with hypernatremia (Answer B) found incidentally on routine screening. Appropriate fluid management with or without desmopressin is an effective treatment.

In some cases, there may be abnormal hypothalamic osmoreception with rare reports of both diabetes insipidus and syndrome of inappropriate antidiuresis causing hyponatremia (Answer E) in the same patient. While anterior pituitary dysfunction can occur, it is less common. In the same series, hypothyroidism (Answer A) was observed in 11% of patients. Hypocortisolism, which could contribute to hypoglycemia (Answer D) occurred in 7% and GH deficiency was observed in 5%. A low IGF-1 level (Answer C) would be expected in the setting of GH deficiency. Growth delay is commonly observed in these children, and it may also be multifactorial and not necessarily a result of GH deficiency. While anterior endocrine dysfunction is less common, a baseline evaluation of ACTH, thyroid, and GH status should be undertaken.

Educational Objective
Describe the spectrum of anterior and posterior hormone deficiencies associated with holoprosencephaly.

Reference(s)

Hahn JS. Holoprosencephaly. *Handb Clin Neurol.* 2008;87:13-37. PMID: 18809016

Hasegawa Y, Hasegawa T, Yokoyama T, Kotoh S, Tsuchiya Y. Holoprosencephaly associated with diabetes insipidus and syndrome of inappropriate secretion of antidiuretic hormone. *J Pediatr.* 1990;117(5):756-758. PMID: 2231210

54 ANSWER: B) *DICER1* syndrome

Thyroid nodules are rare in children, and their evaluation should include assessment for the possibility of an underlying genetic syndrome that predisposes to thyroid neoplasia, particularly if the patient is very young or has multiple thyroid nodules. When a genetic syndrome is suspected, confirmatory genetic testing should be performed because most such syndromes predispose to other benign or malignant tumors for which surveillance may be required.

DICER1 syndrome (Answer B) is associated with tumors of the lung, thyroid, female reproductive tract, kidney, brain, and other organs. The syndrome is caused by inactivating pathogenic variants in the *DICER1* gene, which is involved in microRNA regulation of multiple biologic pathways. Lung tumors arise in infancy or early childhood and range from simple cysts to malignant pleuropulmonary blastomas. Thyroid nodules—often multiple—develop in up to 30% of affected individuals by age 20 years, and thyroid cancer can occur as early as 8 years. Ovarian Sertoli-Leydig–cell tumors or embryonal rhabdomyosarcoma of the cervix may arise in adolescence or early adulthood. Macrocephaly is a common finding.

This patient's findings of multiple thyroid nodules, a functional ovarian tumor, lung cysts, and relative macrocephaly are most consistent with *DICER1* syndrome. Most cases of *DICER1* syndrome are inherited in an autosomal dominant fashion. Consensus recommendations for the care of individuals with *DICER1* syndrome include screening thyroid ultrasonography beginning at age 8 years and every 2 to 3 years thereafter. In children previously treated with chemotherapy for other tumors, thyroid ultrasonography is recommended annually for 5 years, then every 2 to 3 years thereafter.

McCune-Albright syndrome (Answer D) is caused by activating pathogenic variants in the *GNAS* gene, which encodes the stimulatory α subunit associated with multiple G-protein–coupled hormone receptors. Constitutive activation leads to the classic triad of cutaneous café-au-lait macules, gonadotropin-independent precocious puberty, and fibrous dysplasia of bone. Activation of the TSH receptor can cause hyperthyroidism or multinodular goiter. Additional features may include adrenal Cushing syndrome and GH excess.

Carney complex (Answer A) consists of lentigines, myxomas of the heart and other tissues, endocrine neoplasia, and other tumors. Most cases are caused by inactivating pathogenic variants in the *PRKAR1A* gene, which encodes the regulatory subunit of protein kinase A. Skin findings, including lentigines or cutaneous myxomas, are present in most patients. The most common endocrine manifestation is primary pigmented nodular adrenal disease, which causes adrenal Cushing syndrome. Affected patients are at increased risk for thyroid nodules and thyroid cancer, which is often of the follicular type. Testicular or ovarian tumors can occur but are generally not hormone-producing, as was the ovarian tumor in this patient. Lung cysts are not typical of Carney complex.

PTEN hamartoma tumor syndrome (Answer E) encompasses several clinical syndromes caused by inactivating pathogenic variants in the tumor suppressor gene *PTEN*, including Cowden, Bannayan-Riley-Ruvalcaba, and Proteus-like syndromes. These syndromes predispose to benign and malignant tumors of the thyroid, skin, vascular tissue, breast, and other organs; however, tumors of the lung or ovary are not commonly observed. Macrocephaly is common, as is developmental delay or autism spectrum disorder, which were not present in this patient. Thyroid nodules can develop in early childhood and are often multiple; thyroid cancer has been reported in children as young as 6 years.

Familial adenomatous polyposis (Answer C) is characterized by the development of innumerable colonic polyps and eventual colonic carcinoma. This syndrome is caused by autosomal dominant pathogenic variants in the *APC* gene. Affected individuals are also at increased risk of developing thyroid nodules and papillary thyroid cancer, which can occur in adolescence. Tumors of the lung or ovary are not common, and macrocephaly is not observed.

Educational Objective
Diagnose *DICER1* syndrome on the basis of clinical findings.

Reference(s)
Schultz KAP, Williams GM, Kamihara J, et al. *DICER1* and associated conditions: identification of at-risk individuals and recommended surveillance strategies. *Clin Cancer Res.* 2018;24(10):2251-2261. PMID: 29343557

Francis GL, Waguespack SG, Bauer AJ, et al; American Thyroid Association Guidelines Task Force. Management guidelines for children with thyroid nodules and differentiated thyroid cancer. *Thyroid.* 2015;25(7):716-759. PMID: 25900731

55 ANSWER: E) Inhibition of 11β-hydroxysteroid dehydrogenase 1

The action of corticosteroids in peripheral tissues is regulated, in part, by a "shuttle" mechanism of interconversion of the active hormone (cortisol = formerly known as compound F) and the inactive hormone (cortisone = formerly known as compound E), catalyzed by the 11β-hydroxysteroid dehydrogenase (11β-HSD) isoenzymes. The enzyme 11β-HSD1 activates cortisone to cortisol in the liver and adipose tissue, while 11β-HSD2 inactivates cortisol to cortisone in the kidney.

There is evidence that GH indirectly, through IGF-1, modulates cortisol metabolism by decreasing 11β-HSD1 activity. This leads to a decrease in the cortisol-to-cortisone ratio, which, in individuals with limited cortisol production such as patients with hypopituitarism and partial ACTH deficiency, can lead to adrenal insufficiency once GH is administered.

The patient in this vignette was diagnosed with GH deficiency via an arginine-L-dopa stimulation test, which does not evaluate the integrity of the ACTH-cortisol (hypothalamic-pituitary-adrenal) axis as do tests that include insulin or glucagon as one of the stimuli. It is conceivable that, in addition to GH deficiency, this child has partial ACTH deficiency that has not rendered major clinical manifestations. Initiation of GH therapy leads to reduction of an already limited cortisol reserve, triggering clinical manifestations of adrenal insufficiency. Therefore, the mechanism that best explains this patient's presentation is preexisting, unrecognized ACTH deficiency with exacerbation of cortisol deficiency by GH-induced inhibition of 11β-HSD1 (Answer E) (not stimulation of 11β-HSD1 [Answer D]).

Modulation of 11β-HSD2 activity could potentially lead to a similar scenario via an increase in the activity of this enzyme (Answer B). However, GH does not decrease the free cortisol-to-free cortisone ratio in the urine, suggesting that it does not affect renal 11β-HSD2 activity. A decrease in this isoenzyme activity (Answer C) would lead to enhanced activation of cortisone to cortisol and an adrenal crisis would not be expected.

Inhibition of 21-hydroxylase (Answer A) could lead to a drop in cortisol levels and manifestations of an adrenal crisis in individuals with limited endogenous cortisol production such as those with partial ACTH deficiency. However, GH is not known to affect 21-hydroxylase activity.

Educational Objective
Explain the mechanism by which GH decreases cortisol synthesis.

Reference(s)
Stewart PM, Toogood AA, Tomlinson JW. Growth hormone, insulin-like growth factor-I and the cortisol-cortisone shuttle. *Horm Res.* 2001;56(Suppl 1):1-6. PMID: 11786677

Gelding SV, Taylor NF, Wood PJ, et al. The effect of growth hormone replacement on cortisol-cortisone interconversion in hypopituitary adults: evidence for growth hormone modulation of extrarenal 11-beta-hydroxysteroid dehydrogenase activity. *Clin Endocrinol (Oxf).* 1998;48(2):153-162. PMID: 9579226

Walker SB, Weiss ME, Tattoni DS. Systemic reaction to human growth hormone treated with acute desensitization. *Pediatrics.* 1992;90(1):108-109. PMID: 1614758

Kim SH, Park MJ. Effects of growth hormone on glucose metabolism and insulin resistance in human. *Ann Pediatr Endocrinol Metab.* 2017;22(3):145-152. PMID: 29025199

56

ANSWER: C) DXA scan

Adults with type 1 diabetes mellitus have a significantly increased fracture risk compared with the risk in the general population. Recent studies confirm that children and adolescents with type 1 diabetes also have a higher fracture risk. Multiple studies have demonstrated that children and adolescents with type 1 diabetes have lower bone mineral density than individuals without diabetes and that this correlates with future fracture risk. The bone mass deficit in type 1 diabetes may be present at an early stage after diagnosis. Suboptimally controlled celiac disease is an additional independent risk factor for low bone density. Therefore, fracture risk should contribute to the decision to order a DXA scan (Answer C) to evaluate this patient's bone health.

The existence of a low bone-turnover state, characterized by low circulating levels of both bone-specific alkaline phosphatase and C-terminal telopeptide of type I collagen (Answer A), is important to highlight in children with type 1 diabetes, even with optimal glycemic control. This biochemical picture has also been described in young adults with type 1 diabetes. However, studies on bone turnover status of children and adolescents with type 1 diabetes have produced variable results. These markers vary widely in growing children, and the values for bone-specific alkaline phosphatase and C-terminal telopeptide of type I collagen require adjustment for age and sex.

The low bone turnover state might be a reflection of functional GH resistance that may exist in persons with diabetes, but circulating IGF-1 was not particularly low in the studies. There may be an inverse association between bone formation and hyperglycemia and between bone resorption and the age at diabetes diagnosis. The mechanisms that influence bone turnover in type 1 diabetes are possibly mediated through several pathways. Calcium and vitamin D levels are also usually normal, if not better, in children with type 1 diabetes compared with levels in age-matched controls. Thus, measurement of IGF-1, calcium, and 25-hydroxyvitamin D (Answer B) is incorrect.

Skeletal survey (Answer D) may help to evaluate previously healed or healing fractures and fibrous dysplasia. However, this vignette does not suggest any history of fractures or musculoskeletal symptoms and skeletal survey is therefore not the correct choice.

Recommending no further investigation unless the patient has a second fracture (Answer E) is not a valid strategy because it would delay identifying and managing underlying osteopenia.

Educational Objective
Explain the determinants of bone health and fractures in children with type 1 diabetes mellitus.

Reference(s)

Ching Chen S, Shepherd S, McMillan M, et al. Skeletal fragility and its clinical determinants in children with type 1 diabetes. *J Clin Endocrinol Metab.* 2019;104(8):3585-3594. PMID: 30848792

Vestergaard P. Discrepancies in bone mineral density and fracture risk in patients with type 1 and type 2 diabetes—a meta-analysis. *Osteoporos Int.* 2007;18(4):427-444. PMID: 17068657

Hothersall EJ, Livingstone SJ, Looker HC, et al. Contemporary risk of hip fracture in type 1 and type 2 diabetes: a national registry study from Scotland. *J Bone Miner Res.* 2014;29(5):1054-1060. PMID: 24155126

Weber DR, Haynes K, Leonard MB, Willi SM, Denburg MR. Type 1 diabetes is associated with an increased risk of fracture across the life span: a population-based cohort study using The Health Improvement Network (THIN). *Diabetes Care.* 2015;38(10):1913-1920. PMID: 26216874

Vavanikunnel J, Charlier S, Becker C, et al. Association between glycemic control and risk of fracture in diabetic patients: a nested case-control study. *J Clin Endocrinol Metab.* 2019;104(5):1645-1654. PMID: 30657918

Weber DR, Schwartz G. Epidemiology of skeletal health in type 1 diabetes. *Curr Osteoporos Rep.* 2016;14(6):327-336. PMID: 27744554

57

ANSWER: D) Wean treatment and measure 8-AM serum cortisol

This child most likely has adrenal suppression due to the long history of steroid use. Therefore, stopping treatment (Answer A) is incorrect. Measuring cortisol while being on prednisolone (Answer B) is not helpful, as it will not be detected. There is no clear evidence that alternate-day dosing (Answer C) prevents adrenal suppression. Weaning treatment and measuring serum cortisol (Answer D) is easy and may obviate the need for a standard cosyntropin-stimulation test (Answer E).

Glucocorticoid treatment is the mainstay of treatment for many inflammatory diseases in childhood. Prolonged courses of high-dosage steroids taken orally, transdermally, or inhaled could all result in secondary adrenal suppression. Therefore, clinicians should be cautious and screen at-risk patients for adrenal suppression. When treating inflammatory bowel diseases, a 10-week course of systemic glucocorticoids is frequently prescribed to induce remission, and this treatment can suppress the hypothalamic-pituitary-adrenal axis for up to 1 year. The rates of adrenal insufficiency have been reported to be between 20% and 89% in patients with inflammatory bowel disease. In adults, adrenal suppression has been reported with hydrocortisone dosages of 15 mg/m^2 per day and prednisolone dosages greater than 7.5 mg daily taken for 3 weeks or longer. In children, treatment courses as brief as 2 weeks may result in transient suppression of endogenous cortisol production. Four weeks of glucocorticoid therapy suppresses the hypothalamic-pituitary-adrenal axis for up to 8 weeks after discontinuation.

Central adrenal insufficiency is associated with low blood cortisol and ACTH levels. According to a review by Shulman et al and the Lawson Wilkins Drug and Therapeutics Committee, an 8-AM cortisol concentration of 3 µg/dL (82.8 nmol/L) is suggestive of the diagnosis; a value of 18 µg/dL (496.6 nmol/L) essentially eliminates it. Cutoff values are often debated and may be unit and assay dependent. Woods et al point out the utility of using a single morning cortisol measurement as the first screening step for adrenal suppression in patients with asthma to reduce the need for dynamic testing. Alternative screening methods are also possible, with a standard or low-dose cosyntropin-stimulation test being the most popular.

The timing of testing is important, and different centers have adopted various time points ranging from the final phase of treatment (1 to 5 mg prednisolone daily) to months after the course is completed. Weaning regimens are different depending on the units used. The length of time off glucocorticoids before a blood test is performed is also important and is dependent on the half-life of the glucocorticoid in question.

Educational Objective
Develop an approach to identify and test for adrenal suppression due to exogenous glucocorticoid use.

Reference(s)

Sidoroff M, Kolho KL. Screening for adrenal suppression in children with inflammatory bowel disease discontinuing glucocorticoid therapy. *BMC Gastroenterology*. 2014;14:51. PMID: 24661924

Ahmet A, Mokashi A, Goldbloom EB, et al. Adrenal suppression from glucocorticoids: preventing an iatrogenic cause of morbidity and mortality in children. *BMJ Paediatr Open*. 2019;3(1):e000569. PMID: 31750407

Shulman DI, Palmert MR, Kemp SF; Lawson Wilkins Drug and Therapeutics Committee. Adrenal insufficiency: still a cause of morbidity and death in childhood. *Pediatrics*. 2007;119(2):e484-e494. PMID: 17242136

Goldbloom EB, Mokashi A, Cummings EA, et al. Symptomatic adrenal suppression among children in Canada. *Arch Dis Child*. 2017;102(4):340-345. PMID: 28320817

Woods CP, Argese N, Chapman M, et al. Adrenal suppression in patients taking inhaled glucocorticoids is highly prevalent and management can be guided by morning cortisol. *Eur J Endocrinol*. 2015;173(5):633-642. PMID: 26294794

Wood P, Henderson P. Letter: screening for adrenal suppression in paediatric inflammatory bowel disease. *Aliment Pharmacol Ther*. 2018;48(8):884-885. PMID: 30281831

58 ANSWER: C) Fetal karyotyping by amniocentesis

Prenatal screening that is universally available to screen for multiple genetic or chromosomal disorders can also detect fetuses with Turner syndrome. Such screens include prenatal ultrasonography, which may detect increased nuchal translucency, cystic hygroma, congenital heart defects such as coarctation of the aorta and/or left-sided cardiac defects, brachycephaly, renal anomalies, polyhydramnios, oligohydramnios, and growth retardation. Increased nuchal translucency seen in first-trimester ultrasonography and left-sided heart defects are common in fetuses with Turner syndrome or autosomal trisomy syndromes. However, prenatal ultrasonography and triple or quadruple marker first-trimester screening can be normal in such cases, so normal results from these assessments cannot be used to reassure patients (Answer A) when results from cell-free DNA screening are abnormal.

Noninvasive prenatal screening using cell-free DNA extracted from maternal blood is increasingly used to screen for many genetic disorders. It performs well in detecting trisomy 21, 18, and 13 and can also detect sex chromosome aneuploidy. However, currently available cell-free DNA screening has a very low positive predictive value (23%) for Turner syndrome and thus positive results should be confirmed with diagnostic testing prenatally or postnatally. Fetal karyotyping by chorionic villus sampling (10-13 weeks' gestation) (Answer D) or amniocentesis (15-18 weeks' gestation) (Answer C) should be offered to confirm the diagnosis before making irreversible decisions (Answer E) relative to the pregnancy outcome. Repeating the cell-free DNA screen (Answer B) will not determine the diagnosis or help with guiding the next management step. Given the gestational age in this case, amniocentesis is the most appropriate diagnostic test to recommend. Amniocentesis is associated with a low risk of complications such as leakage of amniotic fluid, infection, needle injury to the fetus, and miscarriage. It is important to note that the patient may choose not to undergo any further testing, but rather to continue the pregnancy to term and consider further testing postnatally.

Turner syndrome is a common chromosomal disorder with varying genotypes and phenotypes. It is characterized by complete or partial absence of the second sex chromosome with or without mosaicism in phenotypic females. Common genotypes leading to Turner syndrome include monosomy 45,X (45%-50% of all patients with Turner syndrome); varying degrees of 45,X/46,XX mosaicism (15%-25%); 45,X/46,XY mixed gonadal dysgenesis with a female phenotype (10%-12%); 46,Xi(Xq) or 46,X,idic(Xp) isochromosome Xq or isodicentric Xp (10%); and 45,X/47,XXX or 45,X/46,XX/47,XXX mosaicism with triple X (3%). Patients with small microdeletions of Xp22.3, Xq24 deletion or isodicentric Xq24, or 45,X/46,XY gonadal dysgenesis with a male phenotype are not diagnosed with Turner syndrome.

Educational Objective
Explain the advantages and limitations of various prenatal screening options for Turner syndrome.

Reference(s)
Gravholt CH, Andersen NH, Conway GS, et al; International Turner Syndrome Consensus Group. Clinical practice guidelines for the care of girls and women with Turner syndrome: proceedings from the 2016 Cincinnati International Turner Syndrome Meeting. *Eur J Endocrinol*. 2017;177(3):G1-G70. PMID: 28705803

Wang Y, Li S, Wang W, et al. Cell-free DNA screening for sex chromosome aneuploidies by non-invasive prenatal testing in maternal plasma. *Mol Cytogenet*. 2020;13:10. PMID: 32190123

Meck JM, Dugan EK, Matyakhina L, et al. Noninvasive prenatal screening for aneuploidy: positive predictive values based on cytogenetic findings. *Am J Obstet Gynecol*. 2015;213(2):214.e1-e5. PMID: 25843063

59 ANSWER: C) Free T$_4$, normal; total T$_3$, low; reverse T$_3$, high; high-output heart failure

The infant in this vignette has the classic presentation of consumptive hypothyroidism due to excess iodothyronine deiodinase type 3 enzyme activity, associated with large liver hemangiomas, which express this enzyme. This condition typically manifests in early infancy in babies who harbor a large tumor with high enzyme activity, either with a few large hemangiomas or multiple smaller hemangiomas that overcome the thyroid gland's ability to compensate. TSH levels can range from mildly elevated to concentrations greater than 500 mIU/L. The mechanism was first elucidated in 2000, only after the index patient had died and his hemangioma tissue was analyzed. Type 3 deiodinase is normally present in the brain and placenta, and it catalyzes the conversion of T$_4$ to reverse T$_3$ and the conversion of T$_3$ to 3,3'-diiodothyronine, both of which are biologically inactive.

Heart failure in such cases is high-output failure due to decreased peripheral vascular resistance that occurs because of large arteriovenous shunts in the hemangiomas. Affected patients may also have consumptive coagulopathy depending on the size of the hemangiomas. As noted in the initial report, cardiac impairment from hypothyroidism can exacerbate the congestive heart failure associated with high-flow hemangiomas. Therefore, due to the deiodinase activity, such patients have elevated reverse T$_3$ and low or low-normal T$_4$ and T$_3$, depending on the severity of the hypothyroidism. Thus, the most representative option is Answer C.

Answers B and E list low reverse T$_3$. Answer D lists high total T$_3$ and low-output heart failure. Answer A would be correct as far as the thyroid hormone profile is concerned; however, it lists low-output heart failure.

Due to the inactivation of the thyroid hormones T$_4$ and T$_3$, such patients require higher levothyroxine dosages than would normally be required to treat congenital or acquired hypothyroidism (sometimes given twice daily, and sometimes adding liothyronine) and thus the name *consumptive hypothyroidism*.

Educational Objective
Anticipate that consumptive hypothyroidism can cause high-output heart failure.

Reference(s)
Huang SA, Tu HM, Harney JW, et al. Severe hypothyroidism caused by type 3 iodothyronine deiodinase in infantile hemangiomas. *N Engl J Med*. 2000;343(3):185-189. PMID: 10900278

Kim EH, Koh KN, Park M, Kim BE, Im HJ, Seo JJ. Clinical features of infantile hepatic hemangioendothelioma. *Korean J Pediatr*. 2011;54(6):260-266. PMID: 21949521

Emir S, Ekici F, İkiz MA, Vidinlisan S. The association of consumptive hypothyroidism secondary to hepatic hemangioma and severe heart failure in infancy. *Turk Pediatri Ars*. 2016;51(1):52-56. PMID: 27103866

60

ANSWER: A) Increased leptin, increased insulin, suppressed ghrelin

Hypothalamic obesity is a frequent complication following craniopharyngioma treatment, occurring in up to 50% of patients. In addition to craniopharyngiomas, central nervous system trauma, cranial irradiation, certain genetic conditions, and suprasellar tumors are other etiologies that can lead to hypothalamic damage and dysfunction. The hypothalamus has a critical role in energy homeostasis. Children who develop hypothalamic obesity are usually hyperphagic with impaired satiety. Even if attempts are made at caloric restriction, they demonstrate significant weight gain in the first year after treatment, followed by maintenance of a higher body weight, which is most likely due to alterations in feeding regulation and low energy expenditure. There is altered neural regulation of pancreatic β cells, which leads to increased insulin secretion. This chronic hyperinsulinemia causes increased production of leptin and suppression of ghrelin (Answer A). Leptin levels positively correlate with amount of body fat; thus, individuals with excess adiposity, regardless of cause, have higher leptin levels than do lean individuals. However, when corrected for BMI, leptin levels remain higher in patients with hypothalamic obesity than in those with simple obesity, indicating more severe leptin resistance in these patients.

Congenital leptin deficiency causes very severe early-life obesity characterized by hyperphagia. These patients also have hypogonadotropic hypogonadism and exhibit insulin resistance, not insulin sensitivity. Hyperinsulinemia is the presence of elevated circulating levels of insulin in the blood. Insulin resistance refers to the diminished capacity of cells to respond to circulating insulin. Hyperinsulinemia is commonly seen in the setting of insulin resistance since the pancreas has to produce more insulin in order to maintain glucose homeostasis; however, this is not always the case. Hypersecretion of insulin has been demonstrated in hypothalamic obesity, but many affected patients have normal fasting insulin levels and have been shown to be insulin sensitive, rather than insulin resistant. There is a subset of patients who, in addition to their hypothalamic obesity, also have features of metabolic syndrome, including insulin resistance. Patients with Prader-Willi syndrome have hyperleptinemia similar to what is observed in patients with hypothalamic obesity. Patients with Prader-Willi syndrome show heightened insulin sensitivity compared with what is observed in other obesity conditions. Unlike hypothalamic obesity, however, patients with Prader-Willi have significantly increased ghrelin levels, both fasting and postprandial.

Educational Objective

Identify the alterations in leptin and insulin that occur in patients with hypothalamic obesity.

Reference(s)

Abuzzahab MJ, Roth CL, Shoemaker AH. Hypothalamic obesity: prologue and promise. *Horm Res Paediatr.* 2019;91(2):128-136. PMID: 30884480

Kim JH, Choi JH. Pathophysiology and clinical characteristics of hypothalamic obesity in children and adolescents. *Ann Pediatr Endocrinol Metab.* 2013;18(4):161-167. PMID: 24904871

61

ANSWER: B) Inactivating variant in *CASR*

This patient most likely has familial hypocalciuric hypercalcemia secondary to a heterozygous inactivating pathogenic variant in *CASR* (Answer B). This autosomal dominant condition most often presents with asymptomatic hypercalcemia and an inappropriately elevated or normal PTH, but low urinary calcium excretion. However, it can also present with symptomatic hypercalcemia in the neonatal period, most often when inherited from the father, and is termed neonatal hyperparathyroidism. It is hypothesized that in utero, the fetus's calcium-sensing receptors at the parathyroid glands sense relative hypocalcemia (maternal calcium is actively transported across the placenta) and increase PTH secretion. Medical intervention with hyperhydration, bisphosphonates, and/or cinacalcet is the preferred treatment during infancy, with patients becoming asymptomatic as they grow older despite a higher serum calcium concentration (altered set point). Despite hypercalcemia, affected individuals do not develop nephrocalcinosis because the calcium-sensing receptor present in the thick ascending loop of Henle functions independently of PTH to resorb calcium and maintain the higher serum concentrations. As magnesium is also reabsorbed at the renal tubule through the action of the calcium-sensing receptor, hypermagnesemia is another common finding.

Infants with homozygous or compound heterozygous pathogenic variants in *CASR* can present with severe neonatal hyperparathyroidism with calcium levels as high as 30 mg/dL (7.5 mmol/L). Severe bone disease manifesting as rickets and multiple fractures can also be present. Generally, these patients require total parathyroidectomy, but often surgical intervention can be delayed with the above medical management. The management of postsurgical hypoparathyroidism is slightly different for these patients, as serum calcium levels can be maintained in the normal range given the low concern for nephrocalcinosis.

Activating pathogenic variants in *PTH1R* (Answer A) result in hypercalcemia with low PTH and hypercalciuria and also have skeletal manifestations of short-limbed dwarfism (metaphyseal chondrodysplasia, Jansen type). Ninety percent of patients with inactivating pathogenic variants in *MEN1* (Answer C) develop hyperparathyroidism, but this is secondary to parathyroid adenomas and generally does not present until the second or third decade of life. Inactivating variants in *CYP24A1* (Answer D) and deletion of the *ELN* gene on chromosome 7 (Answer E) result in hypercalcemia with suppressed PTH. Deletion of the long arm of chromosome 7, including the region where the elastin gene (*ELN*) is located, is the cause of Williams syndrome. Additionally, patients with Williams syndrome often have distinctive facial features (broad forehead, short nose with broad tip, wide mouth with full lips) and supravalvular aortic stenosis. Inactivation of 24-hydroxylase (*CYP24A1)* results in elevated levels of 25-hydroxyvitamin D and 1,25-dihydroxyvitamin D. Affected patients can develop nephrocalcinosis.

Educational Objective
Identify inactivating pathogenic variants in the *CASR* gene as a cause of severe hyperparathyroidism in neonates and describe how this can resolve with medical treatment.

Reference(s)
Marx SJ, Sinaii N. Neonatal severe hyperparathyroidism: novel insights from calcium, PTH, and the CASR gene. *J Clin Endocrinol Metab.* 2020;105(4):1061-1078. PMID: 31778168

Cole DE, Janicic N, Salisbury SR, Hendy GN. Neonatal severe hyperparathyroidism, secondary hyperparathyroidism, and familial hypocalciuric hypercalcemia: multiple different phenotypes associated with an inactivating Alu insertion mutation of the calcium-sensing receptor gene. *Am J Med Genet.* 1997;71(2):202-210. PMID: 9217223

62 ANSWER: C) Start oral methimazole
This adolescent with Down syndrome (trisomy 21) has hyperthyroidism due to Graves disease based on his elevated thyroid-stimulating immunoglobulin. Children with Down syndrome are at increased risk for autoimmune conditions, primarily thyroiditis. Hashimoto thyroiditis is more common than Graves disease in this population. In children without Down syndrome, Graves disease is more common in females, but this is not the case in patients with Down syndrome. Pediatric patients with Down syndrome tend to develop Graves disease at a younger age than do children in the general pediatric population.

While thyroidectomy (Answer A) and radioactive iodine (Answer E) are definitive therapies for Graves disease and are valid choices, they are not the best next step in this setting. The American Thyroid Association guidelines indicate that children with Graves disease may be treated with methimazole, radioactive iodine, or thyroidectomy. In choosing the initial treatment, age, clinical status, and likelihood of remission should be considered. Because some patients will go into remission, methimazole (Answer C) is still considered first-line treatment for most children. Since this child has no goiter and has mild hyperthyroidism, he would most likely benefit from methimazole, as recommended for most children with Graves disease.

This child has no tachycardia, no complaints of palpitations, and no hypertension, so propranolol (Answer B) is not indicated. When a β-adrenergic blocker is needed, it should be used in addition to methimazole. This patient is symptomatic and losing weight, and Graves disease is unlikely to resolve spontaneously. Therefore, observing him and repeating thyroid function tests (Answer D) is incorrect.

Although children and adolescents with Down syndrome are at higher risk of developing acute leukemia (in adolescents it would be lymphoblastic leukemia) than children in the general population, there is no increased risk of leukemia described in patients with Down syndrome on methimazole. Higher doses of radioactive iodine, as used to treat well-differentiated thyroid cancer (>100 mCi in adults), have been associated with an increased risk of leukemia, but no such risk has been observed with the ^{131}I doses used for Graves disease. Radioactive iodine use has been reported in children with Down syndrome and Graves disease (in those older than 5 years just like in the general population, due to possible/theoretical risk of cancer in children younger than 5 years). As with surgery, ^{131}I is not considered first-line therapy, but it is a valid option.

Older children and adolescents with Down syndrome may have lymphopenia (both B and T cells), but they are not at higher risk for agranulocytosis due to methimazole than are patients with Graves disease who do not have Down syndrome. Therefore, as in other children and adolescents with Graves disease, methimazole is usually first-line therapy. One could prescribe a β-adrenergic blocker such as propranolol, or atenolol (in case of asthma) if the patient develops palpitations before methimazole is effectively controlling the hyperthyroidism, which usually takes 1 to 2 months. One publication (De Luca et al) suggests that children with Down syndrome are more likely to go into remission than children without Down syndrome, but another smaller series (Goday-Arno et al) does not support that finding. Because this patient has mild hyperthyroidism, a modest methimazole dosage may be started in the range of 5 to 10 mg twice daily (or given as 10-20 mg once daily, as used in adults), which would reduce the likelihood of adverse effects. Once his hyperthyroidism is controlled, the methimazole dosage can be decreased and administered once daily to achieve better adherence.

Educational Objective
Identify important considerations in the management of children with Graves disease and trisomy 21.

Reference(s)

Ross DS, Burch HB, Cooper DS, et al. 2016 American Thyroid Association guidelines for diagnosis and management of hyperthyroidism and other causes of thyrotoxicosis. *Thyroid*. 2016;26(10):1343-1421. PMID: 27521067

De Luca F, Corrias A, Salerno M, et al. Peculiarities of Graves' disease in children and adolescents with Down's syndrome. *Eur J Endocrinol*. 2010;162(3):591-595. PMID: 19955260

Goday-Arno A, Cerda-Esteva M, Flores-Le-Roux JA, Chillaron-Jordan JJ, Corretger JM, Cano-Pérez JF. Hyperthyroidism in a population with Down syndrome (DS). *Clin Endocrinol (Oxf)*. 2009;71(1):110-114. PMID: 18793345

Roberts I, Izraeli S. Haematopoietic development and leukaemia in Down syndrome. *Br J Haematol*. 2014;167(5):587-599. PMID: 25155832

63 ANSWER: C) Baseline 17-hydroxyprogesterone measurement

The most likely diagnosis in this child is premature adrenarche, which is diagnosed by clinical evaluation and exclusion of alternative adrenal pathologies. Premature adrenarche is due to the premature activation of the zona reticularis of the adrenal gland, which results in increased adrenal androgens, most notably DHEA and DHEA-S. One of the main differential diagnoses is nonclassic congenital adrenal hyperplasia. A baseline 17-hydroxyprogesterone value less than 200 ng/dL (<6.1 nmol/L) is reported to have 100% sensitivity to exclude nonclassic congenital adrenal hyperplasia. Cutoff values may vary depending on differences in hormonal assays used at different centers. Measuring 17-hydroxyprogesterone (Answer C) is the most appropriate next step.

In some circumstances (mild symptoms without progression), physicians may choose to follow the child clinically with or without measurement of bone age. In this vignette, there was clinical progression, so further investigations were warranted. Bone age measurement can be helpful, and some clinicians recommend further evaluation if bone age is more than 2 years advanced for a patient's given chronologic age. However, advanced bone age is common in premature adrenarche.

With more frequent use of liquid chromatography–tandem mass spectrometry, increases in alternative steroids such as circulating 11-oxygenated androgens have been described in patients with premature adrenarche. 11-Ketotestosterone may be the dominant circulating bioactive androgen that results in the clinical features seen in premature adrenarche.

Urinary steroid profiles (Answer E) are increasingly being used for the diagnosis of disorders of steroidogenesis, and with growing availability, this assessment will no doubt have clinical utility in the exclusion of other disorders of hyperandrogenism.

Adrenal ultrasonography (Answer A) could be used to assist in the diagnosis of an adrenal tumor, although the study is user dependent. In this child with mild androgenization, the diagnosis is unlikely.

The lack of breast development on clinical examination rules out central precocious puberty, so LH measurement (Answer B) is not necessary at this point.

Measuring TSH (Answer D) could diagnose severe primary hypothyroidism, which has been associated with pseudoprecocious puberty (frequently with delayed bone age) presenting with breast development, galactorrhea, and menarche. This is also referred to as Van Wyk-Grumbach syndrome. The mechanism leading to pseudoprecocious puberty in this setting is not entirely clear, although it is thought to be due to extremely high TSH acting on the FSH receptor, which stimulates the gonads. Clinically, this child does not have breast development; rather, she has advanced bone age and increased height velocity. Thus, Van Wyk-Grumbach syndrome is an unlikely diagnosis and TSH measurement is not the best next step.

Although premature adrenarche is considered a benign variant of maturation that is more common in girls than in boys and is associated with higher BMI, increased susceptibility to polycystic ovary syndrome and insulin resistance have been described in adults. Furthermore, rare disorders can present as premature adrenarche such as cortisone reductase deficiency due to inactivating pathogenic variants in the gene encoding the enzyme hexose-6-phosphate dehydrogenase and cortisone reductase deficiency due to inactivating pathogenic variants in the *HSD11B1* gene. Finally, a recent study highlighted that premature adrenarche is more common among black girls than among white girls and other racial groups. In black patients with premature adrenarche, the age at presentation is younger and there is a lower incidence of organic pathology. Hence, the age definition of premature adrenarche (<8 years in girls and <9 years in boys) may not be appropriate for patients of African American descent, and management may need to be stratified to account for ethnic background.

Educational Objective
Diagnose premature adrenarche and explain why classic definitions may not necessarily be appropriate for all ethnic groups.

Reference(s)

Grandone A, Marzuillo P, Luongo C, et al. Basal levels of 17-hydroxyprogesterone can distinguish children with isolated precocious pubarche. *Pediatr Res.* 2018;84(4):533-536. PMID: 29976972

Rege J, Turcu AF, Kasa-Vubu JZ, et al. 11-Ketotestosterone is the dominant circulating bioactive androgen during normal and premature adrenarche. *J Clin Endocrinol Metab.* 2018;103(12):4589-4598. PMID: 30137510

Lavery GG, Idkowiak J, Sherlock M, et al. Novel H6PDH mutations in two girls with premature adrenarche: 'apparent' and 'true' CRD can be differentiated by urinary steroid profiling. *Eur J Endocrinol.* 2013;168(2):K19-K26. PMID: 23132696

DeSalvo DJ, Mehra R, Vaidyanathan P, Kaplowitz PB. In children with premature adrenarche, bone age advancement by 2 or more years is common and generally benign. *J Pediatr Endocrinol Metab.* 2013;26(3-4):215-221. PMID: 23744298

Şiklar Z, Öçal G, Adiyaman P, Ergur A, Berberoğlu M. Functional ovarian hyperandrogenism and polycystic ovary syndrome in prepubertal girls with obesity and/or premature pubarche. *J Pediatr Endocrinol Metab.* 2007;20(4):475-481. PMID: 17550211

Foster C, Diaz-Thomas A, Lahoti A. Low prevalence of organic pathology in a predominantly black population with premature adrenarche: need to stratify definitions and screening protocols. *Int J Pediatr Endocrinol.* 2020;2020:5. PMID: 32165891

64 ANSWER: E) Initiation of cabergoline and counseling for psychiatric disturbance

This patient has hyperprolactinemia and an area of hypoenhancement of the pituitary measuring less than 10 mm, which is most consistent with a microprolactinoma. Prolactin-secreting tumors account for approximately 40% of all pituitary adenomas. Prolactinomas are rare in childhood, but the incidence increases in adolescence. Reproductive disturbances (amenorrhea and galactorrhea in girls and pubertal delay and hypogonadism in boys) are the most common presentation.

Dopamine agonist therapy is recommended to lower prolactin levels, decrease tumor size, and restore gonadal function in patients with a microprolactinoma and symptoms of hyperprolactinemia, including hypogonadism (infertility, oligomenorrhea, galactorrhea, low bone density). Cabergoline is a long-acting dopamine agonist that is generally recommended over bromocriptine because of better tolerance and greater efficacy in all endpoints. It should be noted that safety and efficacy have not been established in the pediatric population.

Onset or exacerbation of impulse control disorders have been recognized as an adverse effect of dopamine agonist therapy, occurring in 17% of patients treated with cabergoline for prolactinoma in one uncontrolled study of 308 adult patients. A case study documented psychiatric disturbance in several children with prolactinoma treated with cabergoline at a median dosage of 0.5 mg weekly (range 0.25-2.0 mg weekly). In several patients, this necessitated a reduced cabergoline dosage. Given the potential risk of psychiatric disturbance with cabergoline treatment, patients should be counseled regarding this risk when starting treatment (Answer E).

Diagnosis of hyperprolactinemia in an individual with a suspected prolactinoma is straightforward. The Endocrine Society guidelines recommend a single measurement of prolactin obtained without excessive venipuncture stress, as a single prolactin measurement is highly sensitive for hyperprolactinemia. Serial dilution of serum samples is recommended if there is a discrepancy between a large pituitary tumor and mildly elevated prolactin. This eliminates artifact with immunoradiometric assays that can lead to a falsely low prolactin value ("hook effect"). However, dynamic testing of prolactin secretion (Answer A) has not been shown to be superior to measurement of a single serum prolactin measurement.

It is reasonable to defer treatment and monitor microadenomas that are not causing symptoms, as most microadenomas do not increase in size over time. However, the patient in this case has oligomenorrhea and low estradiol, so repeating prolactin measurement and brain MRI without initiating treatment (Answer C) is incorrect.

Visual field deficits are a concern in patients presenting with macroadenoma due to compression of the optic chiasm. However, the presence of visual field defects in individuals with microadenomas would not be expected, as the tumor does not extend beyond the sella. As such, a neuro-ophthalmology examination (Answer B) is not required.

Dopamine agonists are well known to cause fibrotic valvulopathy in a dose-dependent manner and most microadenomas respond to cabergoline dosages well under 2 mg weekly. As there is low risk of cabergoline-associated valvulopathy at dosages used to treat macroprolactinomas, only patients taking a cabergoline dosage greater than 2 mg weekly require annual echocardiography (Answer D). Echocardiography before commencing dopamine agonist therapy followed by echocardiography at 5 years is recommended for patients taking a cabergoline dosage of 2 mg weekly or lower.

Educational Objective
Identify potential precautions and adverse effects associated with dopamine agonist therapy.

Reference(s)
Melmed S, Casanueva FF, Hoffman AR, et al; Endocrine Society. Diagnosis and treatment of hyperprolactinemia: an Endocrine Society clinical practice guideline. *J Clin Endocrinol Metab.* 2011;96(2):273-288. PMID: 21296991

Brichta CM, Wurm M, Krebs A, Schwab KO, van der Werf-Grohmann N. Start low, go slowly - mental abnormalities in young prolactinoma patients under cabergoline therapy. *J Pediatr Endocrinol Metab.* 2019;32(9):969-977. PMID: 31323004

Steeds R, Stiles C, Sharma V, Chambers J, Lloyd G, Drake W. Echocardiography and monitoring patients receiving dopamine agonist therapy for hyperprolactinaemia: a joint position statement of the British Society of Echocardiography, the British Heart Valve Society and the Society for Endocrinology. *Clin Endocrinol.* 2019;90(5):662-669. PMID: 30818417

65 ANSWER: A) Brain MRI

This patient has diencephalic syndrome, which is a rare cause of profound emaciation in infancy characterized by significant absence of subcutaneous tissue despite normal caloric intake. Affected patients do not have vomiting, hepatomegaly, or abnormal liver function tests as observed in patients with loss of subcutaneous tissue due to generalized lipodystrophy. This condition was first described by Russell in 1951. Linear growth is usually maintained or only minimally affected in these children. Other features that can be observed in some children with diencephalic syndrome include hyperkinesis, emesis, and ophthalmologic findings such as nystagmus, optic pallor, or papilledema. Affected children usually attain developmental milestones appropriate for age. Some have hydrocephalus. A high index of suspicion should prompt brain MRI (Answer A), which would demonstrate tumor near the anterior hypothalamus and occasionally a brain tumor in the posterior fossa. Treatment considerations are focused on reducing the tumor burden.

Differential diagnosis of failure to thrive during infancy is broad. However, this child has normal linear growth, no history of hypoglycemia, normal electrolytes and glucose, normal thyroid function, and a normal GH concentration. Thus, adrenal insufficiency or other endocrinopathies are less likely to be the cause of poor weight gain. Cortisol measurement and cosyntropin-stimulation testing (Answer B) are not necessary. The baby is happy and interactive with normal development and no history of fractures. Therefore, there is no need to obtain a skeletal survey (Answer C) or bone age x-ray (Answer D). Referral to gastroenterology (Answer E) will only delay the diagnosis and treatment and hence is not the best next step in this patient's care.

Educational Objective
Identify the characteristic clinical features of diencephalic syndrome as a cause of failure to thrive in young children.

Reference(s)
Fleischman A, Brue C, Poussaint TY, et al. Diencephalic syndrome: a cause of failure to thrive and a model of partial growth hormone resistance. *Pediatrics.* 2005;115(6):e742-e748. PMID: 15930202

Brauner R, Trivin C, Zerah M, et al. Diencephalic syndrome due to hypothalamic tumor: a model of the relationship between weight and puberty onset. *J Clin Endocrinol Metab.* 2006;91(7):2467-2473. PMID: 16621905

66

ANSWER: A) Elevated serum reverse T₃

This infant presents at 6 weeks of age with primary hypothyroidism that was not present on newborn screening, suggesting a postnatally acquired cause. His findings of marked hepatomegaly and a cutaneous hemangioma suggest that the most likely cause is the presence of massive hepatic hemangiomas. These vascular lesions highly express type 3 deiodinase (D3), an enzyme that converts both T_4 and T_3 to the inactive metabolites reverse T_3 and T_2, respectively. Massive hemangiomas, which occur most often in the liver, can express sufficient amounts of D3 to produce consumptive hypothyroidism, which is characterized by elevated levels of reverse T_3 (Answer A), low levels of T_3 (not elevated [Answer C]), and, when severe, low levels of T_4. Serum thyroglobulin levels are increased (not low [Answer B]) due to stimulation by elevated TSH. Because of the rapid degradation of circulating thyroid hormones, management consists of levothyroxine at high dosages, sometimes given twice daily due to its shortened serum half-life. Replacement of T_3 also may be required in severe cases. Hemangiomas can cause severe complications including cardiac failure, but they usually regress over time, leading to resolution of consumptive hypothyroidism.

Exposure to excess iodine—such as from topical iodine antiseptics, iodinated radiocontrast agents, or maternal iodine ingestion—can cause acquired hypothyroidism in infancy. In such cases, the urinary iodine concentration is elevated (Answer E). However, hepatomegaly is not characteristic of iodine-induced hypothyroidism, and there is no history of excess iodine exposure in this case.

Maternal transfer of TSH-receptor antibodies that block TSH-receptor signaling (Answer D) is a rare cause of congenital hypothyroidism, which is unlikely in this patient with a normal newborn screen. Congenital hypothyroidism may be missed on newborn screening due to problems with the screening sample (including obtaining the sample after blood transfusion) or in infants who are preterm, of low birth weight, or are monozygotic twins; however, none of these risk factors is present in this case. Although a sample-handling error cannot be excluded based on the information provided, the physical findings in this patient are not typical of congenital hypothyroidism.

Educational Objective

Diagnose consumptive hypothyroidism based on clinical findings and identify the laboratory abnormalities associated with this diagnosis.

Reference(s)

Huang SA, Tu HM, Harney JW, et al. Severe hypothyroidism caused by type 3 iodothyronine deiodinase in infantile hemangiomas. *N Engl J Med*. 2000;343(3):185-189.
PMID: 10900278

67

ANSWER: D) Syndrome of inappropriate antidiuresis

This hospitalized child who is undergoing treatment for acute lymphoblastic leukemia presented with hyponatremia and bacteremia. His blood pressure and heart rate were normal and there was no evidence of edema on examination, which together suggest a euvolemic state. Hyponatremia occurs commonly in hospitalized patients and has many contributing factors. The kidney's ability to generate and excrete free water is the primary way the body defends against developing hyponatremia. With normal renal function, it is rare to develop hyponatremia from excess water ingestion, due to the ability of the kidneys to excrete large volumes of free water. Similarly, it is rare to develop hyponatremia from large renal losses alone without an excess of free water ingestion. It is arginine vasopressin (AVP), released from the posterior pituitary, that increases water permeability in the collecting tubules of the kidney. In addition to increases in serum osmolality, AVP release can be stimulated by both hemodynamic stimuli (eg, volume depletion, hypotension, congestive heart failure, nephrotic syndrome, adrenal insufficiency, liver cirrhosis) and nonhemodynamic stimuli (eg, pain, stress, nausea, vomiting, medications, central nervous system disease, pulmonary disease, perioperative state, inflammation).

Syndrome of inappropriate antidiuresis (SIAD) is a common cause of hyponatremia in hospitalized children. Patients with SIAD have hypotonic hyponatremia caused by impaired free water excretion due to excess AVP secretion from nonphysiologic stimuli, in the absence of endocrine or renal dysfunction. There are numerous causes of SIAD, but in children it most often results from central nervous system disorders, pulmonary disorders, malignancy, and medications (most commonly the anticonvulsant drugs carbamazepine and oxcarbazepine and the chemotherapeutic agents vincristine and cyclophosphamide). Patients with SIAD are typically euvolemic or have mild volume expansion. However, volume status is often difficult to assess accurately; therefore, SIAD is generally a diagnosis of exclusion. While there is no specific diagnostic test to confirm SIAD, hypouricemia with an elevated fractional excretion of urate is highly suggestive of SIAD. Other hallmarks of SIAD include mild volume expansion with low to normal plasma concentrations of creatinine, urea, uric acid, and potassium; impaired free water excretion with normal sodium excretion that reflects sodium intake; and hyponatremia that is relatively unresponsive to giving sodium without concomitant fluid restriction. Measurement of AVP or copeptin is not useful. Useful biochemical markers in adults include a spot urine sodium concentration greater than 30 mEq/L (>30 mmol/L), fractional excretion of sodium greater than 0.5%, fractional excretion of urea greater than 55%, fractional excretion of urate greater than 11%, and plasma uric acid less than 4 mg/dL (<237.9 μmol/L).

In the workup of hyponatremia, it is important to distinguish true hypoosmolality from pseudohyponatremia (seen with hyperproteinemia or severe hyperlipidemia) or translocational hyponatremia (seen with hyperglycemia, mannitol, hypertonic radiocontrast). Urine osmolality should be measured to determine whether there is impaired free water clearance. Diseases causing decreased circulating volume, renal impairment, adrenal insufficiency, and hypothyroidism must be excluded. The patient in this vignette appears to be euvolemic. He has hyponatremia with true hypoosmolality. His serum uric acid concentration is very low and his urinary sodium excretion is elevated. Although he has bacteremia, his vital signs are not suggestive of sepsis. Therefore, he most likely has SIAD (Answer D) associated with vincristine chemotherapy.

Severe hypertriglyceridemia causes pseudohyponatremia. While this child does have an elevated triglyceride concentration (Answer A), it is not high enough to cause this degree of hyponatremia.

Cerebral/renal salt wasting (Answer B) can be very difficult to distinguish from SIAD, but it would be a more likely etiology if there were evidence of circulatory volume depletion.

Hospitalized patients are at risk of developing hyponatremia if given excessive hypotonic fluids (Answer C). However, this patient was receiving isotonic fluids at a maintenance rate.

Cortisol insufficiency (Answer E) can be associated with SIAD, as glucocorticoids have an inhibitory effect on AVP synthesis. Although this child has a very low cortisol level, this is most likely due to adrenal suppression from the dexamethasone he is currently receiving.

Educational Objective
Identify characteristic clinical and laboratory findings in patients with syndrome of inappropriate antidiuretic hormone secretion.

Reference(s)
Moritz ML. Syndrome of inappropriate antidiuresis. *Pediatr Clin North Am.* 2019;66(1):209-226. PMID: 30454744

Cuesta M, Thompson CJ. The syndrome of inappropriate antidiuresis (SIAD). *Best Pract Res Clin Endocrinol Metab.* 2016;30(2):175-187. PMID: 27156757

68 **ANSWER: C) Start oxandrolone at a dosage of 0.03 mg/kg daily and maintain the current GH dosage**
GH therapy is approved for the management of short stature associated with Turner syndrome, which is usually not due to GH deficiency. Early initiation of GH therapy leads to better final height outcomes than late treatment. Clinical guidelines suggest starting GH around age 4 to 6 years and certainly before age 12 to 13 years. A decline in growth velocity in a patient with Turner syndrome may also be considered as a reason to start treatment at an even earlier age. The GH dosage recommended for Turner syndrome (45-50 mcg/kg daily or 0.315-0.35 mg/kg weekly) is higher than the dosage recommended to treat GH deficiency (25-34 mcg/kg daily or 0.18-0.24 mg/kg weekly). Nevertheless, surveillance of dosage adequacy with measurement of IGF-1 is recommended to avoid overdosing as manifested by an elevated IGF-1 SDS (>+2.0). Therefore, increasing the GH dosage to 0.35 mg/kg weekly (Answer A) is not the preferred strategy given that this patient already has an IGF-1 SDS above +2.0 while receiving a GH dosage lower than that which is recommended for this condition.

Girls with Turner syndrome whose karyotype shows a 45,X complement without mosaicism also have gonadal dysgenesis with lack of pubertal development and lack of estrogen secretion. Sex steroids have a synergistic effect with endogenous GH on linear growth during pubertal development. However, at the same time, estrogen advances growth plate fusion, thus limiting the duration of linear growth. Initiation of estrogen replacement in girls with Turner syndrome, who do not have spontaneous puberty, is recommended around age 11 or 12 years with transdermal estradiol being the preferred route of administration. Starting estrogen at an earlier age (Answer B) may induce undue advancement in skeletal maturation with subsequent limitation of growth potential. Initiation of ultra-low estrogen dosages at an earlier age has been proposed, but this intervention has not reached the consensus guidelines. However, it has been shown that delaying the initiation of estrogen replacement to a later age such as 14 or 16 years (Answer E) does not have an additional beneficial effect on final height as initially thought. This may actually have a negative psychosocial impact because of lack of pubertal changes at this critical age.

Androgens have a positive effect on linear growth during puberty. While estrogens may have a similar role, they also exert a negative impact on final height as a result of their effect on growth plate maturation and fusion. Aromatase inhibitors (Answer D) are capable of blocking the conversion of androgens into estrogens. Hence, the use of aromatase inhibitors has been proposed for the management of short stature in boys in early puberty, but there is no FDA approval for this indication. Aromatase inhibitors would not have this effect in a prepubertal girl with Turner syndrome whose endogenous estrogen production is most likely insignificant.

Oxandrolone (Answer C) is a synthetic anabolic steroid that has been used for the treatment of constitutional delay of growth and puberty, as it induces secondary sexual characteristics, including an increase in height velocity. It is nonaromatizable and, therefore, does not lead to an increase in estrogen levels that would induce growth plate maturation and fusion. Oxandrolone has been shown to increase the final height of girls with Turner syndrome who are treated with GH. The recommended age of initiation is around 10 years and the recommended dosage is 0.03 mg/kg daily and maintained below 0.05 mg/kg daily. In some studies, higher dosages are possibly associated with some degree of virilization.

Educational Objective
List the benefits and caveats of oxandrolone in the management of short stature in girls with Turner syndrome.

Reference(s)

Gault EJ, Cole TJ, Casey S, et al. Effect of oxandrolone and timing of pubertal induction on final height in Turner Syndrome: final analysis of the UK randomized placebo-controlled trial. *Arch Dis Child.* 2019 [Epub ahead of print] PMID: 31862699

Gravholt CH, Andersen NH, Conway GS, et al; International Turner Syndrome Consensus Group. Clinical practice guidelines for the care of girls and women with Turner syndrome: proceedings from the 2016 Cincinnati International Turner Syndrome Meeting. *Eur J Endocrinol.* 2017;177(3):G1-G70. PMID: 28705803

Klein KO, Rosenfield R, Santen RJ, et al. Estrogen replacement in Turner syndrome: literature review and practical considerations. *J Clin Endocrinol Metab.* 2018;103(5):1790-1803. PMID: 29438552

Ross JL, Quigley CA, Cao D, et al. Growth hormone plus childhood low-dose estrogen in Turner syndrome. *N Engl J Med.* 2011;364:1230-1242. PMID: 21449786

Hasegawa Y, Itonaga T, Ikegawa K, et al. Ultra-low-dose estrogen therapy for female hypogonadism. *Clin Pediatr Endocrinol.* 2020;29(2):49-53. PMID: 32313372

69 ANSWER: C) Measurement of ALT

Nonalcoholic fatty liver disease (NAFLD) is a chronic liver disease due to excess fat accumulation in the liver. It has become the most common liver disease in children in western countries. The prevalence of pediatric NAFLD in the United States ranges from 29% to 38% in select studies. Male sex, older age, and ethnicity (Hispanic children have the highest risk) are all risk factors for NAFLD. Although data on the long-term complications resulting from pediatric NAFLD are limited, disease in children appears to be more severe than in adults. It is often asymptomatic and thus screening for NAFLD in at-risk patients is prudent, so that the condition can be recognized and treated before the onset of end-stage liver disease. According to the most recent pediatric guidelines, screening should be considered for all children with obesity aged 9 to 11 years and for children who are overweight who present with other risk factors such as insulin resistance, prediabetes/diabetes, dyslipidemia, or a family history of NAFLD/NASH. However, it may be prudent to screen younger patients who present with severe obesity or those with a positive family history of NAFLD/nonalcoholic steatohepatitis.

While ALT measurement (Answer C) has limitations, including the fact that optimal cutoffs have not been well established, it is inexpensive and is widely available as a screening tool. It has also been shown to correlate with the presence of hepatic steatosis. Recent standards have been proposed for normal cutoff values of ALT ($\leq$26 U/L [$\leq$0.43 µkat/L] for boys and $\leq$22 U/L [$\leq$0.37 µkat/L] for girls). ALT values greater than 2 times the upper normal limit (ALT $\geq$50 U/L [$\geq$0.84 µkat/L] for boys and $\geq$44 U/L [$\geq$0.73 µkat/L] for girls) in overweight/obese children aged 10 years and older have a sensitivity of 88% for diagnosing NAFLD.

AST (Answer B), as well as γ-glutamyl transferase, has not been tested independently for the purpose of screening in pediatric patients. Additionally, elevated AST or γ-glutamyl transferase may represent liver conditions other than NAFLD, particularly if the ALT concentration is normal.

Abdominal ultrasonography (Answer A) is poor at detecting steatosis. Referral to gastroenterology (Answer D) could be considered in the face of an abnormal ALT value, but screening with ALT is a more appropriate starting place. Abdominal MRI (Answer E) has been validated and shown to be accurate for detection and quantification of hepatic steatosis in both adults and children; however, cost, lack of availability, and lack of validated cutoffs limit its current usefulness as a screening tool. Newer noninvasive diagnostic tools, such acoustic radiation force impact, transient elastography, and magnetic resonance elastography, are increasingly being used for the detection of hepatic steatosis and fibrosis, although these still need to be validated in pediatric patients.

Educational Objective
Identify nonalcoholic fatty liver disease as the most common liver disease in children living in the United States and recommend ALT measurement as the preferred first-line screening test.

Reference(s)

Draijer L, Benninga M, Koot B. Pediatric NAFLD: an overview and recent developments in diagnostics and treatment. *Expert Rev Gastroenterol Hepatol.* 2019;13(5):447-461. PMID: 30875479

Vos MB, Abrams SH, Barlow SE, et al. NASPGHAN clinical practice guideline for the diagnosis and treatment of nonalcoholic fatty liver disease in children: recommendations from the expert committee on NAFLD (ECON) and the North American Society of Pediatric Gastroenterology, Hepatology and Nutrition (NASPGHAN). *J Pediatr Gastroenterol Nutr.* 2017;64(2):319-334. PMID: 28107283

Styne DM, Arslanian SA, Connor EL, et al. Pediatric obesity—assessment, treatment, and prevention: an Endocrine Society clinical practice guideline. *J Clin Endocrinol Metab.* 2017;102(3):709-757. PMID: 28359099

70 ANSWER: C) Lumbar spine DXA and vertebral fracture analysis by DXA

Atraumatic vertebral compression fractures alone are sufficient to diagnose pediatric osteoporosis. While many adult guidelines define chronic steroid exposure as at least 3 months or more of greater than 7.5 mg daily of prednisone equivalents, work from the Steroid-Induced Osteoporosis in the Pediatric Population program identified that pediatric patients may present with vertebral compression fractures within 30 days of starting glucocorticoid therapy. Risk factors include greater cumulative glucocorticoid exposure, increased BMI (likely secondary to the cushingoid effect from high-dosage glucocorticoids), and lower bone mineral density. This patient is at high risk for vertebral compression fractures. Strict bed rest (Answer A) can further compromise skeletal health by leading to muscle deconditioning and bone loss from immobility. In fact, physical therapy is still recommended for patients with vertebral compression fractures to strengthen core muscles.

Imaging can help guide the treatment plan, as the presence of 1 atraumatic vertebral compression fracture is sufficient for the diagnosis of pediatric osteoporosis. Bone density assessment by DXA now is important to assess the patient's current bone health, as well as to monitor response to treatment interventions over time. Importantly, vertebral compression fractures can occur even with a normal bone mineral density Z-score (thus, Answer B is incorrect). One also must be cautious interpreting a lumbar spine bone mineral density Z-score result alone without review of the DXA image itself, as a vertebral compression fracture could result in false elevation of bone mineral density. While DXA images can suggest the presence of a vertebral compression fracture, dedicated spine imaging is recommended.

The most recent pediatric position statement developed by the International Society for Clinical Densitometry in 2019 supports the validity of vertebral fracture analysis via DXA (Answer C) to detect vertebral compression fractures in at-risk children when images are interpreted by a clinician with experience in pediatric vertebral development. Anterior wedging may be present as part of normal physiologic development, especially in the midthoracic region where most vertebral compression fractures occur. Reliance on DXA manufacturer software would thus potentially overdiagnose vertebral deformities in children. Vertebral fracture analysis has similar sensitivity and specificity to that of standard spine radiographs to detect moderate to severe vertebral compression fractures (>25%), but requires less than half of the amount of radiation. Vertebral fracture analysis by DXA does have limited ability to detect mild vertebral compression fractures (20%-25% height loss), especially in the upper thoracic spine (T4-T7); however, standard radiographs also have this limitation secondary to the overlying soft tissue and other organs in that region. Therefore, the new guidelines are that vertebral fracture analysis by DXA is a reasonable first-line assessment for patients at high risk for vertebral compression fractures, followed by spine radiograph (Answer D) or MRI only if the vertebrae are unable to be measured accurately. In centers without this expertise, it may be appropriate to obtain standard radiographs initially.

While this child complained of back pain, it is important to be aware that nearly half of vertebral compression fractures in at-risk populations are asymptomatic. Therefore, monitoring an objective measure of spine health should be considered when patients are at increased risk for vertebral compression. Children with sufficient remaining linear growth have the ability to recover the vertebral height loss without the use of antiresorptive agents such as bisphosphonates (Answer E) if risk factors for osteoporosis are mitigated (ie, cessation of glucocorticoid therapy). It is unknown how much growth potential must remain, but given the fact that this child is prepubertal, bisphosphonate therapy may not be necessary if she is able to discontinue the high-dosage glucocorticoid therapy and undergo remission.

Educational Objective
Recommend vertebral fracture analysis by DXA as a reliable method to diagnose vertebral compression fractures if scans are read and interpreted by an experienced clinician.

Reference(s)
Crabtree NJ, Arabi A, Bachrach LK, et al. Dual-energy X-ray absorptiometry interpretation and reporting in children and adolescents: the revised 2013 ISCD Pediatric Official Positions. *J Clin Densitom.* 2014;17(2):225-242. PMID: 24690232

Halton J, Gaboury I, Grant R, et al; Canadian STOPP Consortium. Advanced vertebral fracture among newly diagnosed children with acute lymphoblastic leukemia: results of the Canadian Steroid-Associated Osteoporosis in the Pediatric Population (STOPP) research program. *J Bone Miner Res.* 2009;24(7):1326-1334. PMID: 19210218

Ward LM, Ma J, Lang B, et al; Steroid-Associated Osteoporosis in the Pediatric Population (STOPP) Consortium. Bone morbidity and recovery in children with acute lymphoblastic leukemia: results of a six-year prospective cohort study. *J Bone Miner Res.* 2018;33(8):1435-1443. PMID: 29786884

Weber DR, Boyce A, Gordon C, et al. The utility of DXA assessment at the forearm, proximal femur, and lateral distal femur, and vertebral fracture assessment in the pediatric population: 2019 ISCD Official Position. *J Clin Densitom.* 2019;22(4):567-589. PMID: 31421951

71 ANSWER: D) Assess thyroid function now and aim for a TSH concentration 0.5-1.0 mIU/L; measure thyroglobulin in 2 to 3 months while on levothyroxine

The recent 2015 pediatric guidelines from the American Thyroid Association classify the risk of having persistent cervical disease and/or distant metastases after thyroidectomy with/without cervical lymph node dissection. The mortality risk from thyroid cancer is very low in pediatric patients. The risk assessment is used to guide the management and monitoring of patients with nonmedullary differentiated thyroid cancer and is geared primarily toward papillary thyroid cancer or the follicular variant of papillary thyroid cancer. The American Thyroid Association pediatric low-risk designation is reserved for thyroid cancer grossly confined to the thyroid with N0/Nx (no metastatic lymph node/s found, or no lymph node/s checked) or incidental N1a (microscopic metastasis to a small number of central neck [level 6] lymph nodes). The American Thyroid Association pediatric intermediate-risk designation defines those with extensive N1a or minimal N1b (lateral neck), whereas the high-risk designation defines those with regionally extensive disease (extensive N1b) or locally invasive disease (T4 tumors per the American Joint Committee on Cancer [AJCC] Tumor, Node, Metastasis [TNM] classification), with or without distant metastasis (typically pulmonary). Both intermediate- and high-risk cancers require stimulated thyroglobulin measurement and whole-body ^{123}I scan to better stage them postoperatively and decide whether ^{131}I radioablation and/or additional surgery is required. Thyroglobulin antibodies should be confirmed to be undetectable to ensure that the thyroglobulin level in a routine panel is reliable.

Although this patient's large tumor size would make it more likely for her to be in a higher risk group, her tumor does not manifest any aggressive features such as invasion of the capsule or lymphatic or vascular invasion. She is in the N0/Nx category and is therefore in the low-risk group. As a result, this patient's goal TSH concentration is 0.5 to 1.0 mIU/L, and nonstimulated (basal) thyroglobulin should be measured within 12 weeks of surgery (Answer D).

Patients in the high-risk group and some in the intermediate-risk group who require [131]I (Answer A) receive it after review of the results of the stimulated thyroglobulin measurement and ^{123}I whole-body scan. The TSH cutoffs in Answer B (TSH cutoff is for high risk) and Answer C (TSH cutoff is for intermediate risk) are incorrect. Stimulated thyroglobulin and a whole-body scan (Answer E) are not recommended for patients at low risk.

Guide the management of low-risk papillary thyroid cancer in an adolescent.

Reference(s)

Edge SB, Byrd DR, Compton CC, eds. *AJCC Cancer Staging Manual.* 7th ed. Springer International Publishing; 2010.

Francis GL, Waguespack SG, Bauer AJ, et al; American Thyroid Association Guidelines Task Force. Management guidelines for children with thyroid nodules and differentiated thyroid cancer. *Thyroid.* 2015;25(7):716-759. PMID: 25900731

72 ANSWER: D) Hypophosphatasia

The most notable finding in this child is the low serum alkaline phosphatase concentration. While the reported value is just outside of the reference range, it is important to remember that children have significantly higher levels of alkaline phosphatase than adults, and levels less than 100 U/L (<1.67 μkat/L) should raise concern when there are physical signs of rickets. Hypophosphatasia (Answer D) occurs in 1 in 100,000 live births and is due to loss-of-function pathogenic variants in the *ALPL* gene, which encodes tissue nonspecific alkaline phosphatase. Inadequate action of tissue nonspecific alkaline phosphatase results in accumulation of the substrate inorganic pyrophosphate, which is a potent inhibitor of mineralization. The spectrum of disease includes perinatal lethal, infantile-onset, childhood-onset, and adult-onset forms, as well as odontohypophosphatasia (premature tooth loss alone without a skeletal phenotype). The phenotype is related to the residual function of the enzyme. Skeletal manifestations include craniosynostosis, rickets, bone and joint pain, fractures or pseudofractures, and the hallmark premature loss (before age 5 years) of primary teeth with the root intact. Radiographs show "radiolucent tongues" extending from the growth plate into the metaphysis. The infantile form presents with respiratory issues due to an underdeveloped thoracic cage, hypercalcemia and hyperphosphatemia due to inability to deposit mineral into bone, nephrocalcinosis, and seizures responsive to vitamin B_6. Some children present with weakness, delayed walking, and a waddling gait. Adult forms can present with recurrent metatarsal stress fractures, loss of adult dentition, osteomalacia, and pseudogout. Ongoing data collection suggests that bisphosphonate use in adults with hypophosphatasia may result in an increased risk for atypical femur fractures. In 2015, the enzyme replacement therapy asfotase alfa became clinically available to treat this disorder. Treatment with asfotase alfa results in improved skeletal mineralization, respiratory function, growth, and cognitive and motor function for the infantile and childhood forms, as well as improved bone mineralization, motor function, muscle strength, and patient-reported function in adolescents and adults. While the mother's recurrent stress fractures may be secondary to her training for marathons, it would be reasonable to measure her alkaline phosphatase level. It is also important to ensure age-specific reference ranges are reported, as alkaline phosphatase levels are significantly higher in children than in adults.

The differential diagnosis of low serum alkaline phosphatase is broad and includes vitamin D intoxication, hypoparathyroidism, zinc deficiency, magnesium deficiency, celiac disease, Wilson disease, Cushing syndrome, hypothyroidism, pernicious anemia, osteogenesis imperfecta type 2, and cleidocranial dysostosis. Vitamin D intoxication (Answer A) leads to hypercalcemia, hyperphosphatemia, and low serum alkaline phosphatase; however, serum 25-hydroxyvitamin D values are generally above 100 ng/dL (>249.6 nmol/L). Lower-extremity bowing deformities are not part of the clinical presentation. This patient's PTH was low-normal with a mildly elevated phosphate concentration and normal serum calcium concentration appropriate for the 25-hydroxyvitamin D level. Thus, he does not have hypoparathyroidism (Answer B).

Risk factors for rickets of prematurity (Answer E) include gestational age less than 27 weeks, birth weight less than 2 lb 3 oz (<1000 g), prolonged use of total parental nutrition (>4 weeks), history of necrotizing enterocolitis, and prolonged postnatal steroid use. Biochemical changes of low serum phosphate and elevated alkaline phosphatase present between 3 and 14 weeks of life due to the inability to replicate the extensive skeletal uptake of calcium by the fetus during the third trimester. While physical changes are rare, some cases can manifest with fractures. Although this child was at risk for rickets of prematurity, his symptoms are progressing, whereas rickets of prematurity is self-resolving and there is little evidence for long-term consequences on bone health.

Physiologic bowing (Answer C) is certainly a possibility; however, the alkaline phosphatase concentration is frankly low.

Educational Objective

Diagnose hypophosphatasia in a child with rachitic changes in the setting of low serum alkaline phosphatase.

Reference(s)

Whyte MP. Hypophosphatasia - aetiology, nosology, pathogenesis, diagnosis and treatment. *Nat Rev Endocrinol.* 2016;12(4):233-246. PMID: 26893260

73 ANSWER: A) Inhibin B = 17.7 pg/mL (SI: 17.7 ng/L); antimullerian hormone = 41 ng/mL (SI: 293 pmol/L); FSH = 0.33 mIU/mL (SI: 0.33 IU/L)

The patient in this vignette has a testicular volume less than 3 mL at 15 years of age. The differential diagnosis includes constitutional delay of growth and puberty vs primary or hypogonadotropic hypogonadism. The history of cryptorchidism, hyposmia, and hypogonadism is most consistent with a diagnosis of Kallmann syndrome, which results from a defect in formation of the olfactory placode during embryonic development. This causes loss of olfactory nerve fibers and failure of GnRH neuron migration to the hypothalamus. Low inhibin B, antimullerian hormone, and FSH levels (Answer A) are consistently found in patients with hypogonadotropic hypogonadism due to Kallmann syndrome.

Distinguishing hypogonadotropic hypogonadism from constitutional delay is challenging but can be based on certain features, including absent or diminished sense of smell and the finding of a hypoplastic olfactory bulb on brain MRI. Other findings that are suggestive of Kallmann syndrome include micropenis, cryptorchidism, and synkinesia (mirror movements of the hands). While more than 25 genes involved in Kallmann syndrome have been identified, a genetic cause is not found in nearly half of cases.

In children with hypogonadotropic hypogonadism, inadequate low FSH levels and consequent failure of Sertoli-cell proliferation result in decreased production and secretion of peptide hormones, including inhibin B and antimullerian hormone. As such, inhibin B and antimullerian hormone levels are helpful in distinguishing constitutional delay of growth and puberty from hypogonadotropic hypogonadism. Children with constitutional delay of growth and puberty have normal inhibin B and antimullerian hormone levels before onset of puberty. In contrast, both inhibin B and antimullerian hormone are low in children with hypogonadotropic hypogonadism.

Antimullerian hormone levels peak in the first year of life and stay elevated throughout childhood. Antimullerian hormone levels decrease in puberty due to inhibition by testosterone. Pubertal-aged individuals with hypogonadotropic hypogonadism have antimullerian hormone levels that are low when compared with the normal prepubertal range due to FSH deficiency but are high for age due to lack of testosterone inhibition.

Inhibin B levels remain detectable throughout childhood and then rise in puberty along with FSH levels. Inhibin B concentrations are significantly lower in individuals with hypogonadotropic hypogonadism than in those with constitutional delay of growth and puberty; a cutoff of 61 pg/mL (61 ng/L) has 90% sensitivity and 83% specificity for detecting hypogonadotropic hypogonadism, which makes inhibin B a useful marker for detection.

The following graphs contain data used to establish reference intervals for antimullerian hormone and inhibin B in children and adolescents (*see figures*).

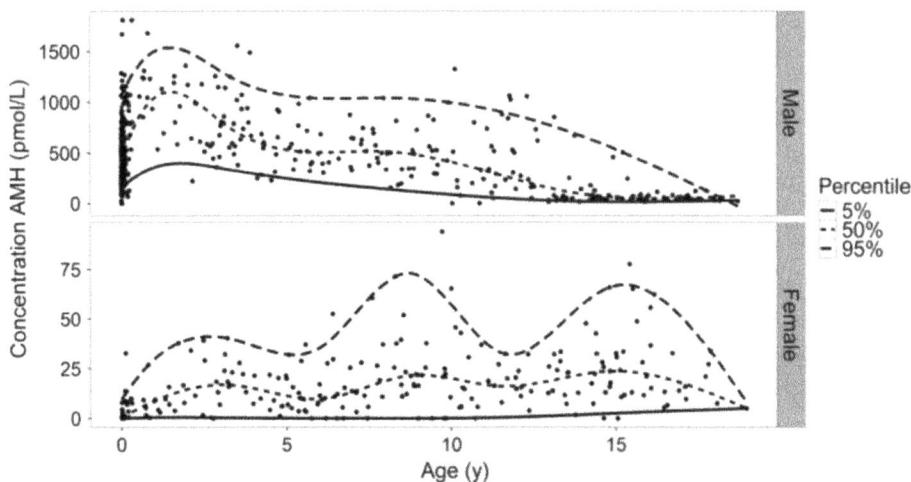

Pediatric antimullerian hormone measurement: male (n = 469) and female (n = 235). Reference intervals established using the automated Beckman Coulter Access AMH assay. Reprinted from Jopling H, Yates A, Burgoyne N, Hayden K, Chaloner C, Tetlow L. Paediatric anti-müllerian hormone measurement: male and female reference intervals established using the automated Beckman Coulter Access AMH assay. *Endocrinol Diabetes Metab.* 2018;1(4):e00021.

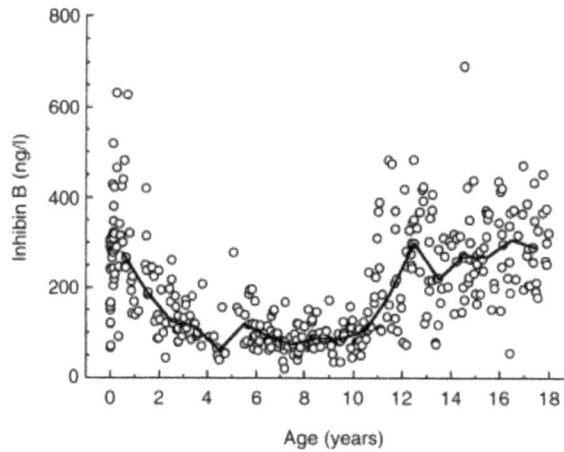

Pediatric inhibin B measurement in 366 boys aged 0 to 18 years. The thick line shows the median for each yearly age group, plotted at the midpoint of each year. Reprinted from Crofton PM, Evans AEM, Groome NP, Taylor MRH, Holland CV, Kelnar CJH. Inhibin B in boys from birth to adulthood: relationship with age, pubertal stage, FSH and testosterone. *Clin Endocrinol (Oxf)*. 2002;56(2):215-221.

Educational Objective

Identify hormone profiles consistent with Kallmann syndrome.

Reference(s)

Condorelli RA, Cannarella R, Calogero AE, La Vignera S. Evaluation of testicular function in prepubertal children. *Endocrine*. 2018;62(2):274-280. PMID: 29982874

Crofton PM, Evans AEM, Groome NP, Taylor MRH, Holland CV, Kelnar CJH. Inhibin B in boys from birth to adulthood: relationship with age, pubertal stage, FSH and testosterone. *Clin Endocrinol (Oxf)*. 2002;56(2):215-221. PMID: 11874413

Grinspon RP, Urrutia M, Rey RA. Male central hypogonadism in paediatrics – the relevance of follicle-stimulating hormone and Sertoli cell markers. *Eur Endocrinol*. 2018;14(2):67-71. PMID: 30349597

Jopling H, Yates A, Burgoyne N, Hayden K, Chaloner C, Tetlow L. Paediatric anti-müllerian hormone measurement: male and female reference intervals established using the automated Beckman Coulter Access AMH assay. *Endocrinol Diabetes Metab*. 2018;1(4):e00021. PMID: 30815559

74 ANSWER: C) Decrease the GH dosage

In June 2000, GH therapy was approved by the US FDA for the management of growth failure associated with Prader-Willi syndrome based on studies showing an improvement in linear growth and body composition (decrease in fat mass and increase in lean mass) in these children.

IGF-1 is a useful indicator of GH dosage adequacy in children with idiopathic GH deficiency. Higher IGF-1 levels have been observed in patients with Prader-Willi syndrome in response to standard dosages of GH when compared with IGF-1 levels in children without Prader-Willis syndrome. The possibility of higher sensitivity to GH therapy is thought to be a possible mechanism. An alternative mechanism has been proposed for this finding. In children with Prader-Willi syndrome treated with GH, most of the IGF-1 is sequestered in the 150-kDa complex with IGFBP-3 and acid-labile subunit, decreasing the proportion of bioactive IGF-1. This has led to the proposal that elevated IGF-1 levels are not a reason to decrease the GH dosage in these individuals because there is no good correlation between serum immunoreactive IGF-1 and bioactive IGF-1 in children with Prader-Willi syndrome treated with GH. However, the clinical consensus guidelines still recommend guiding the dosing of GH in patients with Prader-Willi based on clinical response and recommend maintaining IGF-1 levels within the physiological range. This child's IGF-1 is elevated (SDS >+2); therefore, a decrease in the GH dosage (Answer C) is the best next step. Continuation of the current GH dosage (Answer A) is not the preferred next step despite the reported good response to therapy.

The recommended initial dosage of GH in children with Prader-Willi syndrome is 0.5 mg/m^2 daily with dosage titration to 1 mg/m^2 daily based on clinical response and IGF-1 measurements.

High levels of IGF-1 are associated with lymphoid hyperplasia, which can worsen obstructive sleep apnea. On the basis of several reports of sudden death occurring shortly after initiation of GH therapy in children with Prader-

Willi syndrome, a warning was added to the prescribing recommendations, specifically in patients with preexisting significant obesity and severe respiratory impairment. Polysomnography (sleep study) and otolaryngology evaluation of the upper airway are recommended before initiation of GH therapy. Some authors also recommend a repeated sleep study approximately 6 months after therapy initiation.

While GH, an insulin counterregulatory hormone, increases insulin resistance and the risk of dysglycemia/hyperglycemia, especially in individuals with obesity, the screening laboratory tests in this vignette (random glucose and hemoglobin A_{1c}) are normal and not suggestive of an alteration of carbohydrate metabolism at this time. Thus, an oral glucose tolerance test (Answer D) is not the best next step.

Children with Prader-Willi syndrome may have hypothalamic dysfunction, which can be associated with central hypothyroidism. This child's thyroid function is normal and does not warrant thyroid hormone replacement now (Answer B).

This patient's vitamin D level is normal, so there is no indication for vitamin D therapy (Answer E). Nevertheless, it is advised to ensure adequate maintenance of vitamin D levels through feeds or supplementation.

Educational Objective
Guide the management of GH therapy in children with Prader-Willi syndrome.

Reference(s)
Bakker NE, van Doorn J, Renes JS, Donker GH, Hokken-Koelega AC. IGF-1 levels, complex formation, and IGF bioactivity in growth hormone-treated children with Prader-Willi syndrome. *J Clin Endocrinol Metab*. 2015;100(8):3041-3049. PMID: 26050733

Whitman B, Carrel A, Bekx T, Weber C, Allen D, Myers S. Growth hormone improves body composition and motor development in infants with Prader-Willi syndrome after six months. *J Pediatr Endocrinol Metab*. 2004;17(4):591-600. PMID: 15198290

Barbera J, Voloh I, Berall G, Shapiro CM. Sleep abnormalities and Prader-Willi syndrome. In: Pandi-Perumal, Kramer M, eds. *Sleep and Mental Illness.* Cambridge University Press; 2010.

Miller JL, Shuster J, Theriaque D, Driscoll DJ, Wagner M. Sleep disordered breathing in infants with Prader-Willi syndrome during the first 6 weeks of growth hormone therapy: a pilot study. *J Clin Sleep Med*. 2009;5(5):448-453. PMID: 19961030

Eiholzer U. Deaths in children with Prader-Willi syndrome. *Horm Res*. 2005;63(1):33-39. PMID: 15604598

Carrel AL, Myers SE, Whitman BY, Eickhoff J, Allen DB. Long-term growth hormone therapy changes the natural history of body composition and motor function in children with Prader-Willi syndrome. *J Clin Endocrinol Metab*. 2010;95(3):1131-1136. PMID: 20061431

Chernausek SD, Backeljauw PF, Frane J, Kuntze, Underwood LE; GH insensitivity syndrome Collaborative Group. *J Clin Endocrinol Metab*. 2007;92(3):902-910. PMID: 17192294

Feigerlová E, Diene G, Oliver I, et al. Elevated insulin-like growth factor-I values in children with Prader-Willi syndrome compared with growth hormone (GH) deficiency children over two years of GH treatment. *J Clin Endocrinol Metab*. 2010;95(10):4600-4608. PMID: 20926543

Deal C, Tony M, Höybye C, et al; 2011 Growth Hormone in Prader-Willi Syndrome Clinical Care Guidelines Workshop Participants. Growth Hormone Research Society workshop summary: consensus guidelines for recombinant human growth hormone therapy in Prader-Willi syndrome. *J Clin Endocrinol Metab*. 2013;98(6):E1072-E1087. PMID: 23543664

75 ANSWER: B) *VHL* (von Hippel-Lindau tumor suppressor)

Pheochromocytomas and paragangliomas caused by pathogenic variants in the *VHL* gene (Answer B), associated with von Hippel–Lindau syndrome, have a noradrenergic biochemical profile, unlike tumors associated with *RET* (Answer A), *TMEM127* (Answer C), and *NF1* (Answer D), which show adrenergic predominance. Pathogenic variants in the *SDHC* gene (Answer E) can be associated with tumors that have a noradrenergic biochemical profile, but these variants tend to cause solitary head and neck paragangliomas. The Endocrine Society guidelines for the evaluation and treatment of pheochromocytomas and paragangliomas advocate that genetic testing be considered in all patients independent of a clear family history. This is consistent with other practice guidelines and consensus statements from expert groups, as 40% to 50% of pheochromocytomas and paragangliomas are associated with pathogenic variants in known causative genes. More than 12 genes are associated with pheochromocytomas and paragangliomas (*see table*). Some of these are associated with distinct clinical syndromes and predominant biochemical profiles. The most commonly associated genes in pediatric patients are *VHL* and *SDHB*.

Table. Genes Associated With Pheochromocytomas and Paragangliomas

Gene (symbol, location, and inheritance pattern)	Frequency of pathogenic variants	Syndrome	Biochemical profile
NF1 17q11.2 Autosomal dominant	3% (germline), 20-25% (somatic)	Neurofibromatosis type 1	Adrenergic predominance
VHL 3p25-p26 Autosomal dominant	7%-10% (germline or somatic)	von Hippel–Lindau disease	Noradrenergic
RET 10q11.2 Autosomal dominant	5%-6% (germline or somatic)	Multiple endocrine neoplasia type 2	Adrenergic predominance
SDHx genes Autosomal dominant except SDHD, which is autosomal dominant and paternally inherited (due to maternal imprinting) SDHB (1p36.13) SDHD (11q23) SDHC (1q21) SDHAF2 (11q13.1)	SDHB (8%-10%, germline) SDHD (5%-7%, germline) SDHC (1%-2%, germline) SDHA (<1%, germline or somatic) SDHAF2 (<1%)	Hereditary paraganglioma-pheochromocytoma syndrome	Noradrenergic, possibly dopaminergic, possibly nonsecreting
TMEM127 2q11.2 Autosomal dominant	1%-2% (germline)	Hereditary pheochromocytoma and paraganglioma	Adrenergic predominance
MAX 14q23.3 Autosomal dominant/paternally inherited	1%-2% (germline or somatic)	Hereditary pheochromocytoma and paraganglioma	Adrenergic predominance
EPAS1 (also known as HIF2A) 2p21-p16 Mosaic/somatic	6%-12% (mosaic or somatic)	Polycythemia paraganglioma syndrome	Noradrenergic
FH	1%-2% (germline)	Hereditary leiomyomatosis and renal cell cancer syndrome	Noradrenergic
MDH2	<2% (germline)	Hereditary pheochromocytoma and paraganglioma	Noradrenergic

Table adapted from references (Fishbein 2019, Toledo et al 2017, Favier et al 2015). Additional genes include TP53 <5% (somatic), MET <2% (germline) or <2%-10% (somatic), MERTK <2% (germline), KMT2D <2% (germline or somatic), KIF1B <5% (germline or somatic), IDH2 <0.5% (somatic), H3F3A <2% (mosaic), FGFR1 approximately 1% (somatic), EGLN1/PHD2 <1% (germline or somatic), CDKN2A <2% (somatic), BRAF <2% (somatic), ATRX <5% (somatic). Additional variants in other genes (SCL25A11, GOT2, DNMT3A, and DLST) have been reported but causality is unclear.

The presence of additional features can often help determine which candidate gene to test: for example, retinal angiomas in von Hippel–Lindau syndrome; a thyroid mass in multiple endocrine neoplasia type 2; cafe-au-lait spots, axillary and inguinal freckling, Lisch nodules on the iris, and subcutaneous neurofibromas in neurofibromatosis type 1; and a neck mass in paraganglioma syndromes. A number of algorithms for genetic testing have been developed depending on whether the genetic testing is undertaken by candidate gene Sanger sequencing, gene panel, or next-generation sequencing. In the absence of syndromic features, the pathways account for the presence or absence of metastasis, location of paragangliomas, extraadrenal or adrenal disease, unilateral/bilateral disease, and secretory biochemical phenotypes.

In the case of isolated adrenal disease with a noradrenergic secretory phenotype, *VHL* genetic testing is recommended. Increasingly, the diagnosis of pathogenic variants is through use of gene panels and next-generation sequencing. A consensus statement on next-generation sequencing in pheochromocytomas and paragangliomas was published in 2017, and it recommends the use of a validated targeted gene panel for the clinical genetic diagnosis of hereditary pheochromocytomas and paragangliomas. Although next-generation sequencing is increasingly used in research, there are concerns that without a rigorous pipeline to interpret the data, high-throughput sequencing methods may lead to false-positive results with many variants of unknown significance reported as causative. This could have severe consequences for patients and their relatives who would undergo surveillance/screening accordingly.

Educational Objective

Explain the genetics of pheochromocytomas and paragangliomas and describe the stratification of genetic diagnosis dependent on clinical phenotype, tumor location, and biochemical phenotype.

Reference(s)

Fishbein L. Pheochromocytoma/paraganglioma: is this a genetic disorder? *Curr Cardiol Rep.* 2019;21(9):104. PMID: 31367972

Lenders JW, Duh QY, Eisenhofer G, et al; Endocrine Society. Pheochromocytoma and paraganglioma: an Endocrine Society clinical practice guideline. *J Clin Endocrinol Metab.* 2014;99(6):1915-1942. PMID: 24893135

Hampel H, Bennett RL, Buchanan A, Pearlman R, Wiesner GL, Guideline Development Group, American College of Medical Genetics and Genomics Professional Practice and Guidelines Committee and National Society of Genetic Counselors Practice Guidelines Committee. A practice guideline from the American College of Medical Genetics and Genomics and the National Society of Genetic Counselors: referral indications for cancer predisposition assessment. *Genet Med.* 2015;17(1):70-87. PMID: 25394175

NGS in PPGL (NGSnPPGL) Study Group, Toledo RA, Burnichon N, et al. Consensus statement on next-generation-sequencing-based diagnostic testing of hereditary phaeochromocytomas and paragangliomas. *Nat Rev Endocrinol.* 2017;13(4):233-247. PMID: 27857127

Favier J, Amar L, Gimenez-Roqueplo AP. Paraganglioma and phaeochromocytoma: from genetics to personalized medicine. *Nat Rev Endocrinol.* 2015;11(2):1010-111. PMID: 25385035

76 ANSWER: D) Ophthalmologist

Elevated hemoglobin A_{1c} levels in the double digits are associated with long-term microvascular complications, as demonstrated in the Diabetes Control and Complications Trial and in many studies since then. Recent data in adult populations suggest that the glycemic excursions are as concerning as elevated hemoglobin A_{1c} levels. Even with the same hemoglobin A_{1c} level, patients with much wider glycemic fluctuations have an increased risk of complications.

This vignette is a good example of glycemic variability that can be simply defined as the degree to which the patient's blood glucose level fluctuates between high (peaks) and low (nadir) levels. These patients are at greater risk of developing microvascular complications in the short- and long-term. These complications include, but are not limited to, retinopathy, nephropathy, and neuropathy.

The risk of retinopathy is far greater than any other complications at this stage; therefore, the first referral should be to an ophthalmologist (Answer D). In a published study, the retinopathy risk doubled when glycemic variation worsened.

Referring this patient to a cardiologist (Answer A) could be considered because cardiac autonomic neuropathy, defined as measurement of heart rate variability assessed by 10-minute continuous electrocardiography, is a potential complication. However, the patient is not reporting any symptoms and is able to tolerate exercise.

He is indeed at increased risk of microalbuminuria and nephropathy, which may require consultation with a nephrologist (Answer B). However, his urine albumin is detectable but still within the normal range.

Referral to a neurologist (Answer C) could be considered if he were experiencing any symptoms consistent with neuropathy, which he is not.

Podiatrist referral (Answer E) for annual foot examination is also important, especially for this patient who is an avid soccer player, but it is not the first priority for children with type 1 diabetes without relevant clinical concerns.

Educational Objective

Explain the importance of early referral to appropriate subspecialty care to address potential microvascular complications in an adolescent with suboptimally controlled type 1 diabetes mellitus.

Reference(s)

Virk SA, Donaghue KC, Cho YH, et al. Association between HbA1c variability and risk of microvascular complications in adolescents with type 1 diabetes. *J Clin Endocrinol Metab.* 2016;101(9):3257-3263. PMID: 27186858

77 ANSWER: B) Cell-surface receptor with intrinsic tyrosine kinase activity

This patient has classic features of IGF-1 resistance, including poor prenatal and postnatal growth, short stature, microcephaly, midface hypoplasia, and global developmental delay. Furthermore, results of the whole-exome sequencing confirmed a heterozygous pathogenic variant in the *IGF1R* gene. The IGF-1 receptor is a heterotetrameric transmembrane glycoprotein encoded by *IGF1R*. It consists of an α-subunit, involved in ligand binding, and a β-subunit, accounting for the intrinsic tyrosine kinase activity (Answer B). *IGF1R* is located on the distal part of the long arm of chromosome 15 (15q26.3). Patients with pathogenic variants in the *IGF1R* gene and those who have 15q deletions that include *IGF1R* may exhibit clinical signs and symptoms of IGF-1 resistance. The serum IGF-1 level in these patients can be normal or high, and the phenotype is variable. GH therapy has been shown to have moderate effects when used to treat short stature in these patients.

IGF-1 is one of the important regulators of prenatal growth, whereas GH does not have a vital role in intrauterine growth.

Table. Hormones Involved in Growth and Mechanisms of Action

Hormone	Receptor location	Receptor type	Mechanism of action
GHRH	Transmembrane	G-protein–coupled receptor	Increases intracellular cAMP
GH	Transmembrane	Class I cytokine receptor	JAK2-STAT activation
IGF-1	Transmembrane	Tyrosine kinase receptor	Tyrosine kinase–mediated receptor autophosphorylation and phosphorylation of multiple substrates (IRS 1/2, SHC)
TSH	Transmembrane	G-protein–coupled receptor	Increases intracellular cAMP
Thyroid Hormone	Nucleus	Nuclear receptor	Regulates gene expression

Educational Objective
Describe the physiology of IGF-1 receptor activity and clinical features of patients with IGF-1 resistance.

Reference(s)
Walenkamp MJE, Robers JML, Wit JM, et al. Phenotypic features and response to GH treatment of patients with a molecular defect of the IGF-1 receptor. *J Clin Endocrinol Metab*. 2019;104(8):3157-3171. PMID: 30848790

Hakuno F, Takahashi S-I. IGF1 receptor signaling pathways. *J Mol Endocrinol*. 2018;61(1):T69-T86. PMID: 29535161

78 ANSWER: E) Urinary iodine

This infant presents several weeks after birth with severe primary hypothyroidism that was not documented on newborn screening, suggesting a postnatally acquired cause. The patient's mother reports consuming a significant amount of a traditional Korean soup, which may contain large amounts of iodine from seaweed that can be transmitted to the infant through breastmilk. Exposure of infants to excess iodine, such as from topical iodine antiseptics, iodinated radiocontrast agents, or maternal iodine ingestion, can cause acquired hypothyroidism in infancy. In such cases, the urinary iodine concentration is elevated (Answer E). Excess maternal iodine ingestion from seaweed soup has been reported to cause hypothyroidism in term and preterm infants and is particularly common in Asia. In this case, the infant's urinary iodine concentration was 1830 mg/L (regional median 197 mg/L), and the mother's breastmilk iodine concentration was 3023 mg/L (regional median 45-155 mg/L).

Management consists of discontinuing the source of excess maternal iodine ingestion. There is minimal evidence regarding the time required to normalize the breastmilk iodine concentration, but in one reported case, the maternal urinary iodine concentration was normal 4 weeks after stopping seaweed ingestion. If the infant's hypothyroidism is overt (as in this case), temporary levothyroxine treatment may be necessary.

Increased serum reverse T_3 (Answer A) and low serum T_3 (Answer C) are observed in consumptive hypothyroidism, which is caused by massive hepatic hemangiomas that overexpress the type 3 deiodinase enzyme. This infant has no clinical evidence of such a process, such as hepatomegaly or cutaneous hemangiomas.

Maternal transfer of TSH-receptor antibodies (Answer D) that block TSH-receptor signaling is a rare cause of congenital hypothyroidism, which is unlikely in this patient with a normal newborn screen. In addition, such antibodies generally result in a small (not normal-sized) thyroid gland by blocking the trophic effect of TSH on thyroid follicular cells.

TPO antibodies (Answer B) are diagnostic of autoimmune thyroid disease, which is the most common cause of acquired hypothyroidism in childhood and adolescence. Autoimmune thyroid disease generally does not arise in the neonatal period and is unlikely to be the cause of this patient's hypothyroidism. Although maternal TPO antibodies may be transmitted to a fetus across the placenta, these antibodies are nonfunctional and do not cause hypothyroidism.

Educational Objective
Identify and diagnose hypothyroidism caused by excessive maternal iodine intake.

Reference(s)

Shumer DE, Mehringer JE, Braverman LE, Dauber A. Acquired hypothyroidism in an infant related to excessive maternal iodine intake: food for thought. *Endocr Pract*. 2013;19(4):729-731. PMID: 23512394

Chung HR, Shin CH, Yang SW, Choi CW, Kim BI. Subclinical hypothyroidism in Korean preterm infants associated with high levels of iodine in breast milk. *J Clin Endocrinol Metab*. 2009;94(11):4444-4447. PMID: 19808851

Emder P, Jack MM. Iodine-induced neonatal hypothyroidism secondary to maternal seaweed consumption: a common practice in some Asian cultures to promote breast milk supply. *J Pediatr Child Health*. 2011;47(10):750-752. PMID: 21276114

79 ANSWER: A) Screen for adrenal insufficiency

Autoimmune polyglandular syndrome (APS) type 1 is a rare autosomal recessive condition due to loss of function of the autoimmune regulator gene (*AIRE*), which results in inappropriate expression of organ-specific T cells from the thymus. Classic manifestations include mucocutaneous candidiasis, hypoparathyroidism (80% with mean age of presentation at 9 years), and primary adrenal insufficiency (90% with mean age of presentation of 14 years). Additional endocrine comorbidities may include oophoritis (70%), testicular failure (30%), type 1 diabetes mellitus (30%), hypothyroidism (30%), and hypophysitis (30%). Given her age, weight loss, and symptoms, the most important next step in this patient's management is screening for adrenal insufficiency (Answer A). While the pathophysiology of hypercalcemia in adrenal insufficiency is unclear, it is reported in 5% to 6% of new diagnoses. Proposed mechanisms include decreased glomerular filtration of calcium due to hypovolemia and loss of glucocorticoid inhibition of 1α-hydroxylase leading to enhanced enteral calcium absorption.

The pathogenesis of hypoparathyroidism in autoimmune polyglandular syndrome type 1 is thought to be secondary to development of antibodies against PTH, the calcium-sensing receptor, or the NACHT leucine-rich repeats present in the parathyroid gland. Management of hypoparathyroidism can be especially challenging in patients with gastrointestinal comorbidities. Classic treatment approaches have focused on multiple daily doses of enteral calcium and active vitamin D. In recent years, recombinant PTH has been used to treat adult hypoparathyroidism and bypass the need for enteral absorption. Once-daily injections of recombinant 1-84 PTH demonstrate mean peak serum calcium levels 10 to 12 hours after the dose with sustained increases above baseline for 24 hours despite the half-life of the medication being only 3 hours. Recombinant 1-84 PTH is detected in the serum assay and was already low at the time of hypercalcemia. Reducing her dosage (Answer D) or discontinuing calcium carbonate (Answer E), are potential options to address the hypercalcemia, but neither option addresses the need to rule out adrenal insufficiency. In addition, given the half-life of calcium carbonate, this afternoon dose is unlikely to be affecting the morning serum calcium levels.

While patients with APS type 1 are at increased risk for primary ovarian insufficiency, this patient has started puberty and is progressing at a typical tempo given her Tanner stage 4 breast development. Thus, screening for ovarian insufficiency (Answer B) is not needed now. Hyperthyroidism is a potential cause of hypercalcemia and can present with weight loss, fatigue, and diarrhea; however, the patient does not have tachycardia nor hypertension. In addition, hyperthyroidism is a feature of APS type 2, not APS type 1. Therefore, thyroid function tests (Answer C) are not the best next step.

Describe the presentation of adrenal insufficiency in autoimmune polyglandular syndrome type 1 and explain how hypercalcemia can be a manifestation.

Reference(s)

Winer KK, Kelly A, Johns A, et al. Long-term parathyroid hormone 1-34 replacement therapy in children with hypoparathyroidism. *J Pediatr*. 2018;203:391-399.e1. PMID: 30470382

Tuli G, Buganza R, Tessaris D, Einaudi S, Matarazzo P, de Sanctis L. Teriparatide (rhPTH 1-34) treatment in the pediatric age: long-term efficacy and safety data in a cohort with genetic hypoparathyroidism. *Endocrine*. 2020;67(2):457-465. PMID: 31705387

Winer KK. Advances in the treatment of hypoparathyroidism with PTH 1-34. *Bone*. 2019;120:535-541. PMID: 30243992

80 ANSWER: B) Increase in weight percentile without appreciable changes in appetite or calories

Prader-Willi syndrome (PWS) is a complex imprinted condition with the majority of cases due to deletions in the 15q11.2-q13 region of the paternally inherited chromosome. Obesity, intellectual disability, hypotonia, behavioral challenges, and neuroendocrine dysfunction have been commonly described. In the past, it was thought that there were only 2 nutritional phases associated with PWS (stage 1 with hypotonia and poor feeding in infancy, followed by stage 2 with hyperphagia and rapid weight gain in childhood). However, the nutritional stages are now known to be much more complex than previously recognized. Five main stages have been described with subphases in phase 1 and 2.

Infants with PWS are characteristically hypotonic and have difficulty feeding (Answer E). This phase (phase 1a) can occur between birth and 15 months of age. Infants in this stage may have failure to thrive as a result of feeding difficulties. In late infancy (between 9 and 15 months), there is phase 1b in which infants track along their growth percentile without excess weight gain (Answer D).

Toddlers (median age 2.08 years; age quartiles 20-31 months), such as the patient in this vignette, are most typically described as being in phase 2a in which there is a weight increase that occurs without a change in appetite or calories consumed (Answer B). Whether this weight gain is due to a change in metabolic rate and/or other factors is not known. To avoid excess weight gain at this stage, it is thought that calories consumed must be restricted to 50% to 80% of the recommended daily allowance for age.

In phase 2b, which occurs at a median age of 4.5 years, there is an increasing interest in food, coupled with increased caloric intake and weight gain (Answer C).

Hyperphagia with food-seeking and lack of satiety (Answer A) occurs later than previously thought at a median age of 8 years (phase 3).

It is important to note that not all children with PWS go through all 5 stages, but patients and families should be informed of the possible stages and counseled accordingly regarding appropriate management.

Table. Nutritional Phases Associated With Prader-Willi Syndrome

5 nutritional phases (with subphases) associated with Prader-Willi syndrome	Expected clinical course
Phase 0 (in utero)	Decreased fetal movement, lower birth weight
Phase 1a (infancy)	Hypotonia, difficulty feeding, failure to thrive
Phase 1b (late infancy)	Maintenance of weight percentile along the growth curve
Phase 2a (median age 2.08 years; age quartiles 20-31 months)	Increase in weight percentile without change in appetite or calories consumed
Phase 2b (median age of 4.5 years)	Increase in weight percentile associated with an increased interest in food
Phase 3 (median age 8 years)	Hyperphagia with food-seeking and lack of satiety
Phase 4 (adulthood)	Improvement in appetite control, not as preoccupied with food

Educational Objective

Explain the major nutritional phases associated with Prader-Willi syndrome.

Reference(s)

Miller JL, Lynn CH, Driscoll DC, et al. Nutritional phases in Prader-Willi syndrome. *Am J Med Genet A.* 2011;155A(5):1040-1049. PMID: 21465655

Goldstone AP, Holland AJ, Hauffa BP, Hokken-Koelega AC, Tauber M; speakers contributors at the Second Expert Meeting of the Comprehensive Care of Patients with PWS. Recommendations for the diagnosis and management of Prader-Willi syndrome. *J Clin Endocrinol Metab.* 2008;93(11):4183-4197. PMID: 18697869

81 ANSWER: A) Arginine inhibits somatostatin

Many secretagogues can be used for provocative GH-stimulation testing, including insulin, arginine, glucagon, propranolol, clonidine, and levodopa. GHRH and exercise can also stimulate GH release. Provocative testing is by nature nonphysiologic and the precise mechanisms by which these agents stimulate GH are not fully understood. However, many affect GH release by suppressing somatostatin or stimulating GHRH release.

Pulsatile GH secretion is in part regulated by the hypothalamic regulatory peptides GHRH and somatostatin (somatotropin release–inhibiting factor). GHRH release is stimulated by α2 adrenergic agonists, including clonidine, dopaminergic agonists (eg, levodopa), and exercise.

Somatostatin secretion is stimulated by GHRH, dopaminergic, β-adrenergic stimulation, and GH and IGF-1 feedback. Somatostatin is inhibited by arginine, cholinergic GABAergic stimulation, and insulin-induced hypoglycemia.

Arginine appears to cause GH release by inhibiting somatostatin and thereby increasing GHRH activity (Answer A). Glucagon (Answer B) may work by inducing a relative hypoglycemia following hyperglycemia, although the exact mechanism is not fully understood. Propranolol (Answer C) is a β-adrenergic antagonist, which would be expected to inhibit somatostatin. Clonidine (Answer D) stimulates α2 adrenergic receptors, which would increase GHRH. Levodopa (Answer E) most often increases GHRH.

Educational Objective

Explain the effects and mechanism of action of levodopa, clonidine, glucagon, propranolol, and arginine hydrochloride during testing for GH secretory capacity.

Reference(s)

Melmed S, Polonsky SK, Larense PR, Kronenberg HM, eds. *Williams Textbook of Endocrinology.* 13th ed. Elsevier; 2016.

Rosenfeld RG, Albertsson-Wikland K, Cassorla F, et al. Diagnostic controversy: the diagnosis of childhood growth hormone deficiency revisited. *J Clin Endocrinol Metab.* 1995;80(5):1532-1540. PMID: 7538145

82 ANSWER: A) *SGPL1* (sphingosine-1-phosphate lyase 1)

Pathogenic variants in the *SGPL1* gene (Answer A) have recently been identified as the cause of a new syndrome of primary adrenal insufficiency associated with nephrotic syndrome and multiple endocrinopathies. Pathogenic variants in *MRAP* (Answer B), *POR* (Answer C), *AIRE* (Answer D), and *AAAS* (Answer E) can all give rise to primary adrenal insufficiency, but they are not associated with nephrotic syndrome.

Since the first description in 2017, more than 35 patients carrying a pathogenic variant in the *SGPL1* gene in the homozygous or compound heterozygous state have been reported worldwide. The clinical presentation and phenotypes are variable. Most affected patients have steroid-resistant nephrotic syndrome presenting from birth to 19 years of age. Just over half of all those with *SGPL1* pathogenic variants have glucocorticoid deficiency (with or without mineralocorticoid deficiency). Primary adrenal insufficiency can present from infancy to age 11 years. Some patients have adrenal calcification on imaging. Associated features reported include ichthyosis, neurologic involvement, and lymphopenia. Neurologic involvement is diverse and ranges from early developmental delay, microcephaly, seizures, and sensorineural deafness to late presentation with abnormal gait, peripheral neuropathy, and progressive neurologic deficit. In addition to primary adrenal insufficiency, multiple endocrinopathies such as primary hypothyroidism and gonadal dysfunction have also been described. Dysmorphic features and bone defects have been reported in a few patients. Fetal demise and hydrops fetalis have also been noted in some families.

Deficiency of the SGPL1 protein represents a novel form of sphingolipidosis. Other forms include Fabry disease, Gaucher disease, and Niemann-Pick disease. The SGPL1 protein is an intracellular enzyme that catalyses the breakdown of sphingolipids by cleaving substrate, sphingosine-1-phosphate (S1P), in the final step in the sphingolipid degradation pathway. S1P is a bioactive sphingolipid metabolite that acts on the family of 5 G-protein–

coupled receptors to mediate diverse biologic activities, including angiogenesis, immune-cell trafficking, stem-cell differentiation, and programmed cell death. Inactive SGPL1 leads to an accumulation of sphingolipids and ceramides. Accumulation of ceramides induces apoptosis, while sphingosine is a ligand for steroidogenic factor 1, inhibiting steroidogenesis by maintaining steroidogenic factor 1 in an inactive conformation. More recently, SGPL1 deficiency has been shown to be associated with mitochondrial dysfunction, which may contribute to the pathophysiology of this disorder.

Educational Objective
Identify a new form of syndromic primary adrenal insufficiency due to pathogenic variants in the *SGPL1* gene.

Reference(s)

Prasad R, Hadjidemetriou I, Maharaj A, et al. Sphingosine-1-phosphate lyase mutations cause primary adrenal insufficiency and steroid-resistant nephrotic syndrome. *J Clin Invest.* 2017;127(3):942-953. PMID: 28165343

Lovric S, Goncalves S, Gee HY, et al. Mutations in sphingosine-1-phosphate lyase cause nephrosis with ichthyosis and adrenal insufficiency. *J Clin Invest.* 2017;127(3):912-928. PMID: 28165339

Maharaj A, Theodorou D, Banerjee II, Metherell LA, Prasad R, Wallace D. A sphingosine-1-phosphate lyase mutation associated with congenital nephrotic syndrome and multiple endocrinopathy. *Front Pediatr.* 2020;8:151. PMID: 32322566

Lucki NC, Sewer MB. Nuclear sphingolipid metabolism. *Annu Rev Physiol.* 2012;74:131-151. PMID: 21888508

Maharaj A, Williams J, Brashaw T, et al. Sphingosine-1-phosphate lyase (SGPL1) deficiency is associated with mitochondrial dysfunction. *J Steroid Biochem Mol Biol.* 2020;202:105730. PMID: 32682944

83 ANSWER: E) Methylation analysis of chromosome 11p15

This child has significant short stature with a history of prenatal growth restriction. Target height (midparental height) is at the 25th percentile. This, and the severity of his short stature, makes familial short stature an unlikely cause of his growth pattern. Hypothyroidism, inflammatory bowel disease, and celiac disease are also unlikely given his normal thyroid function, normal erythrocyte sedimentation rate, and negative celiac screen. His IGF-1 concentration is in the midpoint of the reference range for age, and his IGFBP-3 concentration is in the upper half of the reference range, which is not consistent with GH deficiency. Therefore, an arginine-insulin tolerance test (Answer A) for diagnostic purposes is not the best option. Additionally, this child was small-for-gestational-age and did not display "catch-up" growth during the first 4 years of life. He is a candidate for GH therapy based on the diagnosis of being small-for-gestational-age without catch-up growth. A GH-stimulation test would not be required to receive GH therapy.

Although this child is described as having café-au-lait spots, which can be seen in neurofibromatosis type 1 (Answer B), the other clinical manifestations in this case, particularly the significant short stature, are not typical of this condition.

Prenatal and postnatal growth restriction have also been described in individuals with defects in the gene encoding the IGF-1 receptor (Answer D). Elevated IGF-1 levels are described in these individuals and, although not present in all, some dysmorphic features such as microcephaly (as opposed to relative macrocephaly described in this vignette) are seen. Therefore, sequencing this gene is incorrect.

The child in this vignette has clinical manifestations consistent with Silver-Russell syndrome, including prenatal and postnatal growth retardation, prominent forehead, triangular face, asymmetric growth of the extremities, and café-au-lait spots. Multiple types of Silver-Russell syndrome have been reported to date. Approximately 50% of affected children carry an epimutation consisting of hypomethylation of the imprinting control region 1 (ICR1) at the *IGF2/H19* locus on chromosome 11p15 (SRS type 1), while about 10% of affected children have maternal uniparental disomy of chromosome 7 (SRS type 2). A smaller proportion of cases are due to structural aberrations of the short arm of chromosome 11 (SRS type 3). Other less common types of Silver-Russell syndrome have been described with defects on chromosome 8q12.1 (SRS type 4) and 12q14.3 (SRS type 5). Even an X-linked form has been described.

Children with SRS type 1 (caused by hypomethylation of the ICR1 on chromosome 11p15) seem to have the most severe phenotype with smaller size at birth and no significant change in height SDS postnatally when compared with children with SRS type 2 (caused by maternal uniparental disomy of chromosome 7) who have a longer birth length but show a decline in height SDS postnatally. Additionally, children with SRS type 1 (11p15 epimutation) have significantly higher levels of IGF-1 and IGFBP-3 (usually within normal range for age) and these levels increase significantly after GH treatment. This suggests a certain degree of IGF-1 resistance. Children with SRS type 2 (uniparental disomy of chromosome 7) typically have IGF-1 and IGFBP-3 levels that are low for age. The child in this vignette has IGF-1 and IGFBP-3 levels in the normal range, making hypomethylation of the ICR1 on chromosome 11p15 (Answer E) more likely than maternal uniparental disomy of chromosome 7 (Answer C).

Educational objective
Identify the clinical manifestations of Silver-Russell syndrome and recommend testing to confirm the diagnosis.

Reference(s)

Price SM, Stanhope R, Garrett C, Preece MA, Trembath RC. The spectrum of Silver-Russell syndrome: a clinical and molecular genetic study and new diagnostic criteria. *J Med Genet.* 1999;36(11):837-842. PMID: 10544228

Wakeling EL. Silver-Russell syndrome. *Arch Dis Child.* 2011;96(12):1156-1161. PMID: 21349887

Binder G, Seidel AK, Martin DD, et al. The endocrine phenotype in Silver-Russell syndrome is defined by the underlying epigenetic alteration. *J Clin Endocrinol Metab.* 2008;93(4):1402-1407. PMID: 18230663

Abuzzahab MJ, Schneider A, Goddard A, et al. IGF-I receptor mutations resulting in intrauterine and postnatal growth retardation. *N Engl J Med.* 2003;349(23):2211-2222. PMID: 14657428

84 ANSWER: E) *MT-TL1* genetic testing

The case presented in this vignette is characterized by a maternal inheritance pattern and neurosensory deafness that is consistent with maternally inherited (mitochondrial) diabetes and deafness (MIDD). The diagnosis could be confirmed with *MT-TL1* genetic testing (Answer E). The most common *MT-TL1* pathogenic variant associated with this condition is 3243 A>G, but other mitochondrial DNA variants have been linked with a diabetic phenotype suggestive of MIDD.

Wolfram syndrome can present with diabetes as one of its earliest manifestations. Also known as DIDMOAD (diabetes insipidus, diabetes mellitus, optic atrophy, and deafness), Wolfram syndrome is characterized by early-onset diabetes mellitus and optic atrophy (<16 years) with variable presence of neuropsychiatric features, sensorineural hearing loss, and other endocrine features such as diabetes insipidus, hypogonadism, short stature, and/or hypothyroidism. It is caused by autosomal recessive pathogenic variants in the *WFS1* gene (Answer D), which is not consistent with the details in the vignette in terms of inheritance pattern or presenting clinical features.

Monogenic diabetes (maturity-onset diabetes of the young [MODY]) type 3 or type 1, due to pathogenic variants in the *HNF1A* and *HNF4A* genes (Answer C), respectively, could be suspected with the autosomal dominant inheritance pattern in the vignette. However, neurosensory hearing loss and learning disability are not associated features of *HNF1A* or *HNF4A* pathogenic variants.

All the major type 1 diabetes autoantigens are related to the secretory apparatus of the β cell. Assessing zinc tranporter-8 antibodies (Answer A) could be a logical next step in addition to the 3 antibodies tested in the vignette (all undetectable), but this will not lead to the correct diagnosis since the patient has additional clinical clues that should make the learner consider an alternative diagnosis beyond type 1 diabetes. HLA typing (Answer B) is neither cost-effective nor useful in establishing the diagnosis of type 1 diabetes and should not be pursued.

Educational Objective
Consider rare forms of genetic diabetes in the differential diagnosis of diabetes mellitus.

Reference(s)

Bingley PJ. Clinical applications of diabetes antibody testing. *J Clin Endocrinol Metab.* 2010;95(1):25-33. PMID: 19875480

Yeung RO, Hanna-Shmouni F, Niederhoffer K, Walker MA. Not quite type 1 or type 2, what now? Review of monogenic, mitochondrial, and syndromic diabetes. *Rev Endocr Metab Disord.* 2018;19(1):35-52. PMID: 29777474

Mazzaccara C, Iafusco D, Liguori R, et al. Mitochondrial diabetes in children: seek and you will find it. *PLoS One.* 2012;7(4):e34956. PMID: 22536343

85

ANSWER: C) Initiate levothyroxine to maintain TSH <0.1 mIU/L; 2 to 3 months after surgery, measure TSH-stimulated thyroglobulin and perform diagnostic whole-body ^{123}I scan

The key to answering this question is determining the patient's risk category and recognizing the importance of postoperative staging in guiding further management. The patient's risk category is based on the 2015 American Thyroid Association (ATA) Management Guidelines for Children with Thyroid Nodules and Differentiated Thyroid Cancer, which primarily address papillary thyroid cancer. The risk is defined as the likelihood of having persistent cervical disease and/or distant metastases after initial total thyroidectomy with or without lymph node dissection by a high-volume surgeon. The degree of risk is determined by the spread of cancer to cervical lymph nodes (N1a in the central neck compartment, or N1b in the lateral neck) or local spread beyond the thyroid (locally invasive T4 tumors), with or without distant metastases.

Once the risk category is determined, one can follow the guidelines for recommended management and monitoring. This patient had a central and right lateral neck dissection based on preoperative imaging and was found to have extensive N1b disease. Therefore, she has an ATA pediatric high-risk tumor. While it is true that many pediatric patients with high-risk papillary thyroid cancer require ^{131}I, not all do. Postoperative staging includes both TSH-stimulated thyroglobulin measurement and a ^{123}I whole-body scan, as detailed in the pediatric guidelines.

Whole-body scanning helps determine whether there is any cervical uptake outside of the thyroid bed (metastatic lymphadenopathy) or any distant metastases. Whole-body scanning may miss pulmonary micrometastases, which only show up on post-^{131}I scan. When a high-volume thyroid surgeon performs the thyroidectomy, the odds of any significant thyroid remnant are reduced. Documenting a stimulated thyroglobulin value is helpful in patients without cervical or distant metastases on whole-body scanning.

A low stimulated thyroglobulin value (<2 ng/mL [<2 μg/L], assuming negative thyroglobulin antibodies) helps identify which patients do not require ^{131}I. Those with a thyroglobulin concentration greater than 10 ng/mL (>10 μg/L) should have ^{131}I ablation, followed by a posttreatment scan. Those with an in-between thyroglobulin value (2-10 ng/mL [2-10 μg/L]) may benefit from ^{131}I ablation, especially if the tumor has aggressive features such as vascular invasion or is a locally invasive (T4) tumor. Patients with distant metastases require ^{131}I radioablation, but it may be delayed if resectable cervical disease remains.

Chest CT (Answer A), with its associated radiation, is not recommended for all patients at high risk. Furthermore, it may miss pulmonary micrometastases. While it is recommended to maintain TSH less than 0.1 mIU/L in patients at high risk, as one cannot rely solely on unstimulated thyroglobulin measurement at this stage, a whole-body scan is also necessary (thus, Answer B is incorrect). Holding off on levothyroxine replacement right after surgery and administering ^{131}I once the TSH concentration is greater than 30 mIU/L is incorrect, as it assumes that all patients at high risk should undergo radioablation, without postoperative staging, which is not the case. This approach could fail to identify some resectable disease, which may render the ^{131}I less effective in ablating any distant metastases. Furthermore, thyroid cancer is slow-growing, and there is no rush to ablate 2 to 3 weeks after thyroidectomy when the surgical site may be still healing (thus, Answer D is incorrect).

Initiating levothyroxine to maintain TSH between 0.1 and 0.5 mIU/L and performing postoperative ^{123}I whole-body scan (Answer E) is incorrect as well, as it does not include a stimulated thyroglobulin measurement as part of the postoperative staging. While the recommended TSH suppressive level for patients at high risk is less than 0.1 mIU/L, some endocrinologists choose to temporarily keep their patients' TSH concentration less than 0.5 mIU/L ahead of the TSH-stimulated thyroglobulin measurement and whole-body scan, and thus shorten their levothyroxine withdrawal time. After ^{131}I is given, it is important to maintain the TSH concentration less than 0.1 mIU/L.

Initiating levothyroxine to maintain the TSH concentration below 0.1 mIU/L and measuring TSH-stimulated thyroglobulin and performing a diagnostic whole-body ^{123}I scan 2 to 3 months after surgery (Answer C) is the correct management. This approach encompasses the proper postoperative staging and the suppressive TSH level recommended by the pediatric guidelines and does not assume that ^{131}I should be given to all patients at high risk. The use of ^{131}I should be guided by postoperative staging.

Educational Objective
Explain the importance of postoperative staging in high-risk papillary thyroid cancer in an adolescent.

Reference(s)
Francis GL, Waguespack SG, Bauer AJ, et al; American Thyroid Association Guidelines Task Force. Management guidelines for children with thyroid nodules and differentiated thyroid cancer. *Thyroid.* 2015;25(7):716-759. PMID: 25900731

86

ANSWER: C) Start GH replacement therapy at 0.2 mg/kg per week

This patient's height is more affected than his weight, and he has a normal caloric intake. He has no signs or symptoms of malabsorption. His laboratory test results are concerning for possible GH deficiency. Thus, it is not appropriate to provide reassurance (Answer A) or wait until gastrointestinal evaluation is completed (Answer B). He had normal thyroid function and adrenal function when tested, so it is not necessary to repeat these labs again (Answer E). His clinical picture of normal prenatal growth, poor postnatal growth, episodes of hypoglycemia, proportional short stature without dysmorphic features, and delayed bone age plus his laboratory results (low-normal IGF-1, low stimulated GH concentration, otherwise normal pituitary workup) indicate that he has isolated GH deficiency. Patients with isolated GH deficiency are generally started on GH treatment at a dosage of 0.18 to 0.25 mg/kg per week (to minimize the risk of adverse effects), which is then titrated based on growth response. This dosage is lower than the starting dosage for other indications such as idiopathic short stature, small-for-gestational-age with poor catch-up growth, or conditions such as Turner syndrome or Noonan syndrome. The starting dosage of 0.35 mg/kg per week (Answer D) is too high. There is a family history of short stature on the paternal side (the father's first cousin). Thus, it is prudent to consider genetic testing to evaluate for genetic causes of GH deficiency, to assess whether this patient is at risk for developing multiple pituitary hormone deficiency in the future, and to understand the need to test other family members. Therefore, the best strategy is to start GH replacement therapy at a dosage of 0.2 mg/kg per week and consider genetic testing (Answer C).

Several patients with short stature inherited in an autosomal dominant manner have been shown to have a missense pathogenic variant (p.A204E) resulting in complete loss of constitutive activity of the GH secretagogue receptor. The GH secretagogue receptor is a 7-transmembrane G-protein–coupled receptor that is highly expressed in the pituitary and hypothalamus (also known as the ghrelin receptor, as it binds to and is activated by ghrelin). This patient was reported to have compound heterozygous pathogenic variants in the gene encoding the GH secretagogue receptor (*GHSR*). Patients with *GHSR* pathogenic variants are known to have delayed puberty as well (as reported in his father). The patient responded well to GH therapy and had delayed pubertal onset at age 15 years. Although he continued to have 1 to 2 episodes of vomiting and abdominal pain every year, he did not have further episodes of hypoglycemia while on GH therapy.

Educational Objective

Identify the diagnostic challenges in a child with short stature and recall the recommended GH dosage for treating patients with GH deficiency.

Reference(s)

Grimberg A, DiVall SA, Polychronakos C, et al; Drug and Therapeutics Committee and Ethics Committee of the Pediatric Endocrine Society. Guidelines for growth hormone and insulin-like growth factor-I treatment in children and adolescents: growth hormone deficiency, idiopathic short stature, and primary insulin-like growth factor-I deficiency. *Horm Res Paediatr.* 2016;86(6):361-397. PMID: 27884013

87

ANSWER: E) Hypothalamic hamartoma

Precocious puberty, defined as breast development before age 8 years in girls, has been increasing in prevalence since age cutoffs were established in the 1960s. The percentage of girls with precocious puberty is now approximately 10%, with central precocious puberty accounting for 90% to 95% of cases. The prevalence of central nervous system abnormalities is much lower in girls with central precocious puberty than in boys and decreases with age. In one recent meta-analysis, the pooled prevalence of intracranial lesions was 25% in girls younger than 6 years (n = 173) and 3% in girls aged 6 to 8 years (n = 514). In this pool of 1853 individuals, the incidence of tumors was 1.6%.

Hypothalamic hamartomas are considered to be the most common cause of central precocious puberty among girls with central nervous system lesions. These are rare, congenital, benign lesions located in the ventral hypothalamus that are highly associated with gelastic seizures and treatment-resistant epilepsy. The girl in this vignette has central precocious puberty as indicated by the presence of Tanner stage 3 breast development and pubertal gonadotropins. She has a history suspicious for gelastic seizures, which are primarily manifested by sudden outbursts of laughter or crying for no apparent reason and lasting less than a minute. Given her presentation of central precocious puberty with probable gelastic seizures, she most likely has central precocious puberty due to a hypothalamic hamartoma (Answer E).

While idiopathic central precocious puberty is more common than all other causes of central precocious puberty at this age, the presence of gelastic seizures makes idiopathic (Answer C) or genetic causes of central precocious puberty less likely. Many cases of central precocious puberty previously considered idiopathic now have known genetic etiologies, with variants in the *MKRN3* gene (Answer A) being the most common. *MKRN3* encodes the Makorin ring finger protein 3, a protein that normally functions to inhibit the release of hypothalamic GnRH. Variants in the *MKRN3* gene result in loss of GnRH inhibition in childhood, which leads to central precocious puberty. Variants in the *GNAS* gene (Answer B) causing constitutive activation of the G-protein subunit Gsα result in gonadotropin-independent precocious puberty as part of McCune-Albright syndrome. As the patient in this vignette has central precocious puberty, McCune-Albright syndrome is an unlikely diagnosis.

Craniopharyngiomas (Answer D) are also associated with central precocious puberty. As they expand, craniopharyngiomas can disrupt pituitary function and cause central precocious puberty. However, they most commonly affect children between 5 and 14 years of age and are typically associated with findings such as visual field deficits, nausea and vomiting, headaches, growth failure, and diabetes insipidus.

Subsequent workup was notable for a 10-mm lesion consistent with a hypothalamic hamartoma found on MRI and electroencephalography findings of occasional bursts (1-2 seconds) of very high-voltage, semirhythmic delta activity consistent with gelastic seizures, which have been well controlled with anticonvulsant medication. While hypothalamic hamartomas are rare (1:200,000 to 1:600,000), gelastic seizures and precocious puberty are common manifestations. Other endocrine manifestations, including GH deficiency and Cushing syndrome, are rarely reported in this setting. Surgery is not usually required; increased appetite and obesity are common long-term postoperative complications in individuals who require surgical resection.

Educational Objective
Identify gelastic seizures as part of the presentation of central precocious puberty due to a hypothalamic hamartoma.

Reference(s)
Cantas-Orsdemir S, Garb JL, Allen HF. Prevalence of cranial MRI findings in girls with central precocious puberty: a systematic review and meta-analysis. *J Pediatr Endocrinol Metab*. 2018;31(7):701-710. PMID: 29902155

Harrison VS, Oatman O, Kerrigan JF. Hypothalamic hamartoma with epilepsy: review of endocrine comorbidity. *Epilepsia*. 2017;58(Suppl 2):50-59. PMID: 28591479

88 ANSWER: A) Start GH therapy

The child described in this vignette fulfills the criteria to be classified as being small-for-gestational-age based on both weight and length at birth. The etiology of this problem includes placental, fetal, maternal, and environmental factors. Nevertheless, no clear etiology is found in approximately 40% of the cases. Most children born small-for-gestational-age (~90%) undergo linear growth acceleration in the first year of life, so-called catch-up growth that is mostly completed by 2 years of age. However, approximately 10% of children born small-for-gestational-age do not display such acceleration and fail to catch up. GH therapy (Answer A) has been approved by the US FDA for the management of short stature in children born small-for-gestational-age when no catch-up growth has occurred by 2 years of age. The European Medicines Agency has also approved the use of GH therapy in these children starting at 4 years of age. The response to GH therapy in these children is clearly superior, not only in terms of growth velocity but in terms of adult height, when started early (2-4 years of age). Thus, the best course of action is to start GH therapy for this patient.

Data from large-scale international databases for surveillance of efficacy and safety of GH treatment in children with growth disorders show that, on average, physicians initiate GH therapy in children born small-for-gestational-age without catch-up growth at a much older than optimal age (around 8-9 years of age) due to multiple reasons, including parental and primary care physician biases. Late initiation of GH therapy in these children would lead to suboptimal outcomes and be unfavorable from the cost-effective analysis perspective given that larger dosages are needed for larger children. Thus, simply following this patient clinically until age 5 years (Answer E) is incorrect.

A marginal TSH elevation in the presence of normal free T_4 is unlikely to explain the degree of short stature in this child. Therefore, assessing thyroid autoantibodies (Answer B) is not warranted. Additionally, autoimmune thyroid disease (Hashimoto thyroiditis) usually leads to acquired hypothyroidism and the impact on linear growth would not be manifested since birth.

Classic GH deficiency is rare in children born small-for-gestational-age. However, IGF-1 and IGFBP-3 are somewhat reduced in children born small-for-gestational-age (by about 1 SD), as is the case with the patient in this vignette. These levels are not suggestive of GH deficiency. In addition, in the absence of clinical or biochemical data suggestive of GH deficiency, the performance of a definitive test to exclude this condition (GH-stimulation test) (Answer C) is not required to initiate therapy in these children.

Although this patient's linear growth did not show the expected acceleration seen in approximately 90% of children born small-for-gestational-age, the ponderal growth was not unreasonable, as it progressed from well below the 3rd percentile at birth to about the 8th percentile by 35 months of age. The linear growth failure is not linked to poor weight gain and a referral to gastroenterology (Answer D) is not the best answer.

Educational Objective
List the indications for GH therapy in children born small-for-gestational-age who do not display catch-up growth in the first 2 to 4 years of life.

Reference(s)
Houk CP, Lee PA. Early diagnosis and treatment referral of children born small for gestational age without catch-up growth are critical for optimal outcomes. *Int J Pediatr Endocrinol.* 2012(1):11. PMID: 22559301

Clayton PE, Cianfarani S, Czernichow P, Johannsson G, Rapaport R, Rogol A. Management of the child born small for gestational age through adulthood: a consensus statement of the International Societies of Pediatric Endocrinology and the Growth Hormone Research Society. *J Clin Endocrinol Metab.* 2007;92(3):804-810. PMID: 17200164

89 ANSWER: C) Severity of hypothyroidism at diagnosis

Hearing impairment is more common in children with congenital hypothyroidism than in the general population. One population-based study reported the presence of hearing impairment in 9.5% of patients with congenital hypothyroidism. In this study, hearing impairment in patients with congenital hypothyroidism was most often diagnosed between 3 and 19 years of age (median 7 years). Hearing deficits may be detected on neonatal hearing screening (if performed), but not all cases will be detected in this way. Hearing impairment in congenital hypothyroidism is mild to moderate in most cases, and severe in about 10%. For these reasons, long-term management of patients with congenital hypothyroidism should include careful attention to speech and language development, delays in which may indicate underlying hearing deficits. Formal hearing testing should be recommended for any patient in whom hearing impairment is suspected.

The severity of congenital hypothyroidism at diagnosis (Answer C) is a risk factor for associated hearing impairment. This may be related to the key role of thyroid hormone in cochlear development in the prenatal period. Patients with ectopic thyroid have a lower risk of hearing impairment than those with thyroid agenesis or a eutopic thyroid gland, perhaps because patients with thyroid ectopy generally have milder hypothyroidism. Postnatal treatment factors, including timing of treatment initiation (Answer A), rate of thyroid function normalization (Answer B), or treatment adequacy during childhood (Answer D), do not appear to be related to the risk of hearing impairment. This risk is also unrelated to sex (Answer E).

Sensorineural hearing loss in a patient with congenital hypothyroidism and a eutopic thyroid gland can be observed in Pendred syndrome, a rare recessive disorder caused by inactivating pathogenic variants in the pendrin gene (*SLC26A4*). Most patients with Pendred syndrome have goiter, which may not be evident until adolescence or adulthood, and are euthyroid or have mild hypothyroidism, unlike the patient in this vignette. However, it is important to recognize that patients with congenital hypothyroidism of any etiology, particularly if severe, are at increased risk for hearing deficits and require close monitoring and prompt evaluation for hearing concerns.

Educational Objective
Identify risk factors and appropriate screening for hearing impairment in patients with congenital hypothyroidism.

Reference(s)
Lichtenberger-Geslin L, Dos Santos S, Hassani Y, Ecosse E, Van Den Abbeele T, Leger J. Factors associated with hearing impairment in patients with congenital hypothyroidism treated since the neonatal period: a national population-based study. *J Clin Endocrinol Metab.* 2013;98(9):3644-3652. PMID: 23780375

Léger J, Olivieri A, Donaldson M, et al. European Society for Paediatric Endocrinology consensus guidelines on screening, diagnosis, and management of congenital hypothyroidism. *J Clin Endocrinol Metab.* 2014;99(2):363-384. PMID: 24446653

90

ANSWER: E) TSH-producing adenoma

This girl presents with signs and symptoms of hyperthyroidism, goiter, elevated free T_4 and total T_3 levels, and an inappropriately elevated TSH level. When approaching the evaluation of inappropriate TSH secretion and elevated thyroid hormone levels, it is important to rule out genetic causes and interference from medications such as estrogen. Once medication or other laboratory interference has been ruled out, measurement of thyroid function in first-degree relatives is important. This girl is taking an oral contraceptive pill, which most likely contains estrogen. While total T_4 levels may be elevated due to an increase in thyroxine-binding globulin seen with estrogen, the free T_4 level would be normal, as would the TSH level. In addition, this patient appears clinically hyperthyroid. Therefore, medication interference causing abnormal laboratory findings (Answer A) is incorrect.

Graves disease (Answer D) is a common cause of hyperthyroidism and, in fact, this patient's mother had Graves disease. Measurement of thyroid-stimulating immunoglobulins and TSH-binding inhibitory immunoglobulins can be helpful. However, in this setting, the TSH level is expected to be suppressed, so Graves disease is incorrect.

The syndrome of familial dysalbuminemic hyperthyroxinemia (Answer C) presents with elevated total and normal or elevated free T_4 serum values in clinically euthyroid patients with normal TSH levels (euthyroid hyperthyroxinemia). This is an inherited abnormality (autosomal dominant) characterized by the presence of a variant serum albumin that has preferential affinity for T_4. The hyperthyroxinemia can be confused with hyperthyroidism. This girl is clinically hyperthyroid, has a goiter, and has elevated TSH. Therefore, familial dysalbuminemic hyperthyroxinemia is incorrect.

Both TSH-secreting adenomas (Answer E) and resistance to thyroid hormone β (Answer B) have elevated thyroid hormones in common and can present with goiter, but the peripheral response to the hyperthyroxinemia is different. Resistance to thyroid hormone β is due to abnormalities in the thyroid hormone receptor β gene (*TRHB*) and is generally inherited in an autosomal dominant pattern. It can be difficult to distinguish between these 2 entities, highlighting the importance of assessing thyroid function in first-degree relatives.

TSH-secreting pituitary adenomas are a very rare cause of hyperthyroidism with inappropriate TSH elevations and are even rarer in the pediatric population. In most cases, these adenomas are located in the pituitary, but a few instances of ectopic TSH production have been reported in the suprasellar region and nasopharynx. TSH-secreting pituitary adenomas are the rarest of the pituitary adenomas and can be either microadenomas or macroadenomas and may be found incidentally on imaging for other causes. In patients with TSH-secreting pituitary adenomas, cosecretion of GH and prolactin is common. Interestingly, although no values are given for GH or prolactin levels in this vignette, the patient is much taller than her midparental height, suggesting the possibility of excess GH secretion. Measurement of other pituitary function is essential. MRI would be particularly important to perform in this individual.

A thyrotropin-releasing hormone test may be helpful to distinguish between a TSH-secreting pituitary adenoma and resistance to thyroid hormones. TSH rises appropriately after thyrotropin-releasing hormone stimulation in patients with resistance to thyroid hormone but not in most patients with TSH-secreting pituitary adenomas. Measurement of serum α-subunit may also be a helpful diagnostic tool and is elevated in approximately 30% of individuals with TSH-secreting pituitary adenomas.

Educational Objective
Diagnose a TSH-secreting pituitary adenoma and explain the physiologic effects of TSH.

Reference(s)

Tjörnstrand A, Nyström HF. Diagnosis of endocrine disease: diagnostic approach to TSH-producing pituitary adenoma. *Eur J Endocrinol*. 2017;177(4):R183-R197.
    PMID: 28566440

Stanley JM, Najjar SS. Hyperthyroidism secondary to a TSH-secreting pituitary adenoma in a 15-year-old male. *Clin Pediatr (Phila)*. 1991;30(2):109-111.
    PMID: 2007301

91

ANSWER: A) Prefilled syringe, ready-to-inject glucagon, 0.5 mg

Hypoglycemia is a common adverse effect in patients with diabetes mellitus who are receiving insulin therapy. Insulin-induced hypoglycemia emergency is treated with glucagon, which is recommended by the American Diabetes Association and the European Association for the Study of Diabetes for all patients with diabetes on insulin therapy. Glucagon administration can be handled by caregivers after proper education. Until recently, a glucagon kit required mixing of the diluent with the active ingredient to reconstitute 1 mg per mL concentration. The usual adult dose is 1 mg. For children weighing less than 44 lb (<20 kg), one-half the adult dose (0.5 mg) is suggested. The patient in this vignette weighs 33 lb (15 kg) and requires the 0.5-mg dose, not 1 mg (Answer E).

Glucagon is available in a single dose, ready-to-inject liquid preparation that can be used for children older than 2 years. The patient in this vignette is 3 years old and requires the 0.5-mg glucagon injection prefilled syringe (Answer A), not 1 mg (Answer B).

A dry powder inhaler is also available, which can be administered via nasal mucosa at a standard dose of 3 mg (Answer C) to any patient older than 4 years. Since this patient is 3 years old, this option is incorrect. There is no half dose (Answer D), since the applicator administers the standard dose of 3 mg in 1 push.

Educational Objective
Determine the dosage and best way to administer glucagon for hypoglycemia emergencies.

Reference(s)

Carson MJ, Koch R. Clinical studies with glucagon in children. *J Pediatr*. 1955;47(2):161-170. PMID: 13243215

Aman J, Wranne L. Hypoglycemia in childhood diabetes. II: Effect of subcutaneous or intramuscular injection of different doses of glucagon. *Acta Paediatr Scand*. 1988;77(4):548-553. PMID: 3394508

Sherr JL, Ruedy KJ, Foster NC, et al; T1D Exchange Intranasal Glucagon Investigators. Glucagon nasal powder: a promising alternative to intramuscular glucagon in youth with type 1 diabetes. *Diabetes Care*. 2016;39(4):5555-62. PMID: 26884472

92 ANSWER: B) Start supplemental vitamin D and calcium

The child in this vignette fulfills criteria for pediatric osteoporosis in that she has a bone mineral density less than –2.0 and has sustained 2 low-trauma fractures by age 10 years. Potential risk factors for impaired bone health include altered mechanical stimulation due to inadequate weight-bearing activity and nutrient deficiency. The effect of vitamin D supplementation on bone density in children is conflicting, but the best evidence suggests a small beneficial effect in prepubertal girls who receive vitamin D supplementation in addition to adequate calcium intake (Answer B). Review of this child's dietary intake revealed that she is getting only 2 servings of calcium each day, which is unlikely to provide the recommended daily allotment of 1300 mg of calcium. Therefore, supplementing vitamin D alone (Answer A) would not correct the calcium deficiency. While vitamin D and calcium supplementation as primary prevention for falls and fractures is not supported by evidence (US Preventive Services Task Force Recommendation Statement), this strategy is still recommended for patients with vitamin D deficiency and those with an increased risk for osteoporosis. Of the options available, starting supplemental vitamin D and calcium is the best treatment choice for this child.

Anticonvulsant medications have historically been associated with an increased risk for impaired bone mineral density and fractures; however, the evidence for this is primarily with older anticonvulsant medications such as phenytoin and valproic acid through mechanisms of impaired vitamin D metabolism. Newer anticonvulsant medications such as levetiracetam may be associated with low vitamin D, but they have not been shown to have negative effects on bone density. In addition, because seizures increase the potential for falls and trauma-related fractures, stopping this medication could result in increased fracture risk (Answer E).

The patient is of pubertal age, and estrogen exposure is clearly beneficial for improving bone density. However, the incidence of fractures increases around the time of the pubertal growth spurt; thus, induction of puberty (Answer D) may increase her risk for subsequent fractures (albeit temporarily). In addition, it is normal for girls to be prepubertal at this age, so there is no indication to commence puberty even with a low bone density.

Bisphosphonate therapy (Answer C) has been shown to improve bone mineral density in secondary osteoporosis; however, the reduction in fracture risk is unknown. While this patient meets criteria for pediatric osteoporosis, the benefit in fracture risk reduction is likely to be minimal given that her bone mineral density Z-score is just below the normal range. In addition, bisphosphonate therapy is not recommended in the setting of low vitamin D due to the increased risk for severe hypocalcemia.

Educational Objective
Identify risk factors for fractures and falls and manage pediatric osteoporosis.

Reference(s)

Vestergaard P. Effects of antiepileptic drugs on bone health and growth potential in children with epilepsy. *Paediatr Drugs.* 2015;17(2):141-150. PMID: 25567416

Weaver CM, Gordon CM, Janz KF, et al. The National Osteoporosis Foundation's position statement on peak bone mass development and lifestyle factors: a systematic review and implementation recommendations [published correction appears in *Osteoporos Int.* 2016;27(4):1387]. *Osteoporos Int.* 2016;27(4):1281-1386. PMID: 26935424

Weaver CM, Alexander DD, Boushey CJ, et al. Calcium plus vitamin D supplementation and risk of fractures: an updated meta-analysis from the National Osteoporosis Foundation. *Osteoporos Int.* 2016;27(8):2643-2646. PMID: 26510847

US Preventive Services Task Force, Grossman DC, Curry SJ, et al. Vitamin D, calcium, or combined supplementation for the primary prevention of fractures in community-dwelling adults: US Preventive Services Task Force recommendation statement. *JAMA.* 2018;319(15):1592-1599. PMID: 29677309

93 ANSWER: B) Puberty

This child was found to have increased cortisol clearance, most likely due to the onset of puberty (Answer B). Alterations in cortisol dynamics may occur in puberty for many reasons, including changes in 11β-hydroxysteroid dehydrogenase activity (altering cortisol/cortisone conversion), estradiol-related increase in cortisol-binding globulin (altering free cortisol), and GH secretion leading to increased glomerular filtration. Collectively, this leads to reduced circulating cortisol.

The glucocorticoid of choice for the treatment of children with congenital adrenal hyperplasia (CAH) due to 21-hydroxylase deficiency is hydrocortisone given orally 3 times daily. In the case of increased cortisol clearance in puberty, an increase in dosing frequency may be necessary rather than increasing the dosage. A recent publication reported improved cortisol concentrations on a regimen of 4 daily doses.

Obesity (Answer D) increases cortisol clearance due to insulin insensitivity. In this case, the patient had been growing along the same percentiles for weight and height. Other factors, including fatty liver disease (increased cortisol clearance), hepatic metabolism (particularly the cytochrome P450 system), 11β-hydroxysteroid dehydrogenase enzyme activity, 5α-reductase system activity, thyroid hormone levels, cortisol-binding globulin concentration, and numerous medications can all alter cortisol metabolism. All of these factors should be considered when assessing a patient with suboptimally controlled CAH.

Gastritis (Answer C) could lead to poor absorption; however, the child in this vignette was given hydrocortisone intravenously, which would bypass any gut issues.

Drugs interactions (Answer E) should always be considered. Erythromycin is a known inhibitor of CYP3A4 enzyme activity (involved in the elimination of glucocorticoids). Inhibition of CYP3A4 leads to increased glucocorticoid availability. Vitamin D supplementation has no effect on cortisol metabolism. In contrast, CYP3A4 inducers, such as carbamazepine, phenytoin, and phenobarbitone, lead to increased clearance and reduced efficacy of coadministered glucocorticoids and increased risk of adrenal crisis.

Poor regimen adherence (Answer A) is often used to explain suboptimal control of CAH during puberty. However, physiologic changes in puberty that can alter cortisol clearance should always be considered before concluding that poor regimen adherence is the cause.

Educational Objective

Explain how changes in puberty can alter cortisol dynamics and control of congenital adrenal hyperplasia.

Reference(s)

Bryan SM, Honour JW, Hindmarsh PC. Management of altered hydrocortisone pharmacokinetics in a boy with congenital adrenal hyperplasia using a continuous subcutaneous hydrocortisone infusion. *J Clin Endocrinol Metab.* 2009;94(9):3477-3480. PMID: 19567522

Speiser PW, Arlt W, Auchus RJ, et al. Congenital adrenal hyperplasia due to steroid 21-hydroxylase deficiency: an Endocrine Society clinical practice guideline. *J Clin Endocrinol Metab.* 2018;103(11):4043-4088. PMID: 30272171

Charmandari E, Hindmarsh PC, Johnston A, Brook CG. Congenital adrenal hyperplasia due to 21-hydroxylase deficiency: alterations in cortisol pharmacokinetics at puberty. *J Clin Endocrinol Metab.* 2001;86(6):2701-2708. PMID: 11397874

Melin J, Parra-Guillen ZP, Michelet R, et al. Pharmacokinetic/pharmacodynamic evaluation of hydrocortisone therapy in pediatric patients with congenital adrenal hyperplasia. *J Clin Endocrinol Metab.* 2020;105(3):dgaa071. PMID: 32052005

Dineen R, Stewart PM, Sherlock M. Factors impacting on the action of glucocorticoids in patients receiving glucocorticoid therapy. *Clin Endocrinol (Oxf).* 2019;90(1):3-14. PMID: 30120786

94

ANSWER: E) *BRAF* V600E pathogenic variant

Thyroid cancer is the most prevalent endocrine malignancy and is the third most frequent solid tumor in pediatric patients. The most common histologic type is papillary thyroid carcinoma, accounting for about two-thirds of nonmedullary thyroid cancer.

As noted in the vignette, the histopathologic examination revealed classic papillary thyroid carcinoma. In both adult and pediatric patients, the single most common genetic abnormality found in classic papillary thyroid cancer is the *BRAF* V600E pathogenic variant (Answer E), accounting for about 30% to 40% of cases. However, the reality is a bit more complex. Although *BRAF* V600E is the most common pathogenic variant in pediatric patients with classic papillary thyroid cancer, it is observed more often in older adolescents (typically >15 years). *RET/PTC* fusions seem to occur in younger patients and have been associated equally or more frequently with other types of papillary thyroid cancer in the pediatric population, including the diffuse variant of papillary thyroid carcinoma.

RET/PTC fusions (Answer B) (most common *RET/PTC1*) and *NTRK* fusions (Answer D) (most common *NTRK3/ETV6*), as well as *BRAF* pathogenic variants (almost exclusively *BRAF* V600E) all lead to papillary thyroid cancer via activation of the mitogen-activated protein (MAP) kinase pathway. *RET/PTC* and *NTRK* fusions are much more common in pediatric patients with papillary thyroid cancer than in adults, and gene fusions combined are more common in pediatric patients than *BRAF* V600E mutation alone. However, each fusion group on its own is usually not the most common genetic alteration. Furthermore, the *BRAF* V600E pathogenic variant has recently been documented to be the most common genetic alteration in classic papillary thyroid carcinoma in children and adolescents.

The *PAX8/PPARG* fusion (Answer C) is observed in follicular variants of papillary thyroid cancer, not in classic papillary thyroid cancer.

Pathogenic variants in the *RET* proto-oncogene (Answer A) cause multiple endocrine neoplasia type 2. *RET* M918T is the pathogenic variant that accounts for most multiple endocrine neoplasia type 2B cases, while a number of other *RET* variants account for multiple endocrine neoplasia type 2A, with good correlation between genotype and aggressiveness of the medullary thyroid cancer. However, the patient in this vignette does not have medullary thyroid cancer. Although medullary thyroid cancer nodules can have microcalcifications noted on ultrasonography, when medullary thyroid cancer has spread and is associated with cervical lymph node metastases, the calcitonin concentration is elevated. This patient's calcitonin level was normal. As this patient does not have medullary thyroid cancer, a pathogenic variant in the *RET* gene is incorrect.

Another type of differentiated thyroid cancer is follicular thyroid cancer. Patients with follicular thyroid cancer do not commonly present with cervical lymph node metastases. Cervical lymph node metastases are common in papillary thyroid cancer (more so in pediatric patients), as are psammoma bodies on histopathologic examination and microcalcifications on ultrasonography. *RAS* variants have been found in follicular thyroid cancer and follicular variants of papillary thyroid cancer.

Educational Objective

Describe the most common genetic alterations found in children and adolescents with papillary thyroid cancer vs follicular or medullary thyroid cancer.

Reference(s)

Nikita ME, Jiang W, Cheng SM, et al. Mutational analysis in pediatric thyroid cancer and correlations with age, ethnicity, and clinical presentation. *Thyroid.* 2016;26(2):227-234. PMID: 26649796

Cordioli MIC, Moraes L, Bastos AU, et al. Fusion oncogenes are the main genetic events found in sporadic papillary thyroid carcinomas from children. *Thyroid.* 2017;27(2):182-188. PMID: 27849443

Vanden Borre P, Schrock AB, Anderson PM, et al. Pediatric, adolescent, and young adult thyroid carcinoma harbors frequent and diverse targetable genomic alterations, including kinase fusions. *Oncologist.* 2017;22(3):255-263. PMID: 28209747

Bauer AJ. Molecular genetics of thyroid cancer in children and adolescents. *Endocrinol Metab Clin N Am.* 2017; 46 (2): 389-403. PMID: 28476228

Cancer Genome Atlas Research Network. Integrated genomic characterization of papillary thyroid carcinoma. *Cell.* 2014;159(3):676-690. PMID: 25417114

Franco AT, Labourier E, Ablordeppey KK, et al. miRNA expression can classify pediatric thyroid lesions and increases the diagnostic yield of mutation testing. *Pediatr Blood Cancer.* 2020;67(6):e28276. doi:10.1002/pbc.28276. PMID: 32196952

95 ANSWER: E) *ACAN* pathogenic variant

This patient has proportional short stature as evidenced by her normal sitting height to standing height ratio and normal difference between arm span and height. Thus, she does not have features typical of an *FGFR3* pathogenic variant (Answer D), which results in achondroplasia. Classic features of achondroplasia include macrocephaly, short limbs (rhizomelic dwarfism), and significant short stature. Although *FGFR3* pathogenic variants are inherited in an autosomal dominant fashion, most affected patients (about 80%) do not have a family history of achondroplasia but rather have a de novo variant.

Turner syndrome (45,X karyotype) (Answer C) is one of the common causes of short stature in girls. However, this patient does not have features suggestive of Turner syndrome such as a webbed neck, lymphedema, or a congenital heart defect. Also, the history of short stature in her father and paternal cousins suggests the likely presence of an inherited cause of short stature other than Turner syndrome.

Pathogenic variants in the *GNAS* gene (Answer B) result in a rare condition known as Albright hereditary osteodystrophy. Albright hereditary osteodystrophy is inherited in an autosomal dominant manner. Patients with Albright hereditary osteodystrophy may have a wide range of signs and symptoms, including short stature, obesity, brachydactyly, round face, and subcutaneous ossifications. In addition, patients who inherit the disorder from their mother also have evidence of resistance to 1 or more hormones, especially PTH (pseudohypoparathyroidism type 1a). However, patients who inherit the disorder from their father have the Albright hereditary osteodystrophy phenotype, but do not have any hormone resistance (pseudopseudohypoparathyroidism). This patient does not have the classic phenotype of Albright hereditary osteodystrophy such as obesity, round face, or subcutaneous ossifications. Also, there is no evidence of hormone resistance.

Familial short stature (Answer A) is a nonpathologic variant of growth and thus it cannot be considered the cause of short stature in a child with advanced bone age and significant family history of early-onset joint disease. It is important to note that family members with short stature, in this case the patient's father, may have undiagnosed pathologic conditions leading to poor growth.

Her family history of short stature and early-onset lumbar disk herniation and osteoarthritis of the knees is highly indicative of an *ACAN* pathogenic variant (Answer E), which affects aggrecan—a major proteoglycan component of the extracellular matrix in the growth plate and articular cartilage. Patients with *ACAN* pathogenic variants may have mild to moderate dysmorphic features, including macrocephaly, brachydactyly, flat nasal bridge, and midface hypoplasia. Many children, but not all, with *ACAN* pathogenic variants have advanced bone age (as seen in this case), even in prepubertal years, and have a shortened pubertal growth spurt resulting in proportional short stature.

Educational Objective
Identify *ACAN* pathogenic variants as the cause of aggrecanopathies with specific phenotypic features, including short stature in affected patients and their family members.

Reference(s)
Stavber L, Hovnik T, Kotnik P, et al. High frequency of pathogenic ACAN variants including an intragenic deletion in selected individuals with short stature. *Eur J Endocrinol.* 2020;182(3):243-253. PMID: 31841439

Gkourogianni A, Andrew M, Tyzinski L, et al. Clinical characterization of patients with autosomal dominant short stature due to aggrecan mutations. *J Clin Endocrinol Metab.* 2017;102(2):460-469. PMID: 27870580

Sentchordi-Montané L, Aza-Carmona M, Benito-Sanz S, et al. Heterozygous aggrecan variants are associated with short stature and brachydactyly: description of 16 probands and a review of the literature. *Clin Endocrinol (Oxf).* 2018;88(6):820-829. PMID: 29464738

96 ANSWER: E) Orlistat

A number of weight-loss medications have been approved by the US FDA. Such medications can be considered for individuals with a BMI of 30 kg/m^2 or greater or those with a BMI of 27 kg/m^2 or greater who have at least 1 obesity-related comorbidity (eg, dyslipidemia). Most weight-loss medications are only approved for patients who are 16 years old or older. Intensive lifestyle modifications that are age-appropriate and family-based are still first-line therapy. However, pharmacotherapy could be considered for a patient with obesity who has not lost weight despite participation in a formal lifestyle modification program, or in an effort to decrease comorbidities. Pharmacotherapy should only be prescribed by clinicians who have experience using such therapies and are familiar with potential adverse risks. Off-label use of obesity medications in adolescents younger than 16 years is not recommended because of lack of FDA approval, limited efficacy and safety data in children and adolescents, and risks for potential adverse effects.

Orlistat (Answer E) is the only FDA-approved medication for obesity treatment of adolescents who are between the ages of 12 to 16 years. Orlistat can reduce fat absorption by up to 30% through inhibition of gastrointestinal lipases, and it reduces BMI by 0.7 to 1.7 kg/m². However, it has significant gastrointestinal adverse effects, including fatty stools, fecal incontinence, and increased defecation, which lead to its discontinuation in many patients. A multivitamin should be recommended for all patients taking this medication since it can impede the absorption of fat-soluble vitamins.

Phentermine (Answer A) is only approved for short-term weight loss in adults. Some of its potential adverse effects include paresthesias, dizziness, insomnia, and constipation. Octreotide (Answer B) may have a potential role in the treatment of hypothalamic obesity, but it is not an FDA-approved obesity medication. Metformin (Answer C) is not FDA-approved as an obesity medication and its use results in limited reductions in BMI. It is approved for patients 10 years or older for treatment of type 2 diabetes. Liraglutide (Answer D) is a GLP-1 analogue, which is approved for long-term weight loss in adults. It is FDA-approved for the treatment of pediatric patients 10 years or older with type 2 diabetes, but not for weight loss. It can cause gastrointestinal distress, headaches, hypoglycemia, and dizziness, as well as increased risk for possible pancreatitis.

Educational Objective
Identify orlistat as the only medication that is FDA-approved to treat obesity among adolescents younger than 16 years and recognize that intensive lifestyle interventions continue to be the mainstay of treatment for weight management in children and adolescents.

Reference(s)
Styne DM, Arslanian SA, Connor EL, et al. Pediatric obesity—assessment, treatment, and prevention: an Endocrine Society clinical practice guideline. *J Clin Endocrinol Metab*. 2017;102(3):709-757. PMID: 28359099

Kelly AS, Fox CK. Pharmacotherapy in the management of pediatric obesity. *Curr Diab Rep*. 2017;17(8):55. PMID: 28646356

97 ANSWER: A) Decreased energy consumption
Oxytocin is a nonapeptide hormone synthesized by the magnocellular neurons in the paraventricular and supraoptic nuclei of the hypothalamus. A single axon from each magnocellular neuron projects to the posterior pituitary gland where oxytocin is released. Oxytocin is well known to be involved in the regulation of labor, where it stimulates ripening of the cervix and facilitates uterine contraction and clotting post partum. It also stimulates the let-down reflex in lactation. More recently, knowledge of the role of oxytocin in regulation of other physiologic processes has been expanding. Oxytocin has been implicated in psychological and social behaviors such as cognitive empathy, trust, attachment, and anxiolysis. Knockout mice deficient in oxytocin or the oxytocin receptor are obese and have glucose intolerance. Oxytocin administration in these animals reduces food intake (decreases energy consumption [Answer A]), increases energy expenditure [Answer D], and improves glucose homeostasis. However, the increase in energy expenditure seen with oxytocin administration in animals has not been confirmed in humans.

Obese animals are more sensitive than lean animals to the effects of oxytocin administration. In humans, obesity increases plasma leptin levels and promotes leptin resistance. Conversely, obesity decreases plasma oxytocin levels and increases oxytocin receptor expression in adipose tissue and the central nervous system. Exogenous administration of oxytocin decreases food intake and fat mass in animals and humans with severe obesity. Since oxytocin decreases food intake and fat mass in leptin-resistant animal models, it may improve (decrease) leptin resistance (thus, Answer B is incorrect). In addition, oxytocin promotes pancreatic β-cell response to glucose in obese states and improves insulin secretion (thus, Answer E is incorrect). While it may improve fatty liver (Answer C), this would not be the most likely mechanism for weight loss.

In a case report of an 8-year-old boy with craniopharyngioma and evidence of damage to the region of the paraventricular nuclei and supraoptic nuclei, treatment with intranasal oxytocin resulted in a decrease in hunger and hyperphagia. However, the patient continued to have impulsive hedonic food-seeking behaviors. It was postulated that these continued behaviors may have been due to damage to other neuronal brain circuitry involved in the brain reward system. The precise role of oxytocin in the regulation of food intake continues to evolve. Studies evaluating the role of intranasal oxytocin as a therapy for obesity, including in Prader-Willi syndrome, are ongoing.

Educational Objective
Describe the physiologic and pharmacologic effects of oxytocin.

Reference(s)
Hsu EA, Miller JL, Perez FA, Roth CL. Oxytocin and naltrexone successfully treat hypothalamic obesity in a boy post-craniopharyngioma resection. *J Clin Endocrinol Metab*. 2018;103(2):370-375. PMID: 29220529

Olszewski PK, Klockars A, Levine AS. Oxytocin and potential benefits for obesity treatment. *Curr Opin Endocrinol Diabetes Obes*. 2017;24(5):320-325. PMID: 28590323

Maejima Y, Yokota S, Nishimori K, Shimomura K. The anorexigenic neural pathways of oxytocin and their clinical implication. *Neuroendocrinology*. 2018;107(1):91-104. PMID: 29660735

Bhargava R, Daughters KL, Rees A. Oxytocin therapy in hypopituitarism: challenges and opportunities. *Clin Endocrinol (Oxf)*. 2019;90(2):257-264. PMID: 30506703

Spetter MS, Hallschmid M. Current findings on the role of oxytocin in the regulation of food intake. *Physiol Behav*. 2017;176:31-39. PMID: 28284882

98 ANSWER: D) FNA of the thyroid nodule

This adolescent patient with Graves disease has not achieved remission of hyperthyroidism and has evidence of active disease (positive thyroid-stimulating immunoglobulin) after more than 2 years of treatment with antithyroid medication. Therefore, it is reasonable to consider all options for ongoing therapy, including continuing antithyroid medication or pursuing definitive therapy with radioactive iodine (^{131}I) or thyroidectomy. Management should be guided by an informed discussion with the patient of the risks and benefits of each approach. This older adolescent desires definitive therapy and has no contraindication to either radioactive iodine (Answer B) or thyroidectomy (Answer E), so proceeding with either approach would have been reasonable, depending on patient preference, in the absence of a thyroid nodule.

In this case, however, an abnormality on thyroid examination led to discovery of a thyroid nodule. Thyroid enlargement in patients with Graves disease is usually symmetric: significant thyroid asymmetry or palpation of a discrete nodule should prompt further evaluation with thyroid ultrasonography. Thyroid scintigraphy (Answer C) is recommended for the initial evaluation of thyroid nodules in patients with a low TSH concentration to identify an autonomous nodule. Scintigraphy would not be useful in this patient with a normal TSH value; even if methimazole were withdrawn to achieve a low TSH level, scintigraphy generally is not effective for identifying autonomous nodules in patients with active Graves disease due to the background of diffuse thyroid gland autonomy.

The prevalence of thyroid cancer in children with Graves disease may be as high as 1.8%, and a diagnosis of thyroid cancer would affect management decisions about definitive therapy. Therefore, thyroid nodules with concerning features should be evaluated by ultrasound-guided FNA (Answer D) before any decision about definitive therapy for Graves disease. Thyroid ultrasonography should also include evaluation of cervical lymph nodes for potential evidence of metastatic thyroid carcinoma that may alter management. The sonographic features of this thyroid nodule (solid, hypoechoic, calcifications) are concerning for malignancy; therefore, waiting to reevaluate the nodule in 3 months (Answer A) is not appropriate.

Educational Objective
Evaluate thyroid nodules in a patient with Graves disease and include assessment for thyroid nodules in the evaluation for definitive treatment of Graves disease.

Reference(s)
Ross DS, Burch HB, Cooper DS, et al. 2016 American Thyroid Association guidelines for diagnosis and management of hyperthyroidism and other causes of thyrotoxicosis. *Thyroid*. 2016;26(10):1343-1421. PMID: 27521067

Francis GL, Waguespack SG, Bauer AJ, et al; American Thyroid Association Guidelines Task Force. Management guidelines for children with thyroid nodules and differentiated thyroid cancer. *Thyroid*. 2015;25(7):716-759. PMID: 25900731

MacFarland SP, Bauer AJ, Adzick NS, et al. Disease burden and outcome in children and young adults with concurrent Graves disease and differentiated thyroid carcinoma. *J Clin Endocrinol Metab*. 2018;103(8):2918-2925. PMID: 29788090

99
ANSWER: B) Start a GnRH analogue to prevent further pubertal changes

Endocrine Society clinical practice guidelines updated in 2017 made a number of recommendations regarding the treatment of gender dysphoric/gender incongruent adolescents, which included the following:

- Only mental health providers who meet specific criteria should diagnose gender dysphoria/gender incongruence. This includes knowledge of criteria for puberty-blocking and gender-affirming hormone treatment in adolescents.
- Decisions regarding the social transition of prepubertal youths with gender dysphoria/gender incongruence should be made with the assistance of a mental health professional or another experienced professional.
- Adolescents who meet diagnostic criteria for gender dysphoria/gender incongruence, fulfill criteria for treatment, and are requesting treatment should initially undergo treatment to suppress pubertal development.
- Clinicians should begin pubertal hormone suppression after signs of puberty develop. Where indicated, GnRH analogues should be used to suppress pubertal hormones.
- Initiation of sex hormone treatment (partly irreversible) is recommended after a multidisciplinary team of medical and mental health providers has confirmed the persistence of gender dysphoria/gender incongruence and sufficient mental capacity exists to give informed consent, which most adolescents have by age 16 years.

The patient in this vignette has been followed by a qualified mental health professional, has met criteria for gender dysphoria, is in puberty, and has requested treatment to suppress male development. According to the guidelines, she meets criteria to start treatment with a GnRH analogue (Answer B) to prevent further pubertal changes.

Early puberty is an ideal time to start puberty blockers in children with gender dysphoria to prevent or delay the development of undesired secondary sexual characteristics. Pubertal suppression is reversible and enables full pubertal development in the natal gender after cessation of treatment if desired. For those who ultimately choose to proceed with irreversible treatments, early suppression of puberty can help the individual avoid the need for future surgeries and is associated with better physical outcomes. It has also been shown that early access to pubertal suppression is linked to better psychological outcomes and lower suicide risk for transgender patients.

Medroxyprogesterone acetate (Answer C) can be used as an alternative to GnRH analogues to suppress testosterone production. However, this medication is not as effective as GnRH analogues at lowering endogenous androgen production and is associated with adverse effects, including fatigue, weight gain, and increased risk of blood clots.

Starting low-dosage estradiol (Answer A) is not indicated at this age. Guidelines from the Endocrine Society and the World Professional Association for Transgender Health recommend against gender-affirming hormone treatment until approximately 16 years of age. Aside from lack of data studying the effects of this treatment in a younger age group, guidelines require that before starting gender-affirming hormone treatment, an individual must have sufficient mental capacity and maturity to understand the consequences of partly irreversible treatment (which include potential loss of fertility).

Treatment to block pubertal progression is considered reversible and not likely to affect future fertility. Current guidelines do not explicitly recommend counseling on fertility (Answer D) until an individual is ready to consider gender-affirming hormone treatment.

This patient's gender dysphoria may be transient. However, allowing puberty to progress over time (Answer E) may lead to detrimental outcomes for the patient in terms of masculinization, which can increase complexity of gender-affirming treatment and confer a greater risk of psychological harm.

Educational Objective
Provide appropriate guidance for management of gender dysphoria in early puberty.

Reference(s)
Hembree WC, Cohen-Kettenis PT, Gooren L, et al. Endocrine treatment of gender-dysphoric/gender-incongruent persons: an Endocrine Society clinical practice guideline. *J Clin Endocrinol Metab.* 2017;102(11):3869-3903. PMID: 28945902

100

ANSWER: B) L-asparaginase–induced hypoglycemia

This patient has nonketotic hypoglycemia with detectable insulin levels during a hypoglycemic episode. The suppressed β-hydroxybutyrate and free fatty acid concentrations confirm the relative hyperinsulinemic state. He has no history of hypoglycemia and did not experience any blood glucose abnormality until day 18 of induction chemotherapy. The repeated severe hypoglycemia experienced by the patient in this vignette is not a normal response to chemotherapy (Answer E).

The patient is on prednisolone therapy, most likely with a supraphysiologic dosage on day 18 of therapy. With the high steroid dosages used in chemotherapy induction, patients are expected to develop insulin resistance and even hyperglycemia. Hypoglycemia secondary to adrenal insufficiency (Answer A) is a ketotic form of hypoglycemia, which is not the case in this vignette.

Intrathecal injections can cause pituitary dysfunction and disrupt GH secretion; however, GH deficiency–related hypoglycemia (Answer D) is also a ketotic form of hypoglycemia and is not consistent with the patient's presentation or laboratory values.

Hyperemesis induced by chemotherapy can certainly impact nutritional intake (Answer C) and influence glucose levels, but this is not the case in this vignette. Ketotic hypoglycemia is also expected if there is inadequate nutritional intake with suppressed insulin levels.

For more than 30 years, the enzyme L-asparaginase has been commonly used to treat childhood acute lymphoblastic leukemia. Two preparations of L-asparaginase are approved by the US FDA: *Escherichia coli* L-asparaginase (native L-asparaginase) and pegaspargase (a polyethylene glycol-conjugated form of the *E coli* L-asparaginase). Many adverse effects of L-asparaginase have been documented over the years, such as coagulopathy, acute pancreatitis, allergic reaction, hyperlipidemia, hyperammonemia, hepatotoxicity, and hyperglycemia. The case in this vignette is an unusual presentation of hypoglycemia associated with pegylated L-asparaginase-induced hyperinsulinism (Answer B). There are increasing case reports of this phenomena that are directly associated with the timing of L-asparaginase use. The mechanism of elevated insulin level is not well understood. The episodes can last weeks after use, but they resolve with time.

Educational Objective
Determine the etiology of hypoglycemia in a child undergoing induction chemotherapy for acute lymphoblastic leukemia.

Reference(s)

Tanaka R, Osumi T, Miharu M, et al. Hypoglycemia associated with L-asparaginase in acute lymphoblastic leukemia treatment: a case report. *Exp Hematology Oncol.* 2012;1(1):8. PMID: 23211036

Panigrahi M, Swain TR, Jena RK, Panigrahi A. L-asparaginase-induced abnormality in plasma glucose level in patients of acute lymphoblastic leukemia admitted to a tertiary care hospital of Odisha. *Indian J Pharmacol.* 2016;48(5):595-598. PMID: 27721550

PEDIATRIC ENDOCRINE SELF-ASSESSMENT PROGRAM 2021-2022

Part III

This question-mapping index groups question topics according to the 7 umbrella sections of Pediatric ESAP (Adrenal, Bone, Carbohydrate and Lipid Metabolism/Obesity, Growth, Pituitary, Reproductive System, and Thyroid). Relevant **question numbers** follow each topic.

Growth hormone therapy: **55, 68, 74, 86, 88**
11β-Hydroxysteroid dehydrogenase 1: **55**
Hypoglycemia: **12**
Hypopituitarism: **6**
IGF1R gene: **77**
IGF-1 resistance: **77**
Lumbar disk herniation: **95**
Medulloblastoma: **6**
NPR2 gene: **38**
Obesity: **74**
Osteoarthritis: **95**
Oxandrolone: **68**
PAPPA2 gene: **8**
Prader-Willi syndrome: **74**
Precocious puberty: **30**
Prenatal growth restriction: **83**
Prenatal screening: **58**
Pseudohypoparathyroidism type 1A: **20**
Radiation therapy: **30**
Rickets, vitamin D–dependent type 1A: **35**
Short stature: **6, 8, 12, 20, 22, 26, 35, 38, 47, 55, 58, 68, 77, 83, 86, 88, 95**
Silver-Russell syndrome: **83**
Skeletal dysplasia: **26**
Small-for-gestational-age: **88**
Turner syndrome: **58, 68**
Tyrosine kinase inhibitors: **22**

PITUITARY

Adipsia: **24**
Craniopharyngioma: **24, 97**
Galactorrhea: **11**
Growth delay: **32**
Growth hormone/prolactin-secreting pituitary adenoma: **11**
Growth hormone resistance: **32**
Growth hormone–stimulation testing: **81**
Holoprosencephaly: **53**
Hyponatremia: **67**
Hypopituitarism: **97**
Hypothalamic obesity: **97**
Klinefelter syndrome: **44**
Oxytocin: **97**
Precocious puberty: **14**
Prolactinoma: **11**
Short stature: **14, 81**
Somatostatin analogues: **11**
Syndrome of inappropriate antidiuretic hormone secretion: **67**
TSH-secreting pituitary adenoma: **90**
Undernutrition: **32**
Van Wyk-Grumbach syndrome: **14**

REPRODUCTIVE SYSTEM

Amenorrhea, primary: **40**
Amenorrhea, secondary: **18, 64**
Androgen insensitivity syndrome: **27**
Antipsychotic agents: **18**
Dopamine agonist therapy: **64**
Galactorrhea: **5**
Gelastic seizures: **87**
Gender dysphoria: **99**
GnRH analogue: **99**
Gynecomastia: **5, 51**
Histrelin implant: **33**
Hypergonadotropic hypogonadism: **40, 73**
Hyperprolactinemia: **18, 64**
Hypospadias: **27**
Hypothalamic hamartoma: **87**
Kallmann syndrome: **73**
Precocious puberty: **87**
Premature ovarian insufficiency: **40**
Prolactinoma: **64**
Pubertal delay: **33, 73**
Short stature: **33**
Silver-Russell syndrome: **33**

THYROID

BRAF gene: **94**
Consumptive hypothyroidism: **59, 66**
DICER1 syndrome: **54**
Down syndrome: **62**
Goiter: **36**
Graves disease: **29, 36, 49, 62, 98**
Exogenous intoxication: **41**
Hashimoto thyroiditis: **29**
Hearing impairment: **89**
Heart failure: **59**
Hyperthyroidism: **29, 36, 41, 49, 62, 98**
Hypothyroidism: **4, 9, 23, 29, 59, 66, 78, 89**
Liver hemangiomas: **59, 66**
Macro-TSH: **9**
Maternal iodine intake: **78**
Medullary thyroid cancer: **13**
Multiple endocrine neoplasia type 2A: **13**
Newborn screening: **9, 23**
Papillary thyroid cancer: **4, 45, 71, 94**
RET gene: **13**
Thyroid nodules: **17, 54, 94, 98**
Thyrotoxicosis: **36**
Ultrasonography: **17, 54, 94, 98**

www.ingramcontent.com/pod-product-compliance
Lightning Source LLC
Chambersburg PA
CBHW070246230326

41458CB00099B/5261